"An important work that will appeal to and help so many. *Retox* is going to change the health of so many confused souls and show them a way to feel good every day."

—Joel Kahn MD, professor of medicine, Wayne State University School of Medicine, author of *The Whole Heart Solution* and *Dead Execs Don't Get Bonuses*

"If you are in pursuit of happiness and health, you will find a fresh take with Retox—a perfect blend of yoga, food, and attitude!"

—Jason Wachob, founder and CEO of mindbodygreen

"*Retox* provides actionable steps toward a healthy life and, most importantly, balance. This book will help you discover the 'new you' you've been waiting to meet, free of deprivation and negative self-talk."

—Joshua Rosenthal, founder and director of The Institute for Integrative Nutrition

"*Retox* helps you eat your way to creating your strongest, healthiest you."

—Terry Wahls, MD, author *The Wahls Protocol: A Radical New Way to Treat All Chronic Autoimmune Conditions Using Paleo Principles*

"*Retox* is about living healthy and empowered in a world full of doubt and toxicity. This book will move you to practice, to receive the wisdom of your simplest acts of wellness, and give you healthy habits that are both accessible and joyful. If you're seeking full self-acceptance and comprehensive nourishment, I dare you to Retox!"

—Elena Brower, meditation and yoga teacher and author of *Art of Attention*

"With a deep understanding of anatomy and physiology, in *Retox*, Lauren writes a fun and entertaining book that shows both students and instructors ways to maximize the value of yoga."

—Francis X. Mendoza, MD, orthopedic surgeon, New York City

"Lauren's book is a must-have, a real-life approach to living the busy lives we all have AND being healthy. Finally a book with tools for everyday life that are easy to follow and understand."

—Eve, recording artist and actress

"*Retox* is such a fresh take on living. Lauren invites us to live intuitively, a deserved freedom for all of us, especially in a time when there's so much restriction around food and body image."

—Emily Nolan, founder of My Kind of Life

"I love *Retox*. Flat-out funny yet meticulously centered on healthy and achievable, everyday good recipes and tips. Cuts through the crap and gets you eating what you need to be, without the pressure, guilt, or added expense but with all the enjoyment. It illustrates the important balance of leading a healthy life without forgoing the important pleasures in life."

—Seamus Mullen, chef

"Yoga for the modern life! You need to delve deep into Lauren's book. Her insights and information are both illuminating and highly entertaining."

—Mick Rock, celebrity photographer

"In *Retox*, Lauren tells it like it is and actually makes you want to eat what's good for you. She keeps the fun in food."

—Michael White, chef, Altamarea Group

"Lauren vibrates with energy and love; she encapsulates physical and mental well-being. *Retox* is all about this energy. Very inspiring and very practical . . . [Lauren's] brand is one of the most authentic ones in the wellness space."

—Bernard Mariette, CEO, Lolë

"*Retox* brings the sexy to mindful living. Lauren provides us with realistic ways to show up as the best version of ourselves and to fully enjoy this beautiful life we have been given."

—Michael Franti, musician

HEALTHY SOLUTIONS FOR REAL LIFE

RETOX

YOGA • FOOD • ATTITUDE

LAUREN IMPARATO
Founder of I.AM.YOU.

BERKLEY BOOKS, NEW YORK

BERKLEY BOOKS
An imprint of Penguin Random House LLC
375 Hudson Street, New York, New York 10014

This book is an original publication of Penguin Random House LLC.

Library of Congress Cataloging-in-Publication Data

Imparato, Lauren
Retox : yoga * food * attitude: healthy solutions for real life / Lauren Imparato.—Berkley trade paperback edition.
p.   cm.
ISBN 978-0-425-27850-5 (paperback)
1. Hatha yoga. 2. Nutrition. 3. Self-care, Health. I. Title.
RA781.7147 2016
613.7'046—dc23
2015030414

PUBLISHING HISTORY
Berkley trade paperback edition / February 2016

PRINTED IN THE UNITED STATES OF AMERICA

10 9 8 7 6 5 4 3 2

Cover photos: (front) Walt Lindveld; (back) Mick Rock.
Cover design by Rita Frangie.
Interior text design by Pauline Neuwirth.

To Chata, my Chief Inspiration Officer, for your infinite positivity, energy, and pure lust for life. For showing me how to believe, fight, love, and live to life's fullest every moment of every day. I am me because you are you.

CONTENTS

IT'S ALL ABOUT NOW

The past is the present unrolled for understanding;
the present is the future rolled up for action.

—WILL DURANT

I AM A GEEK. A bookworm to the max. When I was young, I would hide in the closet with a flashlight, reading well past my bedtime. I soon realized through the pages and pages of books that history is simultaneously cyclical and evolutionary. We repeat patterns, wars, mistakes, and habits, but each time we advance. We embody an intrinsic desire and ability to transcend, and with it, a recognition and desire for change.

This inherent necessity for change, the type that propels us as individuals and as a society as a whole to the next echelon, almost always comes at the most inopportune times: during periods of societal stress, conflict, and personal duress. It is in these moments that we must sever habits that no longer serve us and thoughtfully learn new ways of behaving; we must break with the old and take a conscious step into the new. We are confronted by such a moment again today, amid modern life's duality of magnificence and anguish, tension and freedom. It is time for us to look at the world, and ourselves, anew.

Life is not as it used to be. On an average day, we wake up early to arrive at work having already handled thirty minutes of emails, conference calls, or urgent texts from a frantic boss or discombobulated kid, and work all day with few, if any, moments to come up for air. We take meals at our desks or in the car, feeling drained long before the day is over, even though we sit still, locked to a chair most of the day anyway. Thousands upon thousands of messages bombard our brain in the form of emails, texts, digital media, and advertising. There is a pressure to endlessly do, even if it is inconvenient to our human nature, functioning body, or mere existence. On the off chance we get some free time, we are forced to decide between what we want to do and what we think we should do for our body, loved ones, home, or even fun. As we crawl into bed, exhausted and already stressed out about the impending alarm the next day, we may take our first true breath—the woken day's last.

This all takes a toll on our tangible, physical body and our intangible mind. We have too many choices, too much information, and not enough time. We have more opportunities than any other generation before us, yet we have never had more excuses to not advance to where we want to be—really be—personally. That said, the norm of today's pace and mandates from modern urban living are unlikely to ease. Instead, we need to get real and construct the life we want and need amid it all.

We know our habits need to change—our world has changed and is ever changing. We also all inherently know we cannot transform nature, but we can, and must revolutionize how we operate within our world. Far too often, we feel overwhelmed, distressed, tired, and confused. We know we need something, but we do not necessarily know what. We thus repeatedly attempt piecemeal solutions that do not work, and we are too tired and besieged to search for ones that do. We want everything premade, preset, distilled down to one step, and even with that, it is hard to make decisions, let alone engrain new routines. Our attachment to daily habits, trendy dogma, restrictive beliefs, and advertising handicap any substantial personal progress, and often hinder our basic understanding of the scope of change that is actually needed.

It may sound paradoxically simple and impossible at the same time, but the solution to all the stress, pain, anxiety, insomnia, stomachaches, low energy, down moods, and the twenty modern-life challenges I address in this book is to change our inside world, not fight our outside. No month-long retreats few of us can afford. No hour-long meditation sessions few of us have time for. No restrictive diets that drain us rather than energize us. What we need are concrete, manageable ways to nourish ourselves in between and during our challenging moments—while we are at our desks, entertaining a client, feeding the kids, the morning after an indulgent night, or before bed after a stressful day of juggling too many balls in the air.

We need a solution that is timeless, efficient, and functional. A solution based on science, anatomy, psychology, philosophy, biochemistry, and the life we really lead.

What we need is to Retox.

Retox is a transformation, a rethinking, reforming, reinventing, reconstructing of who you are and how you can truly be, inside and out. It goes to the essence of what living is about—it is living itself.

Retox is about adding things in that will make you strong in body, mind, and life. It is about harnessing all you and the world have to offer, and then adding a splash of simple, straight-up, doable tips and solutions to make it all even better. It is not about depriving or regulating yourself or your lifestyle, but instead about embracing it all and flourishing within it. Retox gives you the tools to thrive no matter what life throws at you; it is your key to success.

Retox is the next step, for you and our world. It is about detoxing the past methods that have not worked, or that are too daunting or demanding to ever be considered permanently realistic, and then adding in new ways to be the best *you* you can be on any given day, all right smack in the middle of the life you really lead. Retox does not change your world. It makes you better within it.

To Retox means to cleanse to get dirty. Rest to rage. Meditate to work. Breathe to energize. Eat to flourish. Sweat to focus. Sleep to party. I Retox to live.

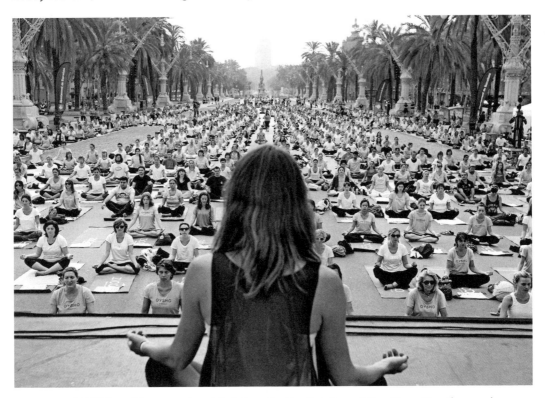

Bringing I.AM.YOU. and Retox to the global stage for the first time at Free Yoga. Two thousand people, Barcelona.

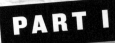

PART I

Detox to Retox

TIME TO GET OFF THE WAGON

The way to get started is to quit talking and begin doing.

—WALT DISNEY

DETOXING AND ELIMINATING LIFE'S PLEASURE FOR THE SAKE OF PURITY OR subscribing to a nutritional orthodoxy is counterproductive. Deprivation only leads to overcompensation, and more often than not, stress and misery. It's a setup for failure because we cannot, and should not, sustain a state of scarcity—and who would really want to? Following a step-by-step restrictive program that overpromises a "new you" is stressful and soul crushing; when we don't reach our goals, we blame ourselves instead of the system. Transforming and restructuring your life completely is unrealistic. Unless we retreat to a cabin on some mountaintop, we won't escape the new normal. And even then, general life stressors such as interactions with your loved ones, body image, and simple day-to-day subsistence chores will still haunt you. Such is twenty-first-century life. Escaping isn't the answer. Retoxing is.

Purity is the dream. Pollution is the norm. Modern urban life is unavoidable for most of us. Mental and physical toxins have seeped into every aspect of our existence, stress has permanently permeated our culture, and I am just going to say it for all of us—sometimes we just want to sit back, have a drink, chill the F out, and not think about it all. I get it. But what if I were to tell you that I had a way for you to take it all on, and feel better than you may have ever imagined? The answer is Retox. Retox is about opening yourself up and throwing yourself in so you can be whole. Retox is about you and your life—the life you're living now, the life you want to love.

Let's be honest: No one, including me, really believes the world needs another yoga, diet, or self-help book. I promise you this is not that. What we do need is a framework that integrates them all into one streamlined solution, a solution that can be applied anytime, anywhere, to the life you really lead, to the day-to-day issues you actually face. One that distills the true value out of each wellness and self-betterment theory and instills them into your actual life with a straight-up dose of reality, so that we as individuals and society can efficiently and realistically improve, and rock it.

That's Retox.

Retox embraces the nitty-gritty details of the real, down-and-dirty, manic, and ecstatic journey that is life today. It allows you to live it without the aches, stresses, and ailments— both mental and physical—that can come with an active lifestyle, and provides you with a new sense of vitality as well. It adds accessible goodness, so you can easily overcome life's most common challenges. Retoxing is like pouring yourself your favorite cocktail over and over.

Retox strips yoga down to its most scientific and anatomical features, offering practical tips for fast relief. It mixes in Tibetan yoga philosophy as a logic-based psychology to build mental strength and agility. It then adds in realistic, doable, and non-dogmatic nutritional tips that quite simply make you feel better. Retox is a 360-degree, multidimensional solution that is palpable and efficient. And it's served up by someone that lives the life you do—me.

You should most definitely expect to find me dancing stiletto-clad on a table, sipping champagne, sometimes into the wee hours of the night. The next day, you will probably see me again at sunrise jetting across a city sidewalk, croissant and coffee in hand, ready to take on a jam-packed workday. I am an absolute lush—of life—as indulgent as I am disciplined.

What makes my ride feasible, both in my life now as an entrepreneur and in my first career path on Wall Street, are the simple practices that sustain my body, sanity, and overall wellness. I call them Retox cocktails because they combine potent ingredients from millennia-old traditions with today's science, and they can be imbibed in the midst of your daily routine. They are one part yoga, one part nourishment, and one part mindset, stirred together with a dose of reality, each designed to address a specific life challenge. I deconstruct the causes of what you may be experiencing, and offer up a remedy, a holistic, 360-degree solution that won't make you look weird, feel annoyed, or roll your eyes.

I personally get squeamish around barefoot yoga cliques, unwarranted hugs from random people I do not know, master starvation cleanses and elimination diets, rules for eating that go against two thousand years of humanity, repeated *om shanti*s. And above all, the phrase "Let go."

I like to keep it real, focusing on facts and science. Anatomy. Biology. Physiology. Ancient philosophy texts. Real life. And instead of drifting through a sea of rules that promise a better body and a magical life, I use simple tenets as a base to take charge, to Retox, within the life we have.

A California girl raised on athletic fields, basketball courts, running trails, and in swimming pools, I traveled east for the classrooms of Princeton, and after graduating moved to New York City to take on the Wall Street trading floors at Morgan Stanley. Throughout my early years in the city, I was an avid athlete and a running addict, averaging sixty miles a week after my extensively long days on the floor, attempting to stay as true to my fitness-oriented California roots as possible in the urban jungle I had come to love. I worked hard, played hard, and sweated harder—pretty much all on a daily basis.

I came to yoga reluctantly at first, borderline hating it, biased by visions of unshaven Berkeley hippies and fears of statically wasting time. Yet one day, as I walked up the Bowery in my dad's navy blue 1970s-era Adidas shorts, I noticed that my legs appeared significantly larger than those of my skinny rocker boyfriend. Double the size, to be precise. How could that be? I was running all the time, swimming, and eating carb free. Yes, I was working fifteen-hour days, but that did not explain what I was staring at beneath those vintage shorts (and this was before the spin craze).

We went to dinner outside at the Bowery Bar, where I proceeded to spaz out silently in my mind about what life was doing to my body. After turning down a basket of chips and salsa, a blasphemy for a Cali native, my boyfriend interrupted my mental laments and asked what was wrong. I sheepishly pointed out my legs, to which he matter-of-factly told me to go to yoga. I looked at him and rolled my eyes. As if.

So infuriated by his inane suggestion, I decided to prove him wrong and give yoga a shot. The next morning, I threw on my basketball clothes—huge mesh shorts and a XXL T-shirt—and grabbed a double espresso. I had read somewhere that it would up my heart rate and make me sweat in those "easy" yoga classes. I chugged it, walked into the studio, and sat down for class. Bad idea.

I'll spare you the details, but it was awful, and hard, so much so that I faked a cramp and walked out halfway through, soaking in sweat, tangled in my mesh, and bewildered. Not to mention feeling totally dejected by the sea of models and dancers making it all look so easy. In disbelief about the severity of my ass-kicking, I returned to a yoga class at the same studio a week later. This time I survived. Barely. Then I went back three days later. And then a day later. And then another day later. And then and then and then . . . Long story short, I was suddenly practicing yoga seven days a week and, by the way, not running at all. What had the world come to?

That said, the classes all felt mildly creepy to me. The chanting, the New Age talk between asanas, and what was to me an aura of holier-than-thou. I simply wanted to make my legs ZZ Top–able, and definitely did not go to my first class in search of a new faith or religion. Nor was I yearning for a new family or support network. Luckily, I had not suffered any personal traumas that I sought to overcome; I was injury free and happily employed. Rock and roll was and still is my "Kumbaya," and endorphins have been my only ever drug addiction.

Yet balancing my intense and quickly developing Wall Street career with my health and busy social and family lives was challenging and stressful. I was subject to insomnia, digestive issues, weight gain, anxiety, and an expanding list of symptoms, depending on the day. But yoga seemed to be helping. In fact, the very yoga I scoffed at ultimately ended up improving my body, mind, and life. After months of daily practice, I realized that when learned through a diagnostic, anatomical lens, yoga can be one of the most effective tools available. I decided to dive all in.

Quite ironically, I ended up immersing myself in yoga studies. Daily classes, weekly workshops, monthly lectures, and a comprehensive reading of the ancient original yoga texts and anatomy books. I began to practice yoga no matter where I was, whether it was on a business trip or family visit. And this was long before it was trendy and accessible. I invented routines that combined my knowledge and passion for athleticism and anatomy, and for an extra edgy kick, I would drop a killer Music Mix. I had become a yoga addict and a closet yoga PhD student, with spunk.

Unsurprisingly, my practice placed me face-to-face with the dreaded meditation. My teachers urged me to meditate an hour every morning, repeating mantras to the tune of "There is no stress, the stress is me" (BS—do they live in the real world?) or "Peace and love for all beings" (sure, but how is that helping me right now?), or as mentioned, my most hated "Inhale, let; exhale, go" (as if that would help). I was already waking up at 5 a.m. to be on the trading floor by 5:30. Did they really think I had an extra hour to lop off on top of that? Let alone one to be spent sitting still with my eyes closed talking to myself?

I hit a roadblock, one that none of my teachers seemed to be able to finagle me around. So I decided to unearth my Princeton geekdom and go to the source, seeking out the original books on yoga meditation and theory as well as their current teachers. This academic venture landed me in the world of Tibetan philosophy, a logic-based approach to thought and, quite frankly, existence. Through this lens, meditation was simply a brain-muscle exercise, one that linked breath with thoughts and served to make the mind stronger and more agile. This I could relate to, and apply to my nitty-gritty New York City life and career.

With Tibetan philosophy as the base, meditation was no longer intimidating, mantra no longer superfluous. It was simply a tool for my mental fortitude, one that I needed to get through the endless hours of mania on the trading floor and city sidewalks. Like the yoga poses themselves, meditation made me stronger, from the inside out, and paved the way for me to take on and create the career and life I dreamed of. I liked it.

I now had a new approach to dealing with my body and mind. Yet there was one piece missing—food. And let me tell you, the trading floor's dependence on bacon breakfast sandwiches, White Castle burgers, Starbucks, gluttonous business dinners, and most other fast-food gems, paired with a Manhattan starter budget, did not make this one easy. I thought I knew what to eat, but I had forgotten how. When I was growing up, Mom made dinner every night of the week, with a traditional steak night on Sundays. The rest of the time we ate pretty much everything and were always healthy. My list of favorite meals was a mile long, including everything from pizza to paella, but always started off with salad.

My lettuce fervor made my early twenties and early yoga-going transition to vegetarianism quite easy. It started as an experiment, one I cloaked as financial to my friends and family. But in reality I went veggie because of a lecture I heard at the yoga studio. The expert insisted that doing yoga while consuming animal products was a futile practice, one that would leave you suffering and in agony. She went on to say that health, true health, was unobtainable if not a vegan, especially in the toxic world of today.

It seemed a bit far-fetched, but did leave me curious. Yoga was, after all, making me feel amazing, and this while eating meat. So what if I just cut it out for a bit, as an experiment . . . ? Could it make this feeling even better? I was willing to try. Worst case, I would be saving more money for cocktails out, the ultimate New York gambling chip.

The experiment was only meant to last two weeks, but instead it lasted almost seven years. My mind loved it, but what I did not know is that my body was hating it. My nails and hair were brittle, my stomach was bloated after every meal, and I was sick all the time, all of which I blamed on my job, not my diet.

I was a committed vegetarian, but that doesn't mean I didn't miss meat. I remember once waking up in the middle of the night, wide-eyed and unable to go back to sleep. I had been dreaming of hamburgers. Juicy, beefy burgers with all the fixings. The dream was so vivid that I was jolted wide awake, salivating. But come daytime, I did nothing about it except stare at everyone's meat around me. Beef was officially bad and I was legitimately a vegetarian. Yet looking back at my anti-meat willpower, I can now see that I was in reality a bona fide yogavore, nothing more.

No matter what I told others, especially the dudes surrounding me on the floor, I knew that deep down the only reason I had become a vegetarian was because of the societal pressure, one that I initially encountered in yoga and from there ran into in every blog, magazine, and lecture. I was past being a simple vegetarian; I was a yoga-going, vegetable-only-eating yogavore, a sheep in the cauldron of food doctrine followers. I had fallen prey to the exact cults I had so hated, the latest victim to their dogma. I had allowed myself to believe that by eating in a restrictive way I had unlocked the path to long-term health, not to mention acceptance by the "cool kids" at the yoga studio. I wore my vegetarianism as a badge of honor; I was a health-conscious and consciously healthy human being. What I did not realize for years, though, is that the trendy yogavore diet I had espoused was breaking me down, one cell at a time.

Then one day, as I sat on the bench outside my local pastry pimp having breakfast, a fellow sat down next to me. He introduced himself, and I, upon glancing at him, quickly realized he was one of the world's most renowned yoga teachers. We struck up a conversation, talking about the philosophy of yoga and the best classes in the city. I told him a bit about myself and my journey to yoga, and when I finished he said, "So you are a vegetarian even though you play with the Wall Street devils. It must be difficult. I would imagine that you are surrounded by meat eaters, as those that take advantage of people every day must consume animal flesh." I think my eyes actually popped out of my head. Was he serious? All I could mutter back was "Not really . . ."

His holier-than-thou, judgmental attitude was ridiculous. What a load of crap. And was I buying into that by being vegetarian? Well, no way. No more dogma for me. I was not raised to follow people and trends blindly, but rather to think critically and reason deductively. This random encounter made me carefully consider my dietary choices. I eventually realized that I was only sticking to vegetarianism because I thought I had to, not because I actually wanted to anymore.

The next day, I went out for a burger. From that first beefy bite on, I dove deep into nutritional studies, determined to figure out what diet was best for me. I learned about major nutritional and dietary theories, as well as the body's biochemical properties. I read scientific studies and perused book after book promoting one eating style or another. I concluded that some ways of eating were optimal for my body or my life; some were completely unrealistic. So I decided to base my personal diet on hard scientific facts, not societal whims, and most important, to listen to my body to determine which foods made me feel good and strong.

It was all finally coming into place. I had the yoga to abate my physical dilemmas, the Tibetan philosophy to apply for my mental resilience, and a way of eating that followed what my body was telling me, not what the world wanted me to ingest, or not, for that matter. Had I discovered the secret to well-being that everyone was looking for?

I must have, because people started asking me for advice. The dudes on the floor, my friends, even people at the yoga studio started asking me questions, questions about how to have more energy, how to lower cholesterol without taking pills, how to avoid headaches, and of course, how to lose weight. At least once a day at work I would hear, "Hey, Cali Girl, what do you have to help my . . . ?" At first I didn't really think much about it; I was always eager to help others and share my knowledge. But soon I realized that these people were coming to me, a mid-twenty-year-old female in finance, for wellness advice because they had nowhere else to turn. They Googled all day and went to experts all week, but they had yet to find someone who could speak their language. I, in turn, distilled all the mumbo jumbo and served them solutions that actually worked within the context of their commute, job, family, and social life. Maybe I was on to something . . .

At the same time I started teaching yoga to my friends for free. I figured that I would do the whole Wall Street thing until I was about forty, quit to start a finance-related business, pop out a kid or two, and then teach yoga once a week on the side as a hobby. Easy peasy. For whatever go-getter hyperdrive reason, it seemed appropriate to start educating myself on the next level, now. First I convinced my boyfriend to let me teach him once a week—he had encouraged this whole yoga thing to begin with, after all—and then I signed up for an official yoga teacher training course on the weekends. After a while, word got out among our friends that I was making my boyfriend tremble in sweat, and that it was actually kind of fun. So I decided to take it up a notch and corralled a small group of friends into my loft on Saturday mornings, offering them class and brunch on me if they then critiqued my teaching over the Bloody Marys. They, bless their muscles and souls, said yes.

Their comments were rough—they criticized my voice intonation, speed, audibility, intensity (usually too intense), linguistics, on and on and on—but they were real comments, from real people across all backgrounds and fitness levels. They kept coming back, and with them always someone new, usually someone I did not know. Soon my loft was packed with dozens and dozens of people for this class I was teaching, this yoga that "was not like other yoga," they would say. Sweaty partakers would come up to me afterward noting that this was different, that it really created a palpable change, that it was cardio and therapeutic, that it was cool, that it was non-dogmatic, that it was the best class they had been to in the city. That, as yoga haters, or people new to yoga, or people totally over the yoga scene, they could relate to my vibe. So they showed up on Saturdays, and I kept teaching them. *Cool*, I thought. *This is a good starting off point for when I actually do this on the side when I'm forty.* Ah, the best-laid plans . . .

The more crowded my classes got, the more I studied. I wanted to know what I was talking about; I needed to know what I was talking about. I really did not want to be another teacher spewing more of the same clichéd yoga lines—you know, "Blossom your heart and crack it open to the sky." I was so over that. So I turned up my academic intensity, pursuing anatomy certificates and advanced yoga teaching certificates simultaneously. I sought out the best Tibetan scholars, and was named "Goddess of the Sun" in the Sakya tradition of Tibetan yoga philosophy by revered teacher Jetsun Luding. If I was going to do it, I was going to do it well. Even if it was just preplanning for my hobby in ten to fifteen years. I got technical about the anatomy, anal-retentive about injury prevention, and scholarly about the philosophy. I started a weekly email, highlighting the psychological or physical theme for Saturday's class, and adding in a nutritional tip or two, and became obsessed with planning the next experience at the loft. It was all I could think about.

Lo and behold, Lehman Brothers crashed, sending my work world into utter disarray, not to mention my personal savings and career outlook into the abyss. The trading floor was a minefield, blanketed in cross tides of stress, fear, and depression. Despite rounds of layoffs, Morgan Stanley promoted me that winter, touting my ability to keep my cool as well as protect the firm and my clients' interests simultaneously, especially in the tumultuous environment. I was elated. But distracted. The once daily "Hey, Cali . . ." became hourly, and the requests for help were more dynamic— what to do for anxiety, feelings of uncertainty, insomnia? Word had also leaked that I was

9

teaching free yoga classes on weekends, and some colleagues even started to come. "Different and hard" is all they would report back on Monday, "not typical yoga." *Nice*, I thought. I knew my NYC yoga teachers had taught me very well, namely Schuyler Grant, Elena Brower, Yogeswari, Dharma Mittra, and the ephemeral Lady Ruth, but I was elated to hear that what I was offering leveraged all I had learned, and continued to learn, from them and took it to a new place, a sweaty, funkified, original one.

I resolved to officially take on two jobs. The first, my paying, serious Princeton-bred one: Vice President in Fixed Income at Morgan Stanley. The second, my side project: a lens for yoga and wellness that real people with real lives could not only relate to, but easily extract value from on a regular basis. But then it hit me. The success of my first job was entirely linked to the existence of my side project. I had not been fired, and instead was promoted; I was respected internally, loved by clients, and doing well, all while feeling physically and mentally better than ever. I had managed my digestive issues, was pain free, and unduly energetic despite my regular dose of four hours of sleep a night. The success of my career was reliant on the vivacity of my passion project. They were irreversibly intertwined. This was too significant to keep to myself.

So on tax day 2009, I showed up to work and quit. My superiors thought they had misheard me. "No," I said, "I am serious. I am actually quitting to start a yoga-centric wellness business." They told me to take some time to think about it, looking at me with pity, as if I had finally lost it. My parents, on the other coast, definitely thought I had cracked, likely fearing I was tossing away my expensive education and converting religions. Neither was true. I had to do this.

After years of daily study, I had discovered a tactic to refine all the wellness babble out there and package it in a manner that was palpable and effective, one that created change in the inconvenient moments we most need it. It was now up to me to share it so that everyone could feel just as outstanding, no matter where or when.

I.AM.YOU. was born.

I.AM.YOU., the platform for Retox, is a 360-degree lifestyle approach based on yoga, nourishment, mindset, and music, aimed at helping us modern-life warriors take charge of our happiness and health. It appeals to not only yoga and wellness junkies devoted to their own health and spirit but also to those of us who are willing to prioritize our careers, social lives, and families over our health if need be. We wear leather, eat meat, rock out, indulge, and sometimes let ourselves get exhausted in the service of something bigger. And we need concrete fixes that allow us to thrive in the midst of it all.

Urban and natural. Heels and kicks. Flamenco and punk. Grunge and suits. Tutus and hoodies. With a mixture of ancient science and traditions paired with modern-life experiences, I.AM.YOU. and Retox teach you to heal yourself so you can heal the rest. On the mat, in the office, and on the street. With a thorough and intense physical, scientific, philosophical practice, I.AM.YOU., and now Retox, help you find *you* inside *you*. Deconstruct who you think you are to reconstruct who you are to be.

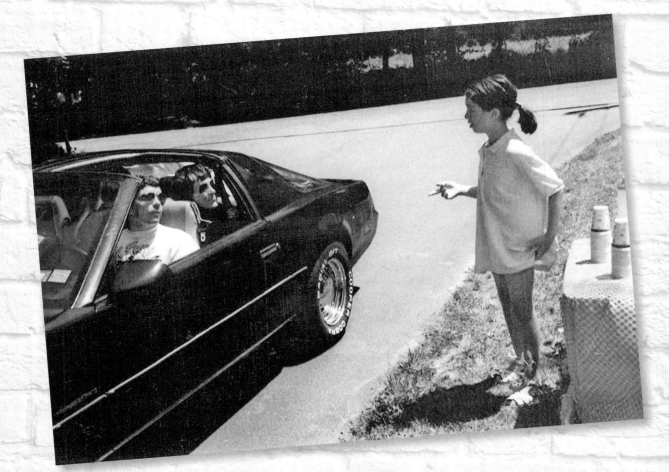

An entrepreneur since the beginning.

02

RETOX REDUX

The mind is its own place, and in itself can make a heaven of hell, a hell of heaven.

—JOHN MILTON

YOGA IS OFFICIALLY EVERYWHERE. FROM CHASE BANK TELEVISION SPOTS TO Tampax ads to laptop names, it seems that everywhere you look there is someone doing Tree pose or Up Dog in attempt to sell pretty much anything. The yoga gear industry has capitalized on this and exploded, with yoga socks, yoga props, yoga vitamins (the ones claiming increased flexibility for your Splits pose are my favorite), yoga jackets, yoga DVDs, yoga wine; and the list goes on. Whether you find value in yoga or not is irrelevant—they will sell it to you.

It did not used to be this way, though. Back when I started doing yoga, long before this craze, I had to keep it secret from my colleagues at work and barely mentioned it to my friends. I would hide my yoga mat close to the elevator so no one would connect it as mine, and deliberately scurry out of the office on my way to class avoiding all mat-carrying sightings. I could not afford to be the only woman in the group, let alone the yoga girl. So I kept to myself, for myself. As I mentioned earlier, just about six and a half years ago, when I resigned my job at Morgan Stanley, my colleagues looked at me as if I was falling into the abyss. Now

13

most of them own shares in one yoga-related company or another, and do yoga at least now and then, if not regularly. Yoga is mainstream, in your face, and here to stay.

But what is yoga, really? Is it merely a conduit to sell us more stuff in the name of relaxation and Zen? Is it a way to stretch and get happy? Or is it the latest version of soft porn, with bikini- and lingerie-clad women seductively posing for social media day and night? Yoga, true yoga, is thankfully much, much more.

Arguably one of the world's oldest traditions, yoga dates to 2500 BC, when the Indus Valley civilization that ruled the lands that are now India, Tibet, and Nepal depicted images of the first yoga poses on various recently discovered artifacts. In AD 400, the first yoga book was written by Patanjali, a doctor, philosopher, and dancer. In *The Yoga Sutras*, or as I refer to it the Bible of yoga, he outlines the steps taken to achieve enlightenment. To Western yoga-goers' surprise, it says nothing about the asanas, or poses of yoga, themselves, and is instead entirely focused on the mind, and with it its inner workings and need for meditation. In 1400, Swatmarama, another Indian scholar, wrote the *Hatha Yoga Pradipika*, a more well-rounded approach that includes fifteen yoga poses, nutritional suggestions, and techniques for meditation and sexual arousal. It was not until 1965 that the poses we all obsess over so much came to the forefront of yoga literature. B.K.S. Iyengar penned *Light on Yoga*, an encyclopedia of all the yoga poses and their variations. In it, he includes some medicinal and scientific notes, but little anatomy.

Since then, yoga has taken on a mind of its own, or perhaps I should say, Western world's own. There are too many styles and theories for me to write about here, but throughout them all one thing is consistent: yoga's definition as *union*, stemming from the Sanskrit root "to yoke."

Yoga is the connection between breath and movement, thought and action. It is a philosophy, a science, and above all, a practice that links your body to your mind, your tangible self to your intangible self. That is what got me so hooked. After years and years, miles and miles of running aimlessly, I finally began to sweat with a purpose, one that took care of my insides as much as it toned my outside. The switch to yoga gave me the long, limber legs I wanted as well as the perfectly functioning digestive system I sorely missed. Not to mention even more energy than I already had. I quickly realized that this was not just a workout or a get-flexible tool; it was an intricate system for full-body betterment, one that addressed my muscles as much as my mood.

According to yoga theory, we all have two bodies, the physical and the energetic, or more easily understood as the external and the internal, the tangible and the intangible. The tangible body is made up of the *you* you can touch—muscles, ligaments, tendons, bones, organs, tissues. The intangible body is made up of the *you* you know is there but cannot put your finger on. It is considered the subtle body, one ensconced deep within your framework and is in charge of how you feel, think, and perceive. Consider waking up in the morning: Why do you wake up in a great mood one day and a horrible one another? That's the intangible body at work. Traditional Chinese Medicine bases its principles on this intangible body, using needles to move energy from one main channel to another. Similarly, the intangible body is represented in yoga theory as thousands of energy channels and three main ones: the left, right, and center, called the *uma* in Tibetan.

The goal of yoga in its most traditional sense is to reach enlightenment. To me this means becoming healthy, happy, and successful, becoming one's true self, free of the need of external validation. Enlightenment is obtained, they say, when all the energy is running in the one central channel of your body. Yoga is merely a tool to get it there. How does yoga accomplish this? Either via the tangible body or the intangible mind.

Think of a clogged sink. You have two ways to fix it: either by banging on the outside of the pipe and tinkering on it with a wrench, or by pouring some Drano down the pipe. The yoga poses, or asanas, are akin to knocking on the outside of the pipe. As you do the poses, you lift, bend, twist, reach, lengthen, squat, jump, balance, and more, all with the outside body being the primary focus. Yet each pose affects not only the external you, but your inside as well, much like the specific placement of an acupuncture needle. When a full yoga sequence or class is designed correctly, the combined series of poses is like a full acupuncture treatment, moving energy out of the side channels and into the central channel. The positions create access to the intangible you. The original point of the poses was not to lift your butt or tone your abs, rather entirely about shifting the internal flow of energy inside you.

So if the poses are the pipe clanking, what is the Drano? This magical potion is all about the mind. Your thoughts move your energy inside your body just as the poses do. Consider a moment you have gotten angry and sworn at someone—how did you physically feel after? I am guessing perhaps you had a stomachache or burning sensation in your chest and/or abdomen. And I bet you experience a totally different feeling when you get an amazing piece of news or a happy surprise. You probably feel light, maybe even effervescent from the inside. Your thoughts, and from there your perceptions, reactions, and emotions, dictate the inner you. Good thoughts move energy to the central channel; bad thoughts keep energy tangled in the side channels. In real yoga, how you think is as important as how you move. (Don't worry, we will discuss this more thoroughly in a bit.)

Breath, in and out through the nose, is the tonic that unites the tangible and the intangible. The yoga breath is called *ujjai* and is hands down the most important part of the yoga practice. Traditionally in and out through the nose, lips closed, it serves as the connecting medium between the all of you, inside and out, outside and in. Without proper breath, yoga does not work the way in which it was designed.

In fact, Western doctors and scientists have recently shown that breathing through the nose, yoga-style, helps create smooth brain waves, mimicking states of relaxation. Breathing through the mouth, on the other hand, encourages erratic brain waves, ones more in line with extreme thought or behavior. The breath affects your brain, and from there everything else. Without proper breath through the nose, yes, you will move around, stretch, and hopefully sweat, but it will not necessarily be yoga,

15

rather just another calisthenics class. Yoga, real yoga, is unconditionally tied to the breath. It just does not work without it.

Breath is what historically has made yoga so powerful. It is the link between inner and outer, outer and inner. Unfortunately, the vast majority of studios, teachers, and methods pay little to no heed to this historical cornerstone, focusing instead on mastering a handstand or zoning out. But Retox is firmly grounded in this true essence of yoga. If yoga as intended has worked for thousands of years, why ignore it? Why do all these "weird" moves on a two-by-five-foot rubber mat if they are not actually creating any meaningful difference?

I care about how it all works, so that it actually works for you. The breath, the selection of postures, and, from there, your alignment within each one. The placement of your arms in a Warrior pose, the position of your knees in a Chair pose, the angle of your neck in a headstand. Anatomy matters. Luckily I am its biggest nerd.

The human body is magic. The way it is constructed, from the arteries to the muscles to the organs to the skin that holds it all together, and the way it functions are singlehandedly *the* universal miracle. Anatomy is the study of the structures of the human body; physiology is the study of how all the structures work together. I have long been obsessed with both.

Back in my competitive sports days, I would spend just as many hours in the training room as on the practice court. Part of this, of course, was due to my plethora of injuries. As frustrating as those injuries were—I hated being sidelined—I also embraced what they taught me. They each created a pathway for me to learn about a joint or muscle group in depth, how it works, what its contradictions are, and how to make it stronger. I would volunteer hours a week taping ankles, running stim machines, and shadowing the therapists and trainers as they led us banged-up athletes through endless exercises and therapies. I just thought it was the coolest thing ever. I loved it so much I set up a personal training business one summer, splattering the town of Woodside with flyers and ads, eager to help people get stronger and healthier from the muscles, out. I guess we can call that foreshadowing . . .

This fascination with anatomy and physiology naturally played into my yoga experience. Beginning with that first semi-fatal class in my basketball garb, I paid acute attention to the musculoskeletal and physiological implications of each pose, the poses I could do and the ones that were a pipe dream. Yes, I was breathing and attempting to be in the moment, but I was also doing a hands-on study of the anatomy of yoga through the lens of a die-hard athlete and anatomy geek. As I practiced, I could feel the muscles and joints interacting in a whole new way, one in which traditional sports or workouts could not access. I also began to notice some risks—poses that I am pretty sure my five-foot-eleven, lanky athletic frame should not be in, alignment requests that seemed contrary to what the human body should do, and most dangerous, repeated strain on the ligaments, which should never be stretched.

The whole thing was fascinating to me. I would go to class, sweat it out, and then run home to scour over my anatomy book as I waited for dinner to be delivered. The next day I would go back and hold that image of the muscle or joints in my mind as I approached the very same pose. From there I tried to optimize it, engaging what needed to be engaged, releasing what needed to release, and protecting what could be in harm's way. I effectively dissected the yoga poses, one by one, day by day. When I finally started giving myself my own classes, often referred to as self-practice, I also entered from an anatomical lens. I would flip open the anatomy bible, *The Atlas of Human Anatomy*, pick a muscle group, joint, or physiological element, stare at it until it seemed ingrained in my brain, and then develop a class focused entirely around that anatomical part. This habit made my body and my yoga practice so much stronger, not to mention safer. I took what I was learning from my amazing teachers and ancient yoga texts and geekified it with some straight-up science. That's Retox.

The human body was created as an optimized machine, one that knows how to sustain, heal, and protect itself, to replenish and revitalize itself, inside and out. We have to respect that. Knowing how it works is essential to knowing how to move. Physical yoga can be dangerous. I am not saying it *is* dangerous and you should run away from it now; I am saying that, like walking down the street in high heels, it *can* be dangerous. The majority of poses, if taught or done incorrectly, can and do inflict harm on a joint, ligament, or connecting tissue. The potential for injury is great, but with a strong foundation in anatomical knowledge, it does not have to be.

The human body is the human body; we each get one, and they all work in the same way. Having said that, we are all unique. My body was not necessarily built to be able to do what yours can and does easily. Nor should it. Yet my body does know when something is bad for it, even if the yoga teacher does not, and most typically sends me that message through a pain or injury, one that no amount of meditation can take away. And believe me, I have experimented with this.

A few years ago, I hurt my shoulder in a diving accident. It was bad, really bad, but I was in denial for many months after the incident, attempting to holistically heal myself before heading to the surgeon for what I knew in my gut would be a big deal. I continued practicing with my yoga teachers, informing them of the injury, and asking them to help me practice in a way that would make it better. They, as good, compassion-filled yogis, fervently agreed. Yet after weeks of going to their classes, I realized I had placed myself in the center of the lion's den. They had me doing all the same poses as usual, saying that if I meditated through it the injury would go away, and that "the practice heals all." I was skeptical and knew better intellectually and anatomically, but I was desperate.

Guess what? The injury did not go away. In fact, it only got worse. Despite what they were telling me to do, I was not supposed to be binding (clasping) my arms behind my back, breathing through Up Dogs, or doing headstands. As I was doing it all, I knew I was screwing myself up more, but I had fallen prey to my own career and industry. After six months of pain and agony, my husband forced me to the surgeon, who not only performed an entire reconstructive shoulder surgery, but educated me on how the injury happened, and how yoga had made it worse. Since his impeccable work and my pain-free recovery, this doctor, rated the top orthopedic surgeon in America, has taken dozens of hours to confer with me on all the nitty-gritty elements of anatomy and yoga. There in his fluorescent-lit office, we have dissected the poses one by one, going through the anatomical risks, benefits, and contradictions of each. We have compared the poses to body types and ailments, physical goals and limitations. In fact, as a result of this process, there are many poses I simply do not teach anymore, let alone do myself. Turns out that from a strict medical, orthopedic perspective, they are not all great for everyone. Shocker. Thanks to this insight, I now just say no to certain yoga pose trends, and I feel even more confident guiding classes with an intense anatomical focus. If it ain't broke, why break it?

This is where I diverge from traditional yoga, as well as where I extract further value from it. I respect the sciences of anatomy and physiology, and I use them to my, and now your, advantage. I look at the body as both the cure and the cause, the self-sustaining source of betterment and the potential source of harm. In doing so, I have created an approach to yoga that can actually make you stronger, leaner, more flexible, more relaxed, and everything else you hope it will, but in a way that is safe and truly effective.

What sets Retox and I.AM.YOU. apart are an intense respect for the tradition of yoga—its union of inner and outer bodies, tangible and intangible—and the laser focus on anatomy. This yoga is technical. And thus it works.

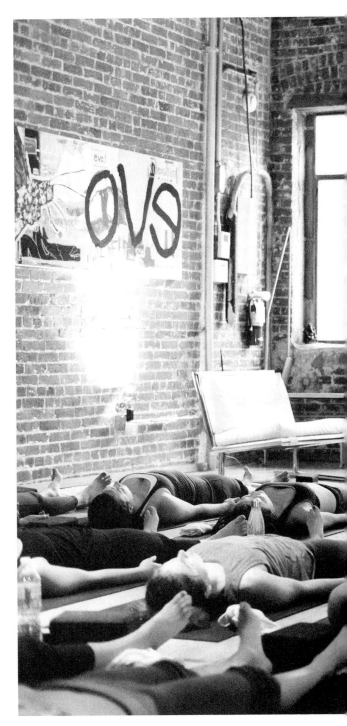

18 **The seeds for RETOX are planted. I.AM.YOU. Studio, New York City.**

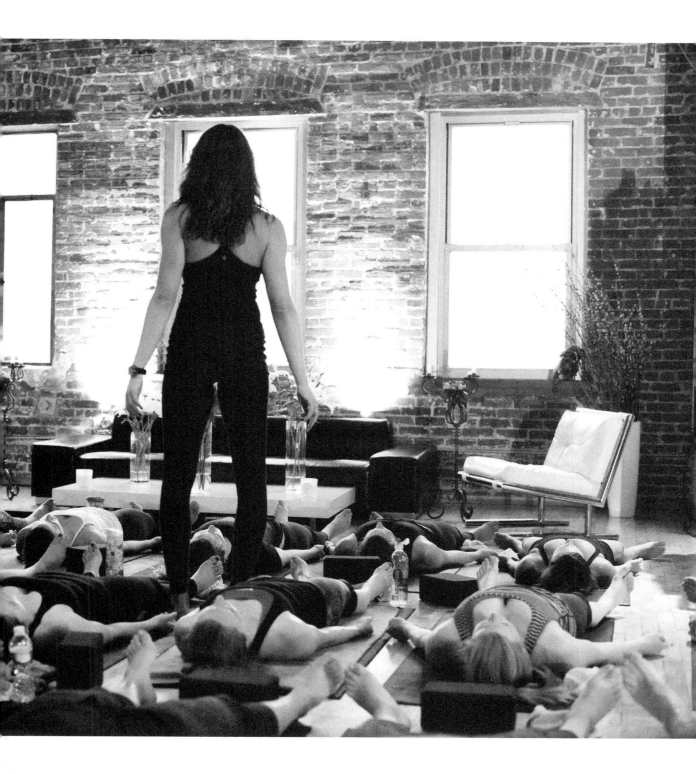

SLAM DUNK

One of the most fascinating things about yoga—real yoga—is how societies approached it. In India, yoga was highly linked with religion, specifically Hinduism. The yoga texts were and still are considered religious books, the poses a calling to a deity up above. Adults and children, mostly men, were encouraged to practice the yoga poses as a way to prepare to sit and meditate or pray.

However, in Tibet, an equal yet less known birthplace of yoga, one was not allowed to do yoga poses until one had mastered meditating. That is right. You could not do a Warrior pose until you managed the workings of your mind. The belief was that without the mind in shape, the body did not matter, or even worse, you ran the risk of injury and illness. In fact, it's been said that Tibetan monks had to meditate for twenty years before ever being allowed to do one pose.

This focus on the power of the mind wasn't really all that foreign to me. I grew up in California, after all. Matt Blanchard, my middle school basketball coach, was the first person to introduce me to meditation—although I didn't know it at the time. Every day we would end our two-hour practice by sitting in a circle on the edge of the court to "see." He would have us close our eyes and notice our breath. Then we would have to visualize ourselves shooting a jump shot and getting nothing but net. At the free-throw line, sinking two in a row. At the boards, seizing the critical rebound. Winning the game. There I sat, knees up by my chin (I was too inflexible to sit cross-legged), mentally picturing the results I wanted to have on the court. Day after day, year after year, Matt had me visualize my Jordan-inspired success. Lo and behold, I was meditating.

As I alluded to earlier, meditation is not a complex practice, nor should it be daunting. Years later in New York City, when I came face-to-face with meditation again, still in my basketball shorts and equally inflexible, I recalled these pubescent visualization practices, and realized I had actually been meditating for a decade, just in a way that was applicable my personality, goals, and life.

Meditation used to get a supremely bad rap, mostly because it was mistakenly thought to be too esoteric or simply New Age mumbo jumbo. Now it is widely accepted, referred to as mindfulness or conscious thinking. I take it up a philosophical and psychological notch, and call it mindset.

Mindset is a brain-muscle practice. It is training the mind to work the way you want it to, so you can feel and live the way you dream of. It is not about sitting aimlessly, but rather about visualizing and from there creating your ideal you and your ideal world, from the inside out.

How? The Tibetan yoga philosophers, the original meditation, mindfulness, and mindset gurus, say that there are over 84,000 *nadis*, or strains of thought, each represented by an energy channel in the intangible body. These are categorized by the way your mind turns, which is generally in two ways—one in which it has correct perceptions, and the other in which it has incorrect perceptions. Correct perceptions are simple to grasp—when you have them, you are happy, healthy, successful. Incorrect perceptions, on the other hand, are intangible

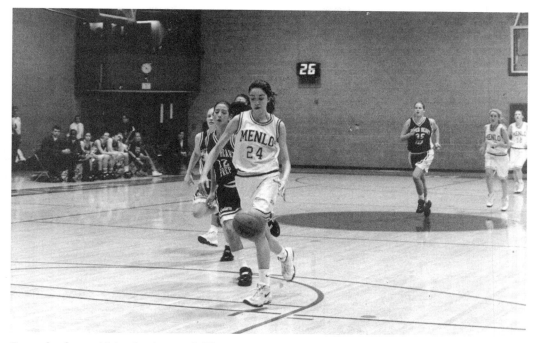

Game day for my high school team. California.

mental assessments that form an experience that makes you suffer, mildly or intensely. The goal of mindset is to train the muscle of your brain to always turn in a way that creates correct perceptions, so that you then live in a body and life free of suffering. (Suffering, by the way, can imply something as banal as missing the train.)

If you change your thoughts, you can change your energy. If you change your energy, you change your intangible body. Changing your inner body shapes your outer body, and from there, you create your world.

Your mind, the thing we all know is there but cannot touch, is at the core of it all. It is your true essence, molded 100 percent from your perceptions. Every time your eye sees something, your mind has a minuscule mo-

ment to see it and then label it. These labels, which we will discuss later in depth, are your perceptions, the very things that construct you and the world you live in. Think about that raging maniac of a woman who is your boss. To someone she is an amazing mother and a loving wife. It is not her, but rather your perception of her, that dictates your experience.

There is a tiny gap of time between what your eye sees and what your mind perceives.

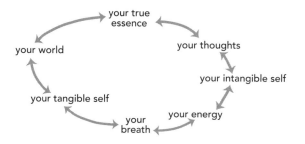

The goal of Tibetan yoga philosophy is to make you agile enough to insert yourself in that space and create the labels you actually want, and from there, your perceptions and experiences. It's not about ignoring your thoughts or letting them go. It's about being able to harness them, taking control of the seeds that are planted and how they will bloom.

But to change your thoughts you need to practice, just like you would practice your jump shot. That is what mindset is for. It is a training camp for your brain, a series of drills for the muscle of your mind. Mindset keeps you in shape for the daily game that is modern life, and if you're lucky, winning the championship, too.

IT'S FOOD; EAT IT

Do you really think our ancestors thought as much about what they ate as we do now? If they had, we would all be dead. Food is food. It has been around longer than we have as humans, in all its natural glory. The problem is not food, but rather our relationship to it.

I often think about my grandmother, my best friend and Chief Inspiration Officer. She is eighty-seven, happy, fit, and healthy as a horse. She eats three to five meals a day, all with bread. Hamburgers are a religious experience for her—a couple weekly is the norm, as is dessert after lunch and dinner. Her plate is equally loaded with fruit and vegetables, but she never overthinks about what she eats. She focuses on food for vitality, and makes a point out of thoroughly enjoying every bite. That's how she was raised. As a result, she is free of all medical issues, takes absolutely no pills, is more energetic than all of us put together, and is ready to take on the world at any given moment. Don't we all want that?

How do you approach food? Are you eating blindly, too impatient to feel what your body is asking for? Or are you hopping on some dietary bandwagon, too lazy to actually think it through? Are you married to your bad habits, unable to make a change? Or just too tired and overwhelmed to think about it at all?

I do not want you to be consumed by what you eat. What I do want is for you to forget about the religion of food and focus on the inherent value of it. Take heed of its fueling nature rather than its harming one. Embrace its therapeutic properties. Food is energy, and it is medicine. In fact, the majority of the herbs used as prescriptions in Traditional Chinese Medicine stem from one natural food source or another—orange peels, grains, dried greens, to name a few. We need food, all sorts of food to make us strong, energetic, and alive. What we do not need is to obsess over it.

Obsessing over food is exhausting, and just so not fun. Yet we as a society have a deep-seated desire to continually grasp hold of the latest food doctrine, ride its wave, and then jump to the next one. This endless tale of dietary trend jumping is merely feeding the food industry and its multimillion-dollar corporations, while killing our chances to be sane, healthy human beings.

Who are you following anyway? The advertising machine or your body? The Hollywood spokesperson or the person in the mirror? The industry that wants you to spend or the you who wants to live?

22

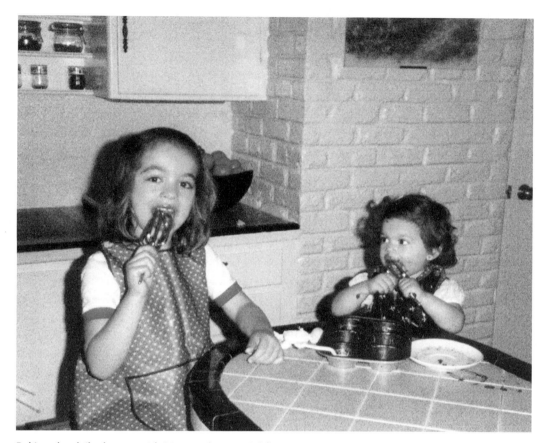

Baking the daily dessert with Mom and sister. California.

In the past thirty years, we have gone from fat free to carb free. Wheat everything (hello, obvious gluten allergies in the making) to meat everything. Gluten free to dairy free. Low fat to full fat. It's a loop created not by our body's actual needs or evolution, but by an industry searching for new sources of revenue and egos longing for a new pedestal. If we actually listened to what our body wanted and needed during this time, we would hear it clamoring for simple, whole foods, the way our ancestors ate and my grandmother eats every day.

Yet year after year, fad after fad, we fixate on what we should not eat, somehow defining our self-worth by how much we eliminate and how regimented we are able to be. But would it not be better for the standard to be how we actually feel?

The detox hysteria is a perfect example of an inane diet trend. Ninety percent of the people who come to me after completing some cleanse or another have a cold, are just recovering from the flu, feel weak, and/or have regained all the weight they lost. Yet they take the plunge, again and again, usually because they feel they have to.

That said, there are two types of toxins— the tangible ones and the intangible ones. Tangible toxins come in various forms, all related to what we physically put into our body. These encompass everything from alcohol to processed foods to pollution, chocolate, chemicals, and more. They are generally referred to as exotoxins. We as a society obsess over these toxins, which often result in people doing the aforementioned painful fasts and juice cleanses on the one hand, and elimination of products and real foods on the other.

Intangible toxins come in the form of emotions—anger, stress, worry, grief, sadness, and extreme excitement, primarily. These are sometimes referred to as endotoxins. In Traditional Chinese Medicine, each of these emotions is processed by a specific organ—stress in the liver, fear in the kidneys, worry in the spleen, for example. These toxins are eliminated in the same way the ingested tangible ones are and are equally toxic to our system.

So when someone is juice fasting to get clean (that is, attempting to eliminate physical toxins from their system) but stressed or angry because of the challenge and logistics of it all, life, or really just because they are starving, they are actually *adding* a plethora of toxins *to* their body, and not advancing in any "cleansed" direction at all. Essentially they are starving themselves for no reason. I gotta ask, what's the point?

Even if you eliminate all the physical toxins from your diet and surroundings (which, by the way, is impossible), you can still create toxins with your mind. These toxins, intangible as they may be, will equally affect your tangible physical body, and elimination diets and restrictive food programs aren't the solution. Retox is.

With Retox we eat to live. There is no "cheating" because it is all just food. Or at least, it should be. Millions of people would kill, fairly literally, for the access we have to whole foods today. Turning them down because you think you have to is an insult to those in need, and the very cells keeping you alive. I am not saying to go on a fast-food binge, but rather to take food for what it is. Food is medicine. It is fuel. It is the essence of what keeps you going, in the most literal of ways. I will guide you through it, so that all you have to do is eat it.

03

KEEPING IT TOGETHER

We must free ourselves of the hope that the sea will ever rest.
We must learn to sail in high winds.

—ARISTOTLE ONASSIS

SWEAT. EAT. BREATHE. THAT'S PRETTY MUCH ALL YOU NEED TO DO. ALAS, IT GETS
so darn complicated these days. Paleo or low fat? Vegan or pescetarian? Should we
cycle, run, do Pilates? But who has time to go to the gym? And when we do, what are
we supposed to do there? Never mind that we're so busy running around, doing everything we "need" to do, we don't even stop for a breath. But moving, eating, and being
happy and healthy need not be complex goals convoluted by competing theories, each
clamoring for your attention and dollars. The whole point of Retox is that life is actually
supposed to be simple. We innately know what we need; the answers are all inside us.
We just have to listen.

Let's face it, though—it can be tough to keep it together. I often feel like I have twenty things competing for my attention and energy at the same time, and I have to juggle them all with a smile on my face, and without getting anxious, downing a bottle of wine at night, or forgetting to do something. That's life today for all of us. And you know what? Sometimes we want to do it all. We want to achieve our goals, be at the top of our game, and yes, have fun! As a result, we may not eat right, move enough, sleep enough, or take time to breathe. We may get overwhelmed, over-worked, and we may overindulge. But that's life when you live it to the max.

In the upcoming chapters, I have decon-structed twenty of the major conundrums that we face during this juggling journey that is modern existence, everything from headaches to stress, iPhone addiction to trouble falling asleep, back pain to endlessly sitting at a desk, feelings of being fat to striving for success. I have a Retox cocktail for each, all of which you can use as you need, perhaps rotating through them, picking one a day in place of, or as an adjunct to, your daily martini. Or you can use them in a more targeted fashion, like a shot for whatever ails you in the moment.

But in this chapter, I offer you a plan for general living, for just being you, and for keep-ing it more than together on any and every given day. I call it the LSP, or Life Stability Plan.

At the center of the Retox LSP is *you*. Who you are, tangibly and intangibly. The goal of the plan is to ensure there are pipelines in place that continually fuel you, so that you can simply take on your day, every day, without having to think about it. The plan includes yoga, nourishment, and mindset, or sweating, eating, and breathing.

Food feeds the cells of your body; thoughts affect the function of your mind. How we feel in any given moment, who we are on any given day, and what we need to sustain ourselves are all connected. What you eat affects how your body feels. How your body feels affects how your mind perceives. What your mind perceives directs your thoughts and your moods. Your moods, in turn, shape what you crave, and the cycle continues, in every possible combination.

To regularly feel like a million bucks, you need to have a go-to, 360-degree LSP, one that understands that every day is different, and, thus, what you need to get on track var-ies. Sometimes that means a steak and a good sleep. Other days may require a solid sweat. And yet others, five minutes of quiet alone time just breathing. It would be absurd for me to suggest one thing that will work to keep you healthy and happy every day; we are just not built like that—although the self-help, well-ness, and diet industries have certainly capital-ized on people believing we are. The Retox LSP takes a macro view and gives you a bit of everything you need to create the best you on any given day.

Consider these as best practices for daily life. Serve it up for yourself every day, then down a Retox cocktail on the side when some-thing specific comes up. You will not only feel different, but you will *be* different, too.

YOGA

I am going to let you in on a little secret, one I am almost certain the multibillion-dollar yoga industry does not want you to know: Yoga has been scientifically shown to reduce base metabolic rate. In other words, it makes you burn less calories per hour while you rest. How can that be, and why would we ever waste hours doing it if all it does is slow your metabolism? Good question, Watson.

Remember earlier when we discussed the true purpose of yoga asana, or poses, as that of directing energy into the central channel of the body? The follow-up to that is that the poses direct the energy with the aim of preparing your body to meditate. When your energy is directed to the central channel, you are healthy, successful, and calm, as previously noted, and thus able to sit for long periods of time. The only hindrance to sitting for long periods of time is getting hungry. (If you only knew how many snacks I have eaten while writing this book . . .) The yoga poses were not necessarily designed to rev up your metabolism; that would have been a meditative, stomach-wrenching disaster. They were instead designed to slow your metabolism so you could sit down, close your eyes, and stay there for hours, maybe even days, at a time.

So when you do yoga today, in a world in which long hours at desks, stress, and murky food sources prevail, you must ensure that it increases your base metabolic rate, not lower it even further. This has been a premise of I.AM.YOU. yoga since day one. That means attention to Sun Salutes and Moon Salutes, the two pose series actually shown to increase metabolic rate. I then add my quintessential I.AM.YOU. Warm-Up Flow, a funkified, modern take on the salutes that combines intense focus on anatomy and cardiovascular exercise. In fact, a study of I.AM.YOU. students wearing heart rate monitors and other health/calorie-tracking devices has shown that this sequencing increased their heart rate and burned up to three times more calories than any other yoga class they took wearing the same monitors.

In addition to this calorie burning, metabolism-boosting, cardiovascular focus, daily yoga must include elements of both strength and flexibility. And, of course, the breath. I have distilled the practice into a Retox cocktail for you, so that you can sweat and move every day, in a way that is efficient for your schedule and your body.

Do not worry about how much time you have. Just turn to these Retox yoga solutions and implement them no matter what, whenever you can. You can do the Desk Fixes at your desk or in the car while you are waiting to pick up your kid; these are each takes on a traditional yoga pose designed to be done at your desk or in a seat. Use the Quick Fixes wherever you are in your day; these are straight-up yoga poses whose anatomical and physiological properties will benefit the issue in question. Do the full sequence as a normal yoga class or workout, or simply in the time you have before dinner, work, or while the baby naps. It is schematic for a full I.AM.YOU. yoga class, tailored to the topic we are addressing. As a general rule of thumb, usually the first and second poses are meant to be held. Then proceed to do the rest of the poses in the first two lines as a flow, usually a Sun Salute or variation, holding only one breath in each. Then hold the rest of the poses for five to eight breaths each, or whatever feels good to you. Are you ready to Retox?

RETOX

DESK FIXES

FOREARM CROSSED BREATH

Inhale, lift your arms up alongside your ears. Exhale, bend your elbows and clasp your forearms on top of each other. Breathe here, imagine the inhaling breath going up your right arm, across your forearms, and the exhaling breath going down your left arm, and then to your center, for three breaths. Repeat in the other direction three times as well. If you have time—if not, then the next time—begin what is traditionally called *khapalabhati.** Inhale to a comfortable level. Begin short, sharp breaths out of the nose, where the inhale is simply a reaction to the exhale, as the diaphragm pumps on the abdominal wall. It should feel somewhere between sneezing and blowing your nose. (If you are pregnant, skip khapalabhati.) Keep these up for a minute, energizing your body with each pump.

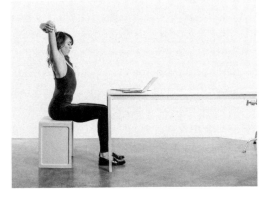

CHAIR FORWARD FOLD

Come to the edge of your chair. Separate your feet hip distance apart. Extend your legs forward and flex your feet so the heels press into the floor. Inhale, sit up tall. Exhale, fold forward, reaching your hands toward your ankles or shins. Let your head hang here and hold for five to fifteen breaths.

GENTLE TWIST*

Inhale, sit up tall. Exhale, twist to the right. Look over your right shoulder. Hold here five breaths, then repeat on the other side.

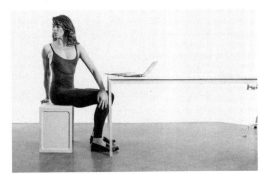

EAGLE ARMS

Open your arms wide out to the sides. Bring your arms toward each other and cross your right arm under your left arm. Bend your elbows, and if you can, wrap your wrists so your palms touch. As you inhale, bring your elbows in line with your chin. Exhale, drop your chin down. Breathe into your upper back and neck for three to ten breaths, then repeat on the other side.

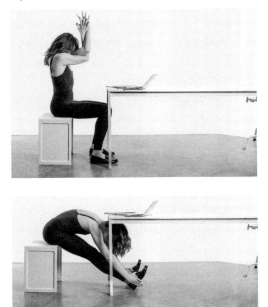

QUICK FIXES

SUN SALUTE A

Start standing with your feet together and your hands touching at your chest. Inhale, reach your arms overhead. Exhale, fold forward, and bring your forehead to your shins. Inhale, extend your spine, look forward. Exhale, bring your hands to the mat, and step or jump into Plank pose, bending your elbows straight back. You can also stay in Chaturanga. Inhale, straighten your elbows, roll over your toes to the tops of your feet and lift your chest, Up Dog. Exhale, push back onto your toes, lift your butt into the air, and press your heels toward the ground, Down Dog. Close your eyes or look at your belly button and hold here five breaths. Then inhale and step or jump your feet between your hands. Exhale, fold forward. Inhale, reach your arms overhead, look up. Exhale, hands to your heart. Repeat five to ten times.

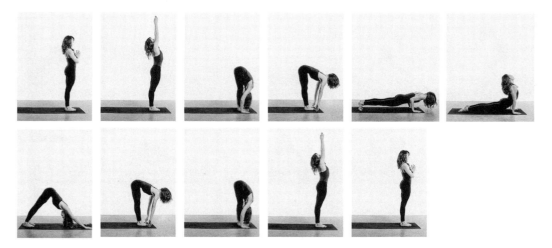

SEATED FORWARD FOLD

Start sitting on the floor, legs straight in front of you. Flex your feet so the heels press into the floor. Inhale, sit up tall. Exhale, fold forward, reaching your head toward your knees. Let your head hang here and hold for five to fifteen breaths.

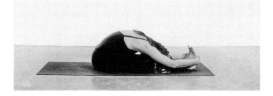

SHOULDER STAND

Lie on the floor. Lift your feet up and over your head and place your hands on your back. Inhale, lift your legs straight up into the air. Look at your toes or close your eyes and breathe here for ten breaths, or up to five minutes.

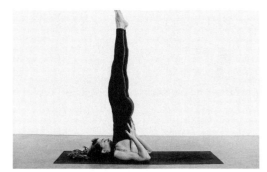

29

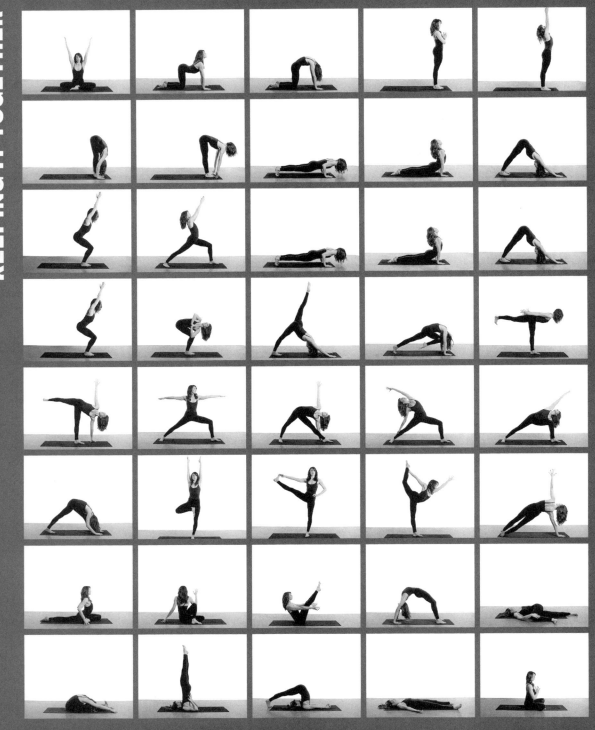

NOURISHMENT

Retoxing is about feeding your insides, eating what you want to eat, enjoying it, and moving on. No guilt. No restrictions. No stress. Retox nutrition is based on six simple tenets. Once you embrace them, you will have freed yourself from overthinking about food, leaving you open to the pure pleasure of eating, and the efficiency of the innate metabolic workings of your body.

NO GUILT

Guilt is an utter waste of energy. Especially when it comes to food. So you ate a big meal and your pants feel a little tight, or you celebrated with an ice-cream sundae. No biggie, as long as you enjoyed it.

Guilt detracts from the satisfaction that is eating, destroying the internal, intangible nourishment of the experience and the food. If you are stressing yourself out with remorse during or after your meal, you are almost ensuring that your body will have an adverse reaction to what you ate. Let your body instead focus on extracting the value out of the food you gave it, and then naturally burn off the rest.

And while we are on the topic, let me just address this whole "indulge" concept. *Indulge* comes from the Latin word *indulgere*, which means "to accede or take pleasure in." *Indulge* is defined as allowing oneself to follow one's will, to yield to an inclination or desire. Yet in the wellness world, indulging is associated with guilt. Why is having chocolate, beef, or pizza indulging? Each has nutrients your body is probably asking for, be it antioxidants, vitamin B, or calcium, to name a few. Is diving into a massive salad indulging? It should be, given what the word means, but oddly in today's society it is not because salad is green. The thing is, your body needs more than just vegetables, and you should not feel shame for consuming something from any other food group. In Retox terms, it is not indulging if your body is telling you to eat it. But that's the key: Listen to your body. Be mindful of what you're eating. Chew and taste and fully savor what you put in your mouth. And guilt is not allowed.

CHOOSE NATURE OVER DOGMA

Aren't you at least a little bit sick of listening to friends babble about gluten, fat, and sugar during dinner, consciously avoiding the carbs and dissecting everything on the menu, driving the poor waitstaff insane? I am! What a waste of time, and not to mention, a total downer! Nutritional dogma has permeated our consciousness, leaving little room for satisfaction. Enough is enough!

Natural foods are overall good foods, even if there is some doctor or celebrity fitness "expert" out there preaching to you that they are not. Let's go through the current nutritional pariahs one by one:

GLUTEN. Gluten has been around in a natural form for thousands of years. Eat it as it was created by Mother Nature, and without making it the centerpiece of all your meals, and you likely will not have a problem. Ingest it in a processed form regularly, as is so common in premade snacks, packaged foods, thickening agents, and more, and yes, you may feel less than well. You can now find gluten and its by-products in hundreds of foods it was never intended to be in—candy, sauces, canned soups,

31

protein and snack bars, to name a few. It is no wonder people have developed allergies.

If you eat gluten solely in its original capacity and do not overwhelm your diet with it, you will likely not have a problem unless you have been medically diagnosed as having a gluten intolerance or allergy. Use gluten as a garnish, not a main course, and as a small proportion of your overall diet, and pay attention to what types of gluten affect you. For example, soy sauce and processed gluten make me bloat and suffer through painful stomachaches. Real grains and pasta make me happy. I have high-quality pasta one to two times a week, bread if I am craving it, and freshly baked croissants and cookies for an often daily treat, but I do not take in any gluten elsewhere. Gluten is a facet of my diet, but by no means do I have it as the centerpiece of every meal.

Look, if you want to be gluten free, great. If you do not, you really don't need to worry about it. Just be honest with yourself, and don't hide your carb-free diet under the "gluten-free" veil; you're not fooling me.

DAIRY. As with most things in life, it all comes down to your individual body. First, see how dairy makes you feel. If dairy gives you a stomachache, avoid it. If it makes you feel strong, as is common in many cultures across the globe, go for it. Then decide how you are going to enjoy it. Choose when and how to have your dairy, and then make sure it fits into the context of your overall daily intake, as a garnish, not a focal point, akin to gluten.

For example, I do not like ice cream, and drinking a big glass of milk gives me a stomachache, but I salivate for cheese and good cappuccinos. So I have dairy in the form of hard cheeses, which I love, and pizza, which I adore. I usually use almond milk in my coffee, unless I am in Italy or know the cappuccino place is legit (I see no point in having a subpar cappuccino). If you keep things balanced and don't go overboard, it will likely all be fine.

ALCOHOL. Clearly with a book called *Retox*, alcohol is not a pariah in my mind. Abusing it, though, is. Feel free to drink if it is right for your body and your mind, acknowledging the health risks and balancing it all with proper food and exercise. As to what type of alcohol to drink, you will just have to keep reading.

MEAT AND EGGS. I touched on this earlier, but being a vegan or vegetarian is not the one-and-only, without-fail solution to permanent health. Meat, in and of itself, is not bad for you. *Homo sapiens* survived exclusively on meat for years, as the trendy Paleo dieters will tell you. The key to eating meat is making sure it is clean, well-treated, and as antibiotic and hormone free as possible. Balance it with ample servings of vegetables, and you will have a healthy and satisfying meal.

I personally embraced red meat's healing properties very soon after quitting vegetarianism. My ob-gyn discovered abnormal cell growth on the lining of my uterus. Specialists wanted to surgically remove it immediately for fear of cancer, but there was a huge risk for my future fertility. I was torn. My Traditional Chinese Medicine doctor, mentors, and primary ob-gyn all suggested I change my diet and see what happened. I was willing to try anything.

I immediately put myself on the "beat this thing" diet, adding organic, grass-fed beef four times a week and eggs with the yolk twice a week to my current diet heavy with spinach, broccoli, and berries. Within six months of eating like this, the growth was gone, and has not come back since. No medicine or surgery needed. My body sent me a very strong message that despite all my spinach, kale, and green goodness, it needed beef and eggs to be healthy. I had no choice but to listen.

Meat is not necessarily bad. You just need to eat it consciously. Focus on organic, grass-fed beef and wild versus farm-raised fish. Be selective about chicken, eating it only if you really want to, or you know it comes from a clean source. Go light on the pork, as it is inherently harder to digest and tougher on the

system. I will go through this in more depth in later chapters, but fire up the BBQ until then!

SUGAR. Your body, especially the brain, needs sugar to function. Period. The end. Glucose, which is known as the most common fuel in living organisms, is a sugar, and the primary source of energy for the brain. Low glucose impairs both psychological and physiological processes, often leading to brain fog, lethargy, poor memory and decision-making, and low energy, among other things.

The richest forms of glucose come via natural sugars, such as fruit and honey. Vegetables and grains do have glucose as well, but not nearly as much. Eliminating sugar, or claiming you have cut out sugar and then dousing every-

THE SWAPERDOODLE

SO WHAT DO YOU DO if you just love it all, all the time? You do what I do: the swaperdoodle. It is a fun way to mix and match what you love with what you crave and need. Just swap out some things so you can enjoy others. Here are some examples:

- ► Skip the sugary frozen cocktail and enjoy your alcohol with club soda and a twist and then have dessert.
- ► Have all-natural margaritas instead of ones from the prefab mix.
- ► Squeeze or crush real fruit into your sparkling water instead of adding fruit juice.
- ► Skip the cheese in your sandwich, but have the fries.
- ► Opt for a salad instead of pizza, but have the ice cream for dessert.
- ► Dive into the steak but have string beans instead of creamed spinach.
- ► Have the egg sandwich for breakfast, but skip the chicken on the salad for lunch.
- ► Crunch on the chips and guacamole, but skip the fried tacos and fried fish.
- ► Have a croissant in the a.m., and veggies in the p.m.
- ► Enjoy the bread basket, but order fish instead of pasta.

thing in agave and having a daily juice, is hypocritical dogmatic doo-doo. As an alive, functioning human being, you need sugar. There is no way around it. What you do not need are fake sugars, such as the ones found in processed and packaged foods. Stick to sugar in its natural form, with some fruit (but not too much! Too much fruit is just as bad), but more vegetables, and if you like, something sweet once a day, and you will be giving your cells the fuel they need for every action. And as you are about to see, feeding your cells is of utmost importance.

So instead of being XYZ-free be +*you*. Eat what you like, not to mention what your body likes, and follow your body's natural ebb and flow. If you want to go meat free for a while, and your body is telling you to do it, by all means go for it. If you want to load up on dairy, do that, too. But listen to what your body is telling you, and you will never have a problem.

Eating in a +*you* way as opposed to a –*free* way will be liberating and help you find your natural body weight, digestive patterns, and self.

GO FOR NUTRIENTS OVER CALORIES

And now we come to one of the most important lessons in the book: Nutrients establish you; calories fuel you. You absolutely need both, and when looking at food, lean toward the higher nutrient choices rather than lower calorie ones.

Let's go back to the discussion of cells earlier in this chapter. Cells make up you and every other living organism; they are the basis of your existence. You are made of trillions of cells, all of which need certain nutrients in order to keep you alive and well. You need to feed your cells, quite literally. If you do not provide them with the nutrients they need, they will not be able to do the work they are supposed to do, which is to keep you alive and healthy. As Dr. Terry Wahls wrote, "What your cells use to fuel the chemistry of life comes directly from what you feed yourself." You must feed yourself on a cellular level, not a calorie-counting one.

Nutrients > Calories

For example, let's say you have the choice of two main courses: grilled chicken or a grilled fillet of beef. Nine out of ten health and diet mongers will tell you to go for the chicken as the low-calorie, "lean source of protein." When you Retox, I ask you to take it one level deeper. Chicken has protein, absolutely, but beef is equally protein packed, and even more, it is loaded with iron, zinc, phosphorous, and vitamin B. In fact, one 3-ounce serving of beef provides the same amount of vitamin B12 as do seven 3-ounce chicken breasts and the same amount of iron as three cups of spinach. So now the question becomes about the quality of the bite. Perhaps you take a moment and assess how you feel—tired, run down, weak, or in need of a boost? Go for the beef as its nutrients are exactly what your body is telling you it needs. The important thing is not to adhere to the calorie count but rather to embrace the nutritional composition of the foods before you.

Let's look at another example. You have a hundred-calorie, fat-free snack bar in front of you. Pick your brand of choice. Do you have that or "indulge" in the three-hundred-calorie avocado? If you look at calorie count alone, you may be compelled to pick the bar. Retox says choose the avocado for its omegas and essential fats. More calories, yes, but many more nutrients. Your body needs the nutrients to build and maintain the mitochondria, or engines, of the cells.

The importance of nutrients has come to the forefront of science under nutrigenomics, or the study of how food affects our genes. Eating certain foods can affect our DNA, and thus shift our genetic outcome, future disease profile, and longevity. Basically, you can literally eat yourself to better health. That's Retox nourishment. I have applied this theory, very much spearheaded by Dr. Wahls, time and time again with my clients.

Let me now share with you two stories to exemplify the power of nutrients as cellular sustenance. The first is of Jeff, a thirty-six-year-old father of two and husband from Philadelphia. He came to me after being diagnosed with multiple sclerosis (MS), looking for meditation lessons to keep the muscle of his mind in check. After a few sessions, I broached the food question, and realized he was eating what could objectively be considered "healthfully," but not in a fashion that could give his cells what they needed to combat the disease. He agreed to let me guide his nourishment, which involved infusing his diet with 90 percent vegetables, mainly dark leafy greens and broccoli. We made sure everything was cooked in garlic and olive oil, and he snacked on berries and tomatoes. The other 10 percent we filled with grass-fed, wild proteins, specifically red meat and salmon. He has had only one MS flare-up in the two years since this shift in diet, and he says he feels stronger than ever.

The second story is of Marie, a forty-two-year-old from Long Island. She was diagnosed with stage four breast cancer out of the blue, having to undergo a combination of intense chemo, radiation, and a double mastectomy. She came to me after her surgeries but pre chemo and radiation, looking to stretch and meditate. I asked her about her diet, and she said she was vegan and gluten free. I asked if she would be willing to experiment with some changes. She thankfully said, "Anything to keep me alive." I started her on one cup of bone broth—made from organic chicken or beef—daily, so that she would not have to chew the animal, but she'd still get the nutrients her cells needed. From there we took out 90 percent of her daily fruit, agave, and other natural sugar sources, and replaced it all with a diet of green, leafy vegetables, tomatoes, and berries. Eventually she added in salmon once a week and red meat once a week, as medicinal cellular doses. Let me tell you, when you see Marie now, you would never guess she had endured what she did. She did not lose one hair, and she is energetic, in remission, and glowing from the inside out.

Nutrients feed cells; cells construct you. So when you decide what to eat, consider the big picture of what you are eating, and the quality of each bite. Go for nutrient-packed foods over low-calorie, fat-free foods. Think of it as feeding your cellular foundation, and from there your current and future healthy being.

BASE OF CLEAN AND GREEN

Now we get into what specifically to eat. First, I really should not even have to be writing this, but I will just in case: Processed food is bad; fast food is worse. Both genres manipulate food from its natural, nutrient-packed, centuries-old genetic makeup and transform it into something that either lasts longer, tastes better, or has some sort of visual or textural sex appeal. I am not saying do not eat them, rather make them rarities, and pick and choose which you want. Tortilla chips with some salsa, cool. Double bacon cheeseburger from that fast-food joint, not so much. You get the drift? Pick your battles, and stick to what is real. You will be so much sexier as a result.

This brings me to your new best friend: water, or as a long-time I.AM.YOU.er calls it, a "celahydration," or celebration of hydration. Make H_2O your beverage of choice, morning, noon, and night. Sure, have a fresh-squeezed juice on the beach, hopefully with one of those little umbrellas in it, but the majority of the time your hydration should be crystal clear. Water oils the machine that is your tangible body, and helps remove all toxins that daily life creates. Lucky for most of us in the developed Western world, it is accessible and free, too.

From there, strive to make 60 to 80 percent of your diet green vegetables. I know that is not necessarily possible every meal of every day, so I want you to look at a three-day average. If you line up your plates at the end of seventy-two hours, shoot for 60 to 80 percent of everything on them to be green. Your body needs the same amount of time to process everything anyway, so have the green when it is available, and don't stress about it when it is not. My friends call me the Queen of Green, and now I want you to be Green royalty, too!

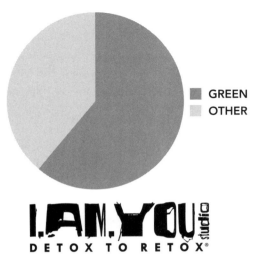

GREEN
OTHER

10- TO 12-HOUR BREAK

It takes, on average, seventy-two hours for your body to fully process something you have ingested. That's about three days. Thus, your body is almost constantly working to digest and metabolize what you give it, which means you also need to give it a break every now and then so it can catch up with you and your life.

Try to leave ten to twelve hours between dinner and breakfast. Meaning, if you finish dinner at 8 p.m., try to not have breakfast until 6 or 8 a.m. the next day. If you have a very late dinner, try to go as long as possible before breakfast, or just keep it to warm liquids such as tea, hot water, and coffee before you get to the ten-hour mark.

This break allows your digestive system to catch up and recuperate, and thus work more efficiently from then on, leaving you feeling more energetic and svelte as well.

THE 2/3 DIRECTIVE

Here it is, the number you have all been waiting for: 2/3. Also known as 66.666 percent, if fractions are not your thing.

When you Retox, aim for two out of every three meals to be "healthy," and one out of three to be whatever you want. (It might be typically healthy, too.) Another way to think about this is having two out of three things on your plate be pure nutrients, akin to the 60 to 80 percent green described above, and the last third can be whatever you like. You can look at this from an overall daily, weekly, or individual meal view. The proportion stays the same.

This is much like the quintessential "no veggies, no dessert" rule growing up. My mom gave us dessert with lunch and dinner every day. But there were two catches: First, we had to bake it fresh. And second, we had to finish our side salad, two vegetables, and either the meat or grain as a main beforehand. Now I have my croissant or pastry in the morning, and leave the rest of the day to nutrient-packed, green-based goodness. No harm, no foul.

RETOX

Those are the habits. Now what do you eat?

Nourishment is not about the dish itself; it is about the ingredients. What you eat creates what you become. The individual food components are the key to your thriving wellness. Which is why RETOX is all about ingredients, and then implementing these into a meal, not making a perfect coq au vin (although if that's your thing, go for it!).

Let's be honest, cooking in modern urban environments is not necessarily a piece of cake. Between going to the store, waiting in line, hauling everything back, prepping, actually cooking, and then the dreaded cleanup, it can all be an expensive, confusing, pain in the . . . Which is why we are Retoxing. The recipes I have provided in the Retox Lab chapters are all straightforward, easy, and legitimately quick. None of that fake ten-minute meal, pseudo-simple, dubiously healthy stuff here. All of the recipes here work for daily life, even if you do not have one of the targeted conditions they are associated with.

That said, Retoxing is not about forced cooking every day. I know that is unrealistic. It is simply about feeding yourself what you need, no matter where or how you get it. If it works for you, cook every day, of course, or maybe just once a week, making enough for the other days. But when you Retox, you are free to eat out and order in as much as you want. Just focus on the Retox Refuge below.

This Retox Refuge provides you a base with which to either make meals on the fly, without mess or hassle, or focus your ordering in or eating out on. Stock these items in your home regularly, and scan menus for them before you order, and nourishment will become second nature.

RETOX REFUGE

Baby spinach

Lettuce: red leaf, romaine, Bibb

Avocado

Tomatoes

Zucchini

Bell peppers

Broccoli, fresh or frozen

Lemon

Clementines or oranges

Cantaloupe

Blueberries

Onions
Garlic
Corn tortillas
Almonds
Quinoa
Black pepper
Mint
Popcorn,
   homemade or
   LesserEvil Buddha
   Bowl brand

Chamomile tea
Olive oil
Balsamic vinegar
Free-range eggs
Salmon, wild
Ground, lean,
   grass-fed beef
Almond milk

RETOX DINING

I eat out a lot . . . probably 50 percent of the time; the other 50 percent of the time, I make the recipes you will see in coming chapters. I do not feel guilty about it because I feel great, and I know how to order, which is what I am going to help you with now.

MANAGE YOUR MOOD. Dining is a shared experience. If you start whining about the menu, service, or food, everyone will have a bad time, which likely defeats the purpose of coming together to eat. The same goes for interrogating the staff on the food sources. Do it nicely, enjoy the experience of eating, and you will leave fully nourished, inside and out.

ALWAYS ORDER A SIDE OF GREENS. No matter what, no matter where, there is always something green on the menu.

TRY NOT TO MIX PROTEINS. We will get into this further later in the book, but attempt to order only one main protein in your meal. Meaning, if you have something with fish as a starter, go vegetarian as a main. Or if you get something with beef as a main, go vegetarian for your starter. Mixing proteins adds additional stress to your digestive system and could leave you feeling sluggish the next day.

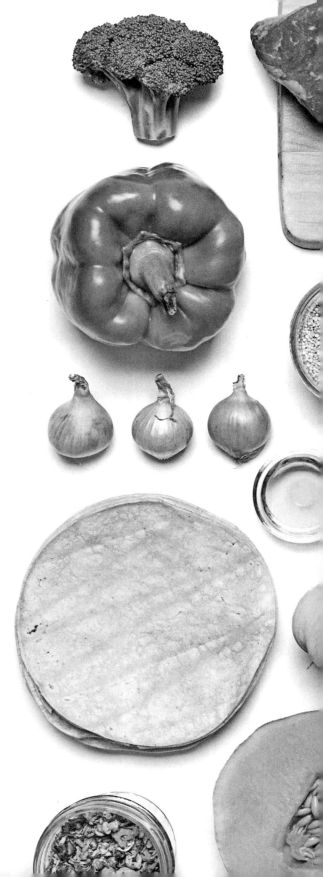

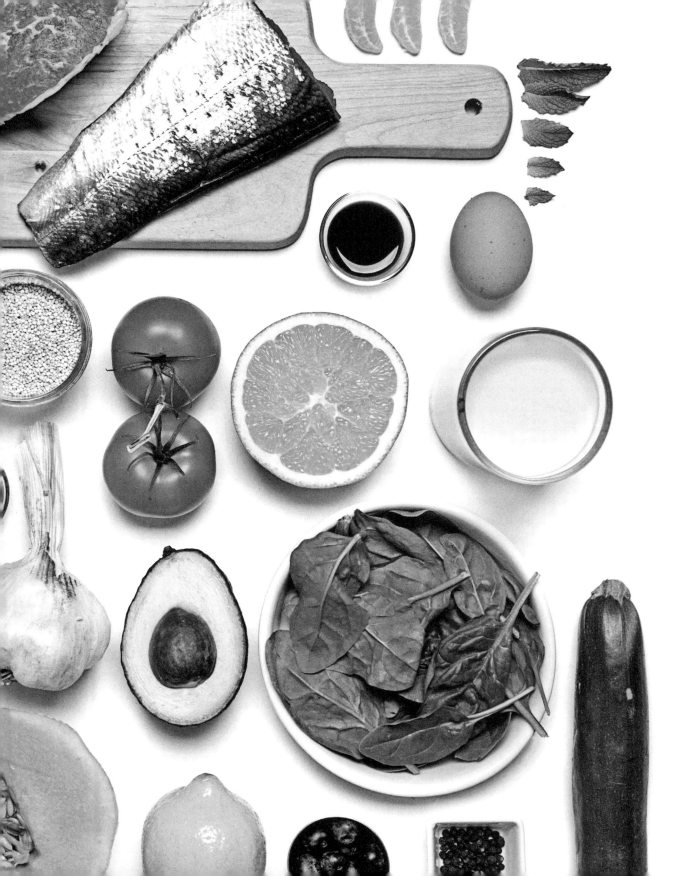

DON'T PANIC ABOUT ORGANIC. You probably (hopefully) will not drop dead right then and there if the food sources are not organic, so just enjoy your meal. That said, you do need to be conscious, without creating a scene, of what comes from where. When the menu says "white fish" or just fish, make sure you ask specifically which kind. Many "white fishes" are farm raised in China in less than optimal conditions—tilapia, hake, cod, and pollack being common contenders. Make sure the fish is wild and the beef is grass fed. Even better if they tell you where they get their beef. I would prefer you to shy away from the chicken, as you really do not know how it was raised or arrived to you these days, and always load up on the greens.

HYDRATE. Make sure you get some water, ideally tap with no ice, upon sitting. Use that as your focal beverage, and then if wine and cocktails come, match them one to one with the water.

SWAP OUT THE SIDES. Unless you know those fries taste like they belong on a café table with an up-close and personal view of the Eiffel Tower, swap them out for a side of string beans, which give the same handheld pleasure of french fries, or a side salad. Do the same for other forms of fried potatoes and grains that are not integral to the dish, or your nourishment on that day. Doing this suddenly removes your likely silly guilt and makes a dish like the burger a 50 percent green meal.

BE WARY OF HIDDEN INGREDIENTS. Of course at a restaurant you can never really know how they make every single dish, but there are some pesky patterns. Asian places tend to load up on MSG and difficult to digest oils. Mexican places often thicken guacamole

with cream and cheese. Large Italian chains often precook the pasta, effectively turning it into Wonderbread when they then recook it for your specific order. Lunch chains regularly add sugar, ketchup, honey, and other sweeteners and thickeners to their salad dressings. They also usually go for the lowest quality oil. Similarly, they add flour, forms of processed gluten, cream, and sugar to soups you may think are simple and clean. Diners, cafeterias, and busy restaurants often use powdered eggs instead of real, fresh ones. Look things up if you can, ask some polite and gentle questions, and let Retox hone your palate to be able to pick out these roadblocks on your own.

So what do you order? There are tips for this throughout the rest of the book, but here are some guidelines:

MEXICAN. Focus on what has corn tortillas and is not fried. That usually means tacos, and I would lean toward vegetable, beef, or fish, but only if you know the quality and source as mentioned above. Forgo the cream and cheese on the tacos, and just add extra salsa if you need. For quesadillas, get them vegetarian and without cream or guacamole, but with extra salsa or pico de gallo. Order the chips—I'm only human—but make sure the guac is made from fresh avocados, not cream (you can tell if there are chunks and if the color is a pure green, not a green-white like a 1950s kitchen tile sample), and ask for extra salsas. Focus on dipping in the salsas and every few chips dip in the guac. Forget about the beans and rice. That is precisely where you will get bogged down. Stick to lean proteins, veggies, and corn tortillas, and you will realize Mexican can actually be a really healthy option.

ITALIAN. With a last name of Imparato, there is just no way I am going to tell you not to order pasta. What I will say is, make sure you order a vegetable-based starter, like antipasti, salad, or soup. If you are going to have a vegetarian pasta, you can even get crudo or carpaccio. Go light on the bread basket so you can really enjoy the pasta, and go for the pastas that are not stuffed or dense. Avoid raviolis and tortellini filled with cheese, and gnocchi, which are essentially little bombs to your system. Look for spaghetti and angel hair, rigatoni, penne, and the dozens of other pasta shapes a great sauce will accentuate. You might think a vegetable risotto is a good gluten-free option, but that is not necessarily healthier as many risottos have a base of cream, butter, and cheese. Better to have a pasta al pomodoro, which I will actually teach you to make later on. Always order a green salad as a side, and maybe even an additional vegetable. Italy knows how to do it all well, so just explore and enjoy.

PIZZA. One of my favorite food groups! Make sure you order a salad with your pizza, and stick to plain or vegetarian toppings. Have water and enjoy.

STEAK HOUSES. Back in my vegetarian years, my friend and I would go to steak houses for our weekly date night, and I would just get the vegetables. Aside from Italian restaurants, there is no better vegetable-friendly establishment in which to eat. Go crazy with the salads to start, just get them without the bacon, and have asparagus, green beans, salads, and sautéed greens with whatever you order as a main. Stick to no sauce or a pepper or chimichurri sauce—whichever is not cream based. Enjoy some mashed potatoes; there is no better combo than steak and mashed potatoes, just order the green around it all.

BURGER JOINT. Get the burger, ideally without cheese, bacon, or mayo, and get that side of greens! If it is a bad bun—and we all know what a disappointment that can be—use half of it, or none. If the fries are exceptional, get some, but double down on the greens later that day.

MIDDLE EASTERN/TURKISH. So many veggies and olive oil, and so much grilling, it is a Retox dream. Go light on the hummus and yogurt-based starters so your system does not get bogged down, and swap out the fried items like falafel for something fresh and grilled.

THE NEIGHBORHOOD LUNCH SPOT. Eating out is not always epic. Work often does not allow that, except maybe in Europe. Grab-and-go lunch spots are often our weekday mainstay, and they can be really easy to clean up. For you sandwich eaters, be conscious about what you are putting in between the bread. Do you really love that roast beef or ham? Or could you just have turkey to get you through the day? Choose clean lunch meats—ideally store-roasted turkey, say no to the mayo, add vegetables like avocado, tomato, lettuce, onion, and maybe even cucumber and sprouts, Cali-style. Leave the beef for high-quality mains at a proper restaurant or home, skip the pork, and consider not including cheese. Will it really make so much of a difference to the taste anyway if you go without that one slice of random cheese? I think not. If you are getting a salad, ask for olive oil and vinegar as your dressing, and watch them pour the real, pure olive oil.

41

THE BREAKFAST JOINT. The best breakfast in New York City is on the corner of Forty-seventh Street and Broadway, right in front of the Morgan Stanley office. It is a simple coffee cart run by my Greek friend Akos. Most people look at all the powdered creamers, bagels, and pastries in its windows and walk straight by, but when you Retox, you know how to find the good stuff—real, organic eggs made on the griddle. Make sure that your breakfast place gives you real eggs. You can have the whites or the whole egg, but make sure they are fresh and not liquid out of a carton, like so many quick breakfast spots offer.

RECIPES

Use these as your go-to meals—they're easy, delicious, and so nutritious!

Retox Scramble

2 cups baby spinach

1 teaspoon extra virgin olive oil

1 clove garlic, minced

2 eggs

Salt and pepper, to taste

Wash spinach and dry thoroughly. Heat the oil in a small nonstick frying pan over medium heat. Add garlic and cook until just starting to brown. Add spinach and cover, allowing to cook for about 5 minutes or until wilted. Meanwhile, crack the eggs into a bowl. Whip them with your fork until they become fluffy. Add a pinch of salt and pepper, if you like. When spinach is cooked, add eggs to the pan and let cook, stirring occasionally, until just set, about 2 minutes.

Retox Fruit Bowl

¼ cup blueberries

1 teaspoon ground flaxseed

½ cantaloupe, seeded

Mix berries and flaxseed. Spoon into cantaloupe. How great that you can eat the bowl!

Retox Bowl

Retox Bowls are an amazing choice for lunch or dinner. You can include whatever veggies you want. It is hard to mess them up! Use the vegetables of your choice—mix and match—just make sure you use two different vegetables, the more colors the better. My favorites are broccoli, red peppers, string beans, asparagus, and peas.

½ cup cooked brown rice or quinoa

1 cup cooked vegetables

1 cup baby spinach or kale

2 teaspoons extra virgin olive oil

1 tablespoon freshly squeezed lemon juice

Freshly ground black pepper, to taste

½ avocado, sliced

1 organic egg, fried (optional)

Add a base of brown rice or quinoa. Top with the vegetables and add a handful of baby spinach or kale. Dress with olive oil and lemon, and add pepper to taste. Top with sliced avocado, and an egg, if desired. Enjoy!

Retox Salad

If I could simply provide you with dozens of salad recipes, I would; I just love salad that much. That said, my editor, and you, would probably kill me. So instead, I'm offering the framework of a good salad and you can pick the specifics.

3 cups salad greens of your choice

½ cup green vegetables of your choice

½ cup non-green vegetable of your choice

1 teaspoon sliced almonds, or nut or seed of your choice

Salad dressing (see note)

Pick a base of your favorite leaf—spinach, romaine, kale, iceberg, butter, Bibb, arugula . . . you name it. Maybe even pick two leaves and blend together. Add in two additional green vegetables, cooked or raw—cucumbers, broccoli, green peppers, etc.—and another colored vegetable (beets, carrots, cherry tomatoes, red cabbage, etc.). If you like crunch, toss in some nuts or seeds.

NOTE: Either dress the salad with olive oil and vinegar, olive oil and lemon, or use this basic Retox Dressing: 2 parts olive oil, 1 part red wine or balsamic vinegar, dash of black pepper, and 1 teaspoon Dijon mustard. Shake or stir, pour over the salad, and enjoy.

Retox Tacos

Here's another loosey-goosey recipe. You really can customize this dish to your liking. Tacos are one of the easiest and quickest ways to Retox; I eat them at least three times a week. The beef, fish, or spinach is the centerpiece of your taco.

3 ounces beef, thinly sliced and grilled *or* 5 ounces wild white fish, sliced and grilled *or* 3 cups of spinach, sautéed in 2 teaspoons olive oil and 2 cloves garlic, minced

1 medium tomato, chopped

½ red onion, diced

Juice of ½ lemon

Salt, to taste

½ avocado

2 corn tortillas

Cilantro, optional

Romaine lettuce, optional

While your centerpiece of choice is cooking, mix the tomato and red onion in a bowl with a sprinkle of lemon and salt, if you like. Smash the avocado in another small bowl with a dash of salt. When the centerpiece is cooked, warm up the tortillas in a pan or by wrapping in damp paper towel and putting in the microwave for intervals of 30 seconds until warmed through. Spread the avocado on the tortillas, then add the main. Top with the tomato and onion salsa, and maybe even some cilantro. If you are having the fish or beef, you may even add some sliced romaine on top for crunch. Roll up the tacos and have a fiesta!

MINDSET

The endless search for balance. It is almost as universal a quest as trying to lose those last five pounds. We as a society try so hard to be balanced, yet we have never been so askew. You know why? Balance does not exist.

There is no such thing as work-life balance, at least not anymore. If you are striving for it, you are always going to be stressed and unhappy. Keeping it together is about accepting reality, and then creating a Life Stability Plan that enhances your real experience.

Work is life and life is work these days; they are unavoidably intertwined, as we live in a world of 24/7 access and instantaneous information. Unless global society decides to implode itself and goes back to a life we haven't seen since before the Industrial Revolution, you will always be juggling work and life in a way that does not necessarily seem even or fair. Taking care of kids is as much work as it is life, answering emails on a Sunday is as much life as it is work. This is not necessarily the way it should be, but it is what it is. Which is why the endless hunt for balance is over, and a direct shot of Retox is imperative.

RETOX

There are five habits to creating a strong, agile, energetic mind, one that is innately balanced, without the pressure to balance work and life. Do these every day and you will be in constant equilibrium, like the tides of the sea:

SHARE A MEAL. Make sure that one meal a day is shared with someone you care about. This can be a quick walk to get lunch with a colleague who makes you laugh, a dinner with an old friend, or a smoothie standing around the kitchen counter with your partner. Eat in the presence of someone else and you will be truly nourished and fulfilled on the inside.

TALK TO SOMEONE YOU LOVE. Pick up the phone and call your grandmother, text for twenty minutes with your friend across the country, Skype with your dad, or sit down face-to-face with your partner. It will likely change daily depending on your schedule, but make sure you have shared conversation time with someone who you love and who loves you.

NOURISH YOURSELF PHYSICALLY. Sweat it out and feed it up. Just refer to the yoga and nourishment parts of this chapter as to the why and how.

BREATHE IN LIGHT. Take one minute a day to connect to your breath, and from there link your breath to your thoughts, your body to your mind, your you to your world. Start with this:

Take a comfortable seat, wherever you are and however feels best. You can sit at your desk, on the floor, at the table, on the train . . . Just make sure that your spine is reasonably long and you are not totally slouching. Rest your arms gently on your thighs or knees, wherever feels most comfortable, and let your eyes softly shut.

Bring your attention to the tip of your nose, and start to notice your breath. Breathe through your nose naturally, maybe even starting to feel the air flutter across your upper lip on its way in and out. Just sit, relax, and breathe. Once you are comfortable and noticeably breathing, start to follow your breath with your mind, starting with the exhale.

Exhale—inhale, exhale—inhale, exhale—inhale.

Now start to count the breaths, exhale-inhale one, exhale-inhale two, exhale-inhale three . . . Try to get up to ten breaths.

Every time your mind wanders away from your breath to something else, start the count again. If you get stuck, just breathe for a bit without counting, and start again. With each inhale, you permit your brain to disengage so it can reengage. With each exhale, you allow in clarity while energizing your entire being.

If you have time, once your breath is smooth, bring your attention to the top of your head. Look down into your body and see everything that you know to be there. Now start to scan down your body and remove all its internal contents. With your mind's eye, remove the bones, muscles, ligaments, tendons, organs, tissues. Clear everything out so you are just an empty shell of you—you on the outside, empty on the inside. Now fly back up to where you started at the top of your head, and look down into your body again, and fill yourself with a perfect blue light. Like the clear sky or warm sea. Fill every corner of your body with that light. See yourself flooded with this infinite blue light on the inside, radiant on the outside.

This is your blue light body. Come to it once a day, maybe as part of your daily routine or simply when things are tough. It is said in the Tibetan traditions of yoga and philosophy that this exercise will protect you and energize you.

ACKNOWLEDGE. I know you are busy. We all are. But take one second a day to acknowledge where you are. Awake. Active. Alive. Just acknowledge how lucky you are to be alive, and you will be planting the seeds for more great life to come your way. Take a moment each day to say, "Thank you, Life."

Retox Soundtrack:
"Let's Dance" —DAVID BOWIE

Keeping it together. Facing three thousand in Latin America's first-ever mass yoga event, It's Free. Panama. **>**

RETOX

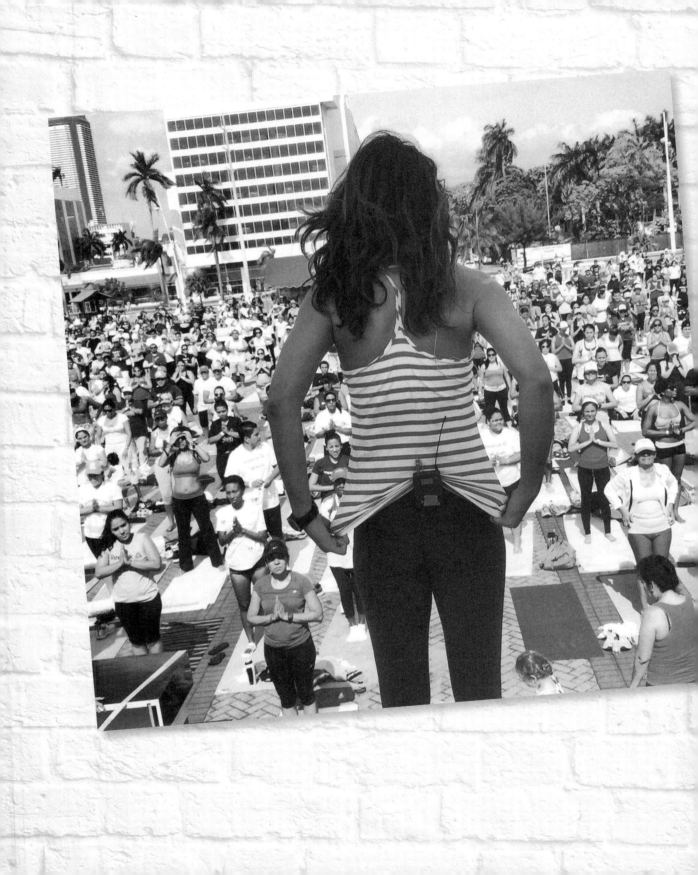

04

DID YOU RETOX TODAY?

The cure for anything is salt water: sweat, tears, or the sea.

—ISAK DINESEN

THE KEY TO LIVING AT THE TOP OF YOUR GAME IS VERY SIMPLE: IT IS SIMPLY Retoxing. So, how do you actually do it?

Start by asking yourself, *Did I Retox today?*

Did you do something for you today? Did you add something into your day that helped you be your best you? Did you engage in some activity, go through a thought process, or eat something to balance, energize, or inspire you? Did you connect with food not as a pariah, but as medicine, or work out the muscle of your mind? Did you pay heed to your body's anatomy and maybe even give it a chance to sweat? Did you do something to reconstruct, repair, or rejuvenate a part of your tangible or intangible being today? Did you plug into you?

I Retox between flights and at dinner parties, before bed and in the car. Retoxing is the habit of becoming the best *you* you can be in any given moment. It is the cure and the solution, the impetus and the inspiration. Retox is happy hour for your body, mind, and life. It is not about retreating, eliminating, or unplugging, rather it's all about adding in what you need on any given day.

Each day has its own rhythm, and each of us has our own beat. Retox is a concert for all of us, and all of you. Just serve up what you crave, like, and know you need to learn to love in the way that is most convenient, and most soothing.

How?

Almost all, if not all, of us encounter these twenty conundrums regularly, or at the very least have suffered from them once before. (Yes, you, too: Men occasionally suffer from PMS. I am almost certain of it.) So I suggest you look at the Retox Lab as your open bar. Peruse and dabble in its varied offerings consistently, be it for something specific or for life and health sustainability.

If you are suffering from an acute problem, perhaps you just focus on that cocktail until it subsides. If you are in between a few of them, alternate between their offerings, having each once or twice a week. If you want to live at the top of your game, cycle through each of the cocktails, having one a day, and then mix and match with what your body or life more specifically demands and craves.

Retox works if you imbibe daily. The thing is, there is so much to choose from, you will never feel restricted. I have provided you with twenty-one full sequence yoga routines, eighty-five Desk Fixes, and seventy-five Quick Fixes for your body. I have created seventy-five recipes that you can make with little to no mess in no time, and suggested dozens of accessible and desirable snacks so that you never get hungry, desperate, or bored. And I have crafted twenty-one mental action plans that merge mindfulness, psychology, philosophy, and straight-up life for your brain and attitude.

Everything you need is right in front of you. The Retox Lab is accessible, convenient, real, and, above all, not daunting. You really cannot go wrong.

Just remember to ask yourself, *Did I Retox today?*

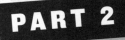

Retox
Lab

GETTING DOMED

HEADACHE RELIEF

AND PREVENTION

Balance starts on the inside

PANAREA, SICILY. SOMETIME BETWEEN LUNCH and dinner, a perfect summer's day, 2011. I lay on top of a boat in my white bikini, overlooking the crystal-clear water, Stromboli's volcanic murmurs faint in the distance. Other than my six friends on the boat, there was not a person in sight, just as an idyllic sea holiday should be. We had spent the morning swimming, sailing, and eating. Having taken up a truly Sicilian sailor routine, we were now resting—after all, it was a very busy morning. Life was perfect, except for one excruciating headache attacking my dome. Like a drummer in a '90s rock band, it was going nuts, banging on my frontal lobe with all its intensity and might.

What had I done to deserve this? I rarely got headaches, let alone one on vacation. Could it have been the sun? Something I ate? That Italian woman who punched me in the skull with her ring a week before at the market near Palermo? (A story for another time.) Regardless, three or four aspirin seemed like the remedy, but with a two-mile swim to shore and our skipper asleep, there was no hope of getting any pills for a while. But it had to stop. Now.

I sat on the back of the boat and tried to think of something that would help. It was tough to think clearly with all the banging, but I started with some breathing techniques, then a couple of modified yoga poses, followed by an ancient tactic inspired by Traditional Chinese Medicine (as explained later). One by one, I applied what I normally reserve as tools for my clients, and one by one, the techniques softened the banging in my head. Not long after, I started to see the distant islands clearly again, felt my jaw unclench, and even uttered a few words to my friends, who were now awake and chattering away. The pressure was slowly abating. Retox was working. I would survive.

Headaches are an interesting phenomenon as they come from and for various reasons. There are those associated with stress and pressure. Those related to a cold or the flu. Those stemming from muscle tension and skeletal alignment. Other from eyestrain and hormonal changes. And those like mine, which have no obvious root.

Although headaches have various causes, and even a combination of different factors, the triggers are almost always what we eat and/or how we think. It often comes down to our food and our thoughts. Yes, the aspirin may relieve pressure in your skull, but a combination of yoga breath and moves, dietary adjustments, and mindset techniques allow you to not only cure the banging in a natural way, but prevent the onset of future heavy metal drum solos as well.

YOGA

Yoga for headaches serves two purposes. First, it gets oxygen to your brain to relieve pressure on the skull and create space for the expanded blood vessels in the head. Second, it helps re-align the vertebrae and releases the muscles and bones that attach your dome to the rest of your body. We will use a combination of *pranayama*, or specific yoga breathing techniques, with poses linked with the basic yoga breath I described in the second chapter. Let's start.

RETOX

DESK FIXES

NECK STRETCHES

Lift your left arm and hold the outer right part of your skull lightly above the right ear. Tilt your head to the left and down, bringing your chin to your upper left chest. Hold here, breathing, then repeat on the other side.

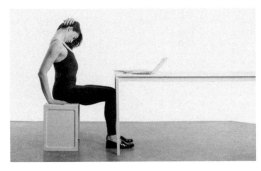

EAGLE ARMS HEAD DROP

Open your arms wide out to the sides. Bring your arms toward each other and cross your right arm under your left arm. Bend your elbows, and if you can, wrap your wrists so your palms touch. Bring your elbows in line with your chin and try to press your forearms together. Hold here three breaths, then drop your head, reaching your chin toward your chest. Hold here three to five breaths.

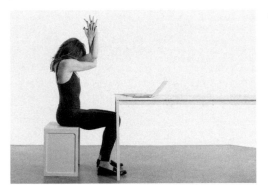

DESK CAT/COW

While seated, place your fingertips on the desk in front of you. Inhale, lift your sternum, stretching across your upper chest. Exhale, round your back like a cat. Repeat and hold wherever it feels good to hold.

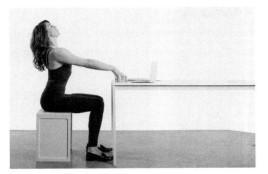

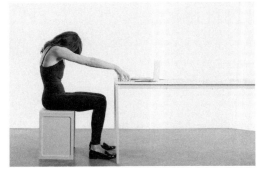

Bonus!

ALTERNATE NOSTRIL BREATHING*

Make a hang ten figure with your right hand. Press your right thumb to your right nostril. Inhale through your left nostril. Hold your left nostril with your pinky. Release your thumb and exhale through your right nostril. Hold your right nostril with your thumb. Inhale through your left nostril. Continue like this for as long as feels good, but try for at least ten rounds of breath.

QUICK FIXES

DOME RELIEF

Start with your hands and knees on the floor, shoulders over the wrists, hips over the knees. Inhale, look up, arching your spine. Exhale, round your spine, bringing your forehead toward your pelvis. Inhale, come to your fingertips keeping the round in your spine. Exhale, place your palms down, keeping the current round of your spine and relaxing your head more. Inhale, arch your back and look up. Repeat five to ten times.

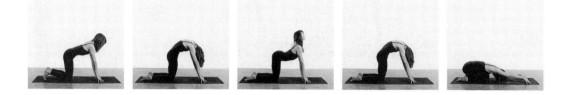

SKULL ROLLS

Start with your hands and knees on the floor, shoulders over the wrists, hips over the knees. Place the top of your head to the floor. Begin to gently roll the top of your head left and right, forward and back, breathing through your nose. Spend some time where you feel the most intense stretch.

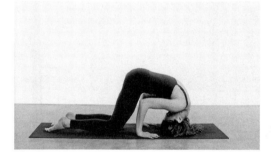

DOME-FREE GARLAND

Stand with your knees slightly bent, your feet together. Come to your tiptoes, bend your knees, and open your knees wide. Drop your head and relax your neck. Either stretch your arms forward or out to the sides, hold the back of your neck, or simply let your arms hang down. Hold here, breathing.

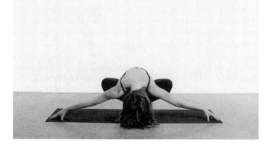

Bonus!

HEAD BATHED IN WARM WATER

Turn on the water in the shower or the tub. Place your head into the warm water and gently massage your skull with the warm water.

57

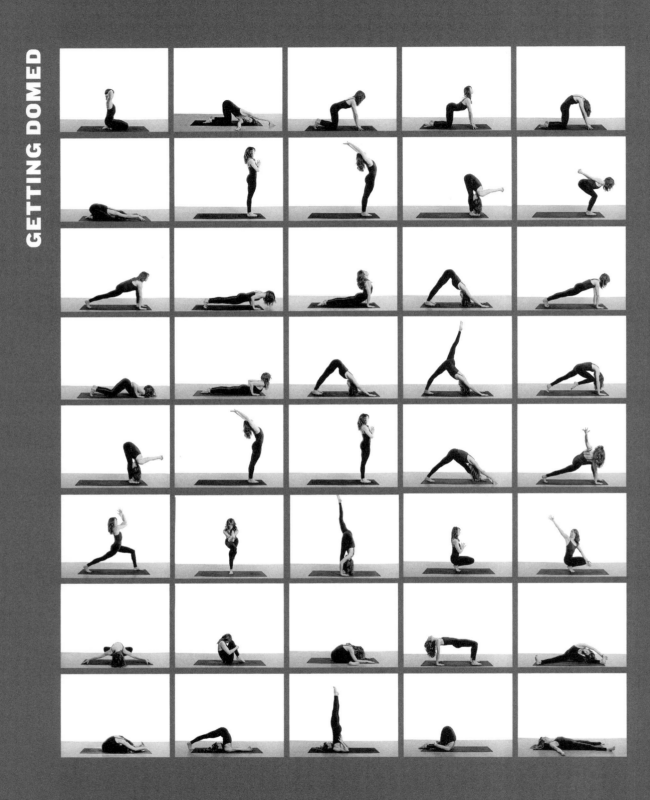

NOURISHMENT

Looking back at that terrible headache in Sicily, I concluded that my headache was triggered primarily by what I had eaten that day: un café latte, a block of cheese, salami, and bowls of fruit freshly picked by the village mamma on my last trip to shore.

Although that headache in Sicily was the first I had had in a long time, there was a time when they were frequent. Through trial and error, I realized that they were triggered by dietary choices. Since then I had avoided excess of dairy, sugar, and spicy foods, but that day on the boat, I had slipped in a major way, tempted by the bounty of Italian treats surrounding me.

Many of my clients are plagued by especially acute headaches, some even with migraines. All headaches usually arrive between two to twelve hours after a trigger, which can be anything from something you ate to something in your environment, so the first step is to assess what caused the headache, both so you can treat it and learn to prevent future ones.

With environmental triggers, usually the only thing you can do is remove yourself from the situations or avoid them altogether. The jackhammering outside your building can eventually cause jackhammering inside your head. Noxious fumes such as paint, nail polish agents, or gas can also bring on a headache. Stress is another culprit. When we're under duress, we tend to clench our muscles, holding the tension in our shoulders, neck, and jaw. Both the yoga poses in the previous section and the mindset techniques to come can help with this type of headache.

Basically, headaches are your body's reaction to something your body does not like. More often than not, that "something" is an allergy induced by food. Your immune system senses the food and then alerts the cells and blood vessels of your body to inflame. There are certain foods than have been shown to specifically trigger inflammation in the head and set off headaches, especially if you already have a propensity for them. By making adjustments to your diet, you can understand these causes and thus learn to control what happens.

Here are foods to avoid and foods to include more of so that you can lower the number of headaches you get to zero over time, and four recipes that can reduce your headache symptoms in the present.

DETOX

Eating any one of the items below can potentially cause a headache. The timing depends on how long it takes for the food to process in your body and how alert your immune system is to that particular entity.

An easy way to determine if any of these foods are triggers for you is to cut them out of your diet for a week or two. If your headaches start to subside, it is likely that one of them is the culprit. To determine which one(s), slowly reintroduce the foods one at a time. By temporarily eliminating them, you may have cured your allergy entirely, but most likely adding them back will help you determine your precise triggers.

FRUIT AND SUGAR. Sugar is an inflammatory agent. Fruit, although natural, is packed with sugar. And sugar is closely associated with expansion headaches. Cut out sugar of all sorts to allow your body to neutralize.

SPICY FOOD. If you throw on too much hot sauce, you might get sweaty and red in the face. This reaction actually starts inside your entire body. Spicy food causes cells to expand including those in your head. This puts pressure on your skull and creates a headache. Try cutting out all spicy foods and literally let your dome chill.

FATTY FOODS. Cheese, avocado, egg yolks, custards, oily dressing, meat, and anything fried goes in this category. Fatty foods are linked to migraines, and we're especially sensitive to them when they are eaten in the mornings as they are more directly absorbed by your empty stomach. You can cut these out altogether or temporarily remove them to get your liver running more efficiently.

DAIRY. While most products for lactose intolerance focus on digestion, some of the more painful ramifications of the inability to process lactose are headaches. Malabsorption or incompletely absorbed lactose has been shown to trigger headaches, so if dairy is an issue for you, you may want to switch to almond, hemp, or coconut milk in your lattes.

MSG. MSG, or monosodium glutamate, is considered as addictive as nicotine. It is not just an additive in cheap Chinese food, fast food, or Doritos. Most fat-free and sugar-free foods have some form of MSG in them to make the food taste better. "Seasonings" and "natural flavorings" on food labels are usually comprised of many additives, including MSG. Ketchup, canned soups, chips, sauces, bouillon cubes, premade broths, and dressings usually contain MSG. MSG is also hidden in gelatin; yeast extract; maltodextrin; hydrolyzed, isolated, and textured soy protein; and calcium caseinate. MSG leads to headaches that often feel like a tight band pressing against the head. By sticking to Retox nonprocessed food suggestions, you should be able to easily eliminate MSG from your diet and from attacking your dome.

RETOX

Food and drink can be as soothing as aspirin when it comes to headaches. Try including these foods on a regular basis, especially when you feel a headache coming on:

WATER. Dehydration is a direct link to headaches. Make sure you sip water continually throughout the day—flat and room temperature.

MINT. An Eastern medicine palliative, mint improves your liver function, reduces inflammation, and calms muscle spasms. Including mint in your daily diet should help you quell your headaches. Try chopping fresh mint and adding it to salads, putting full leaves in a pitcher or glass of water, making a tea, or adding it as a garnish on anything and everything.

GINGER. Ginger works as a strong anti-inflammatory, directly inhibiting inflammation. It reduces pain and muscle spasms. Use ginger in soups, sautés, fresh vegetable-based juices, salad dressings, and in hot water as a tea.

SNACKS

Mint tea
Baby spinach salad
Candied ginger
Sunflower seeds (unless you suffer from migraines)

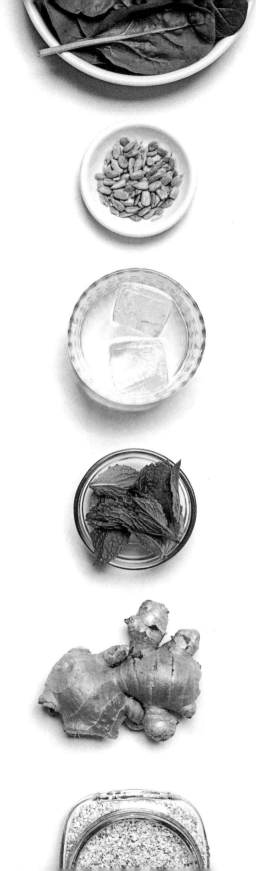

Chata's Carrot Juice

You can use a juicer or a high-speed blender for this recipe.

> 3 large carrots, peeled and chopped
>
> ¼-inch piece ginger, peeled
>
> 1 to 2 mint leaves

Juice or blend carrots, ginger, and mint leaves. Drink at room temperature.

Lemon Water Delight

> ½ lemon
>
> 8 ounces room temperature water
>
> ½ tablespoon baking soda

Squeeze lemon into a glass. Add water and baking soda and stir.

61

Dome-Free Pasta

8 ounces buckwheat pasta

1 (14-ounce) can artichoke hearts (in water)

1 handful fresh mint

½ cup chopped green onion

2 tablespoons sunflower seeds (optional)

4 tablespoons extra virgin olive oil

Bring a large pot of water to boil. Add pasta and cook 8 to 12 minutes, according to directions on the package. While cooking, chop artichoke hearts and mince the mint. When cooked, drain pasta and put in a bowl. Add artichokes, mint, green onion, and sunflower seeds (if using and you don't suffer from migraines). Drizzle with olive oil and toss. You can serve this hot or cold.

Dome-Soothing Soup

1 tablespoon extra virgin olive oil

1 yellow onion, diced

2 cloves garlic, minced

2 (9-ounce) bags baby spinach

1 handful fresh mint, roughly chopped

2 slices ginger, about the size of a quarter, peeled (optional)

1 cup chicken stock (use vegetable stock or water to make this vegetarian)

2 pinches salt

Heat the oil in a pot over medium heat. Add onion and garlic and cook until onion is translucent. Be careful not to burn the garlic. Add spinach, mint, and ginger, if using. As the spinach starts to wilt, add stock or water and salt. When the spinach is completely cooked, remove from heat. Blend with an immersion blender, or put in a blender in batches, and puree until smooth.

MINDSET

On the outside, there are many possible reasons for getting domed, but on the inside, on the mind-side, there is just one: an intangible imbalance inside you.

When your body is in balance there is equanimity, or *upseva*, and you are headache free. When there is an imbalance, akin to when one guitarist is playing louder than the other, the domed drummer lets loose.

The entire purpose of Tibetan yogic inner-body studies is to understand the various elements that need to be balanced. They say there are five winds, or main groups of forces, that run through three energetic channels. Keeping these balanced means attending to the various elements of your day, from how you treat yourself to how you see your boss to how you judge someone's work. Every perception you have and action you take strengthens or weakens one of the winds.

If you can keep the winds more or less in balance, then they can flow correctly and you can become headache free.

RETOX

Close your eyes and rest your palms on your thighs, elbows soft. Sit in silence. If at all possible, sit in a dark place. With your eyes closed, identify where the most central point of pain is in your dome. As you inhale, envision all the air coming up through your right nostril, directly to that point of pain. As you exhale, envision the stream of air coming directly from that point and out of the left nostril.

Inhale now through your left nostril to the point of pain, remembering that your hands are resting and you are solely using your mind. Exhale from that point through your right nostril. Inhale through your right, directly to the point of pain. Exhale out through the left from that point. Inhale through the left, then exhale out the right.

Repeat like this for ten or more breaths. Then just sit and breathe normally through both nostrils. Bring your attention to your dome. Each time you inhale, imagine your skull expanding. Each time you exhale, imagine the inflamed cells receding into clear, expansive, and free form. Repeat like this until your mental vision of your skull expanding is as strong as that of your cells receding and clearing. It might take two, five, or ten minutes.

Do this Retox meditation as long as it takes, or as long as you have. The effects will last long after.

Retox Soundtrack:
"Learn to Fly" —FOO FIGHTERS

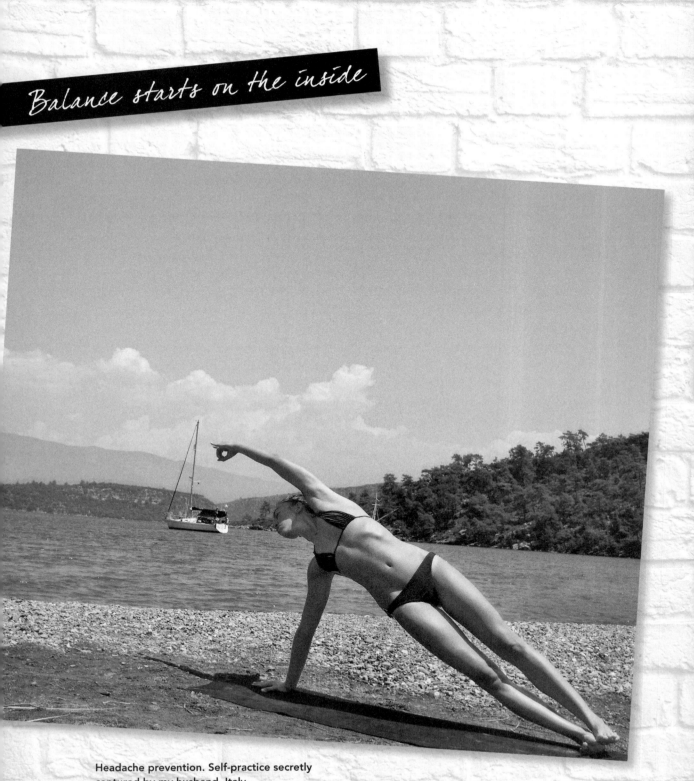

Headache prevention. Self-practice secretly
captured by my husband. Italy.

BACK ATTACK

Dissolve yours by dispelling theirs

ACCORDING TO A STUDY BY the Global Burden of Disease in 2010, back pain is the single biggest cause of disability in the world. Half of Americans admit to having back pain, and 80 percent will suffer from it at least once in their life. Back pain is recorded as the biggest cause of missed days of work; on average, 186 million workdays are lost each year due to back attacks, costing employers $50 billion a year. This is a catastrophe for businesses, and society as a whole, painful in more ways than one.

Over $90 billion are spent on health-care expenses a year to quell Back Attacks, and $26 billion spent specifically in treatment costs. Back pain is the second most common reason for doctor's visits after upper respiratory infections such as colds. The cost of treating back pain increased 65 percent from 1997 to 2005. In that same time frame, spending on back pain relief drugs increased 423 percent. Despite treatments, 62 percent of back-attackees say they still feel pain after twelve months. The spending is increasing, but the recovery rates and return on investment are not, which is why I created a 360-degree Retox approach to Back Attacks.

Back pain itself is merely the screaming, agonizing symptom of an underlying problem. Endless amounts of painkillers, anti-inflammatories, physical therapy sessions, and surgeries are prescribed as remedies, but few address the root cause. Doctors commonly attribute the pain to issues with the vertebrae, back muscles, and tendons, but often miss the true causes hidden one layer deeper. In my experience, there are three main causes for back pain: the pelvis, the mind, and wrong information.

THE PELVIS. The pelvis is a bony structure the shape of a basin (it actually means *basin* in Latin). It connects the base of the spine to the back of the legs. It consists of two (theoretically) bilaterally symmetric pelvic girdles, the sacrum, coxal bones, and coccyx. The muscles and tissues inside the pelvis are known as the pelvic floor.

The strength and stability of pelvic floor muscles are imperative for a healthy back, as is pelvic equilibrium.

When the pelvis is askew or out of its natural equilibrium, it throws off all the muscles, tendons, ligaments, and bones connected to it. These include the lower back muscles, spine, glutes, thigh muscles, and sacral joint, to name a few. In order to prevent back pain, your pelvis needs to be properly aligned and the pelvic muscles must be strong, two things Retox yoga excels in aiding.

I WANT YOU TO TRY THESE two experiments. First, take two scales and place them about six inches apart from each other. Step on them, one foot on each scale, and read the numbers on each. I am willing to guess the numbers on each scale are not the same; mine have ranged from two to twelve pounds different! The difference of weight on each scale represents an imbalance in your pelvis. Now for the second experiment, lie on a flat, hard surface like the floor. Take a wooden board, big book, or tray and place it on the top of your hip bones, aka pelvis. See if the board is even or, most likely, not. This demonstrates a misalignment in your pelvis.

We may not be built to be even kilter all the time, but we should be as close to neutral as possible to avoid Back Attacks. Over three-quarters of the people who come into I.AM.YOU. with back problems have pelvic misalignment and were misdiagnosed until they see me. Retox yoga for Back Attacks targets pelvic alignment and pelvic muscle strength so that we can be as symmetrical and strong as possible.

THE MIND. Statistics suggest that much of the cause of back pain is emotional, especially between the ages of thirty and sixty. Yes, you read that right, my friends—back pain is often in your head. Anxiety, worry, stress, anger, and depression have all been proven to be fiercely intangible causes of Back Attacks. Tension myositis syndrome (TMS), a condition that causes pain due to physiologic alterations to certain muscles, tendons, and ligaments of the postural (back) side of the body because of the biochemical state of mind, also plays a role.

Like Morrissey alludes to in the Smiths' song "Still Ill," the mind can in fact rule the body. We have a natural tendency to cling mentally to back pain, thus reigniting it both literally and metaphorically every time we are angry, stressed, worried, or something goes wrong. If you can redirect the energy and moods from attacking your back, you can relieve the tension and avoid both chronic and acute Back Attacks well into the future. I have a Retox mindset plan to help you do so.

THE WRONG INFORMATION. All too often back pain is diagnosed as quite serious when it is actually unmistakably straightforward and common. Scary exams, addictive prescriptions, and big long words can obfuscate a simple anatomical issue. A simple pelvic adjustment, change in breathing pattern, release of fluid, or shift in thought process can relieve back pain entirely. It just takes someone interested in providing a long-term, 360-degree remedy to notice it, and from there offer doable solutions, which is exactly what I am here to do.

Take Andrew, my poster child for Back Attack recovery for some time now. A thirty-eight-year-old entrepreneur in Manhattan, he works twelve-hour days and travels endlessly for business. Before I met him, he had been suffering an intense lower back pain for eighteen months. He arrived to I.AM.YOU. groggily one morning, unable to sit or stand up straight, and began to recount the doctor by doctor, therapist by therapist diagnoses he had received for his back, which now had him in more pain than ever. I stared at him intently in our first meeting, examining how he stood, sat, and walked, looking for hints from his pelvis, while listening to his story. I proceeded to create a yoga and breath routine for him that focused on pelvic alignment as well as strengthening his pelvic floor and breathing muscles. I taught him a meditation he did at least three times a week at home, and switched around some of his habits that, surprisingly, not one doctor or therapist had pointed out as bad for his back. Within two months, Andrew was 100 percent pain free, using only my Retox methods and avoiding surgery and drugs.

Back pain can be muscular, skeletal, and/or emotional, making a 360-degree solution more important than ever. In the following pages, I outline for you a plan that is both preventative and soothing, so that no matter what brings on your Back Attack that day, you will know how to abate it without the pills, and avoid it from coming again with such force in the future.

YOGA

I am willing to bet that you or someone you know with back pain has been prescribed yoga. The thing is, not all yoga is good for back pain. Yoga for Back Attacks needs to be done with acute focus on anatomy and alignment, and following these cardinal rules:

- Backbends are a total no-no. Seriously, no one cares how sexy you look in one anyway.
- If your doctor said not to do it, do not do it. Forward bends often fall in this camp as well.
- Breathe. The breath is a tonic for Back Attacks. The major muscle for respiration, the diaphragm, connects to the lumbar vertebrae of the spine and the pelvic floor. By focusing on breathing, you automatically strengthen and tone the diaphragm and the muscles it connects to—that is, your back. Make sure you breathe fully and deeply, using your lungs and diaphragm to their fullest capabilities.
- In addition, breathing calmly sends messages to your brain that it is going to be okay. When you are in a bout of pain, trying to avoid one, or in the middle of a yoga pose or stretch for your back, remember to slowly and calmly breathe in and out, letting your body feel that it is all right. When you forget to breathe, your body tenses, inducing even more back pain. Breathe through it to make it better, and it will.
- Embrace the bandhas. Bandha what? *Bandha* is a word I heard my teachers say in class daily, a word that I wrote off as "yogi hippie crap" until I finally experientially understood what it was all about, and how it is one of the most hidden yet powerful tools for alleviating back pain after breathing.

In Sanskrit, *bandha* means "to lock, to hold, or to tighten." It also refers to a lock in and of itself. There are three principle bandhas in the body, and a fourth that ties them all together. The bandhas help you regulate and control all your internal systems (hormonal, sexual, metabolic, digestive) as well as strengthen you pelvic floor and deeper back muscles, which is what we care about here. Each of the three bandhas addresses a different part of Back Attacks. (Note, bandhas should not be practiced while pregnant.)

MULA BANDHA. Mula Bandha focuses on pelvic floor strength and stability. It is also the easiest bandha to explain. Just imagine you are in the middle of a three-hour traffic jam to the airport, the highway has turned into a parking lot, and you have to pee. The muscles you instinctually contract to pull up and hold in what is dying to flood out can be generally considered Mula Bandha, or at least the Mula Bandha region.

In Sanskrit, *mula* means "root," and thus *Mula Bandha* is the "root lock." To find it, sit, stand, or even be in an asana, and if you are a man, contract the area between the anus and the testes. If you are a woman, contract the muscles at the bottom of the pelvic floor, behind the cervix. Initially the anal sphincter will also contract, but with time and practice you will be able to home in on the Mula Bandha region and leave the rest aside.

Now don't freak out! Remember, I thought all this was weird yoga hogwash, too. But the truth is, Mula Bandha should be held throughout your entire yoga practice, and engaged throughout various points of the day. It stimulates the pelvic nerves, the genital system, the endocrine system, and the excretory system, and has also been shown to relieve constipation and depression. More importantly, it activates and strengthens the tough-to-reach pelvic floor muscles. A regular Mula Bandha practice will prevent back pain without anyone even noticing.

UDDIYANA BANDHA.* Uddiyana Bandha focuses on soothing the lumbar region and midback pain, as well as stabilizing the entire back through abdominal strength. In Sanskrit, *uddiyana* means "to fly up, or to rise up." This "flying up lock" is thus all about your insides flying upward. Tangibly that means your diaphragm, stomach, back muscles, and abdominal organs; intangibly it refers to your energy.

To find Uddiyana Bandha, start standing up tall, feet about three feet apart (see photos on page 70). Inhale through your nose and reach your arms up alongside your ears. Exhale out of your mouth and fold forward placing your hands just above your knees. Without inhaling close your lips, straighten your elbows, and feel your abdominal wall and organs push up and back toward your back. It should feel somewhat like a suctioning back and up of everything on the inside. If you are doing it correctly and happen to glance at your profile in a mirror, you should see your waist looking teeny weeny, with the ribs noticeably protruding over and in front of your abdomen or belly button. Retain as such for as long as possible, and exit the bandha via inhaling through your nose and standing up straight, raising your arms up alongside your ears, then exhaling through your nose again as you move your arms down.

Uddiyana Bandha will be one of the most transformative aspects to soothing and preventing Back Attacks. When the abdominal wall presses the organs and tissues of the abdominal cavity backward, Uddiyana Bandha creates a soft massage for the deeper internal muscles of the lower back. It simultaneously strengthens the abdominal muscles needed to stabilize your back. Best of all, it is the sure-fire way to get flat washboard abs without ever doing any crunches. But that is just a Retox perk.

Here is the easiest way to learn Uddiyana Bandha. Try this standing when you get a chance.

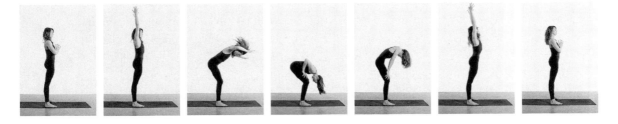

JALANDHARA BANDHA. Jalandhara Bandha focuses on relieving upper back and neck pain. It is pretty much the only double chin you will want, and try, to have. In Sanskrit, *jal* means "throat," *jalan* means "net," and *dharan* means "stream or flow." Thus, in the most basic sense, Jalandhara Bandha can be considered the throat lock that controls the flow of energy in the nerves and blood vessels of the neck.

To find Jalandhara Bandha, sit up tall, either in a comfortable cross-legged position or on your shins with your butt on your heels. Place the palm of your hands on your knees. Inhale slowly and deeply through your nose, then bring your chin toward your neck and lift your sternum ever so slightly. Press down on your hands and straighten your elbows, pull your chin in farther, and retain as long as possible. To exit, lift your chin, inhale the remainder of capacity into your lungs, and exhale. If you felt a nasty double chin or were stressing about someone taking a picture of your profile, you did it right!

Jalandhara Bandha is immensely powerful, as it compresses the sinuses on the main arteries of the neck and in doing so helps regulate the circulatory and respiratory systems, as well as lengthens the posterior muscles of the upper back and neck. Jalandhara Bandha is an instant trigger for mental relaxation as well as stress and anger relief, which will help with the mental aspects of Back Attacks. In addition, pressure on the throat helps balance the thyroid and metabolism, which can help mitigate abdominal weight gain, another common cause of back pain.

MAHA BANDHA. This the big kahuna. *Maha* in Sanskrit means "great," and *Maha Bandha* is the combination of all three aforementioned bandhas.

Sit in a comfortable seat, or on your shins or cross-legged on the floor, palms of the hands on the thighs or knees. Inhale fully through your nose, and exhale completely through your nose. Squeeze, squeeze, squeeze until every last drop is out. Without inhaling, en-

70

gage Mula Bandha, then find Uddiyana Bandha. Inhale a tiny bit and lift your chest, and from there engage Jalandhara Bandha. Retain, pressing your palms down, as long as possible. When you have had enough, lift your head, inhale fully, and release all the bandhas.

Practicing each of these bandhas will help you easily transform back pain into something of the past.

Most people that come to I.AM.YOU. for Back Attack relief have been struggling for quite a while. After endless doctors, pills, therapies, random yoga classes, and chiropractors, they end up at my door, having heard that I had a different approach, the Retox perspective. The poses and routines suggested below have helped countless students tame and prevent their Back Attacks, and they can help you, too. If anything hurts, even just a little bit, skip it and move on to the next thing. Ready?

Bonus!

NEUTRAL SEAT. We often create back pain without even noticing it. When you sit, make sure your feet are firmly on the ground, hip distance apart and not crossed. Place your hands on your lower back and rock forward and back on your sitz bones until you find a place where your palms feel flat against your spine, without a curve. This is neutral. Bring your belly button toward your spine. Lift your sternum. Lift your shoulders toward your ears, then down your back to spread open the front of your chest. Then, place one hand on the back of your neck and move your chin up and down. When the back of the neck is long, release your arms. This is a neutral, Back-Attack preventative spine. Do this until the posture becomes natural.

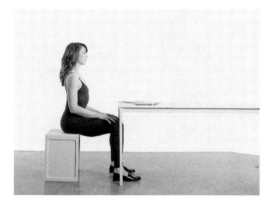

RETOX

DESK FIXES

MOUNTAIN

Stand with your feet hip distance apart. Lift your toes and press your heels into the floor. Engage your quads and pull up on your kneecaps. Bring your belly button to your spine. Lift your chest. Roll your shoulders up toward your ears then down your back. Face your palms forward to wherever feels natural. Drop your toes back on the ground. Breathe. Do this enough until it feels natural. This is how you should be standing.

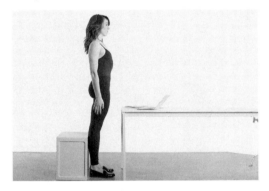

BACK RELIEF LIFTS

Come to the edge of your chair. Place your hands on the seat by your hips or on the armrests. Inhale, lift your butt up, pressing down into your hands, releasing the muscles and tension from the lower back. Stay there for several breaths, as long as it feels good, and repeat frequently.

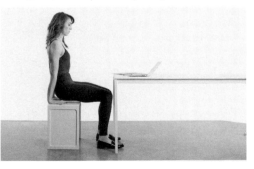

HALF ANKLE TO KNEE

Place your right ankle on your left lower quad, just above the knee. Flex your right foot. Press your right hand down on the inner right thigh or knee. Optionally, fold forward. Hold there, then repeat on the other side.

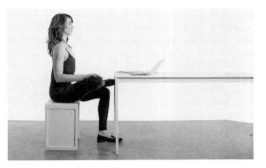

CHAIR FORWARD FOLD

Come to the edge of your chair. Separate your feet hip distance apart. Extend your legs forward and flex your feet so the heels press into the floor. Inhale, sit up tall. Exhale, fold forward, reaching your hands toward your ankles or shins. Let your head hang here and hold for five to fifteen breaths.

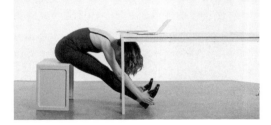

Bonus!

BBB: BACK BODY BREATHING

The connection of the diaphragm to the spine and rib cage make proper breathing imperative to back pain prevention. As you inhale, fill your back lungs and expand your diaphragm completely. Imagine the air inflating your back body. Exhale, grow taller. Repeat like this as often as possible until it becomes natural.

QUICK FIXES

CAT/COW

Start with your hands and knees on the floor, shoulders over your wrists, hips over your knees. Inhale, look up, arching your spine. Exhale, round your spine, bringing your forehead toward your pelvis. Repeat five to ten times daily.

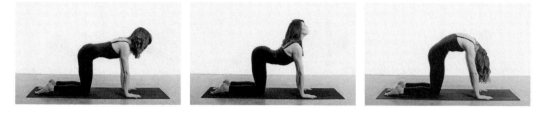

90-DEGREE LEGS AND ABS

Lie on the floor. Make sure your entire back and shoulder blades are touching the floor. Lift your legs to 90 degrees, but keep your back on the floor. Relax your face and shoulders and breathe. If you are feeling strong, start to lower your legs toward the floor, but only as much as you can while keeping the entire back on the floor. This may only be a couple of inches. Either lift and lower ten times or hold here at 90 degrees for ten to twenty breaths.

DIAMOND

Sit on the floor and bring the soles of your feet to touch, heels about one to two feet away from your body. Fold forward, trying to reach the forehead to the heels of the feet or arches. Breathe here, stretching your lower back for eight to twenty breaths.

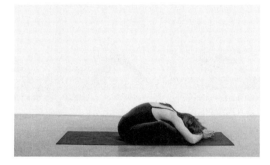

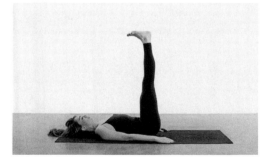

73

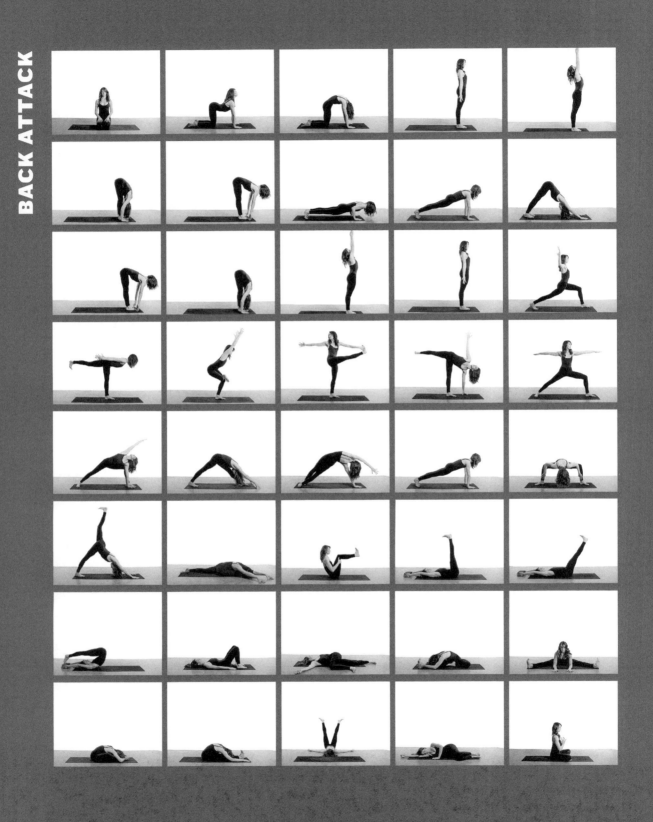

NOURISHMENT

When I lived in Florence, Italy, in my early twenties, I dated a few Italian men. They taught me about Florentine art, grappa, how to be proud of the elegant lady hidden behind my Cali-tomboy persona, and the importance of never, ever having a cappuccino after a meal. They also helped me become fluent in Italian, starting with the phrase *mal di schiena*. *Mal di schiena* is a nondescript back pain that every Italian man I met suffered from. The cure? A quick ride on their Vespa home to Mamma, where she would make *pastasciutta*, or perfectly al dente pasta in a homemade sauce, with a healthy side dish of TLC. I'm not sure what the mammas put in their sauce, but whatever it was, it worked—just like Retox nourishment will work for you.

I break down Retox nourishment for Back Attacks into twelve points: The first six have to do with habits, the next six with food.

DETOX

Fix these habits and you are on your way to fewer Back Attacks:

CIGS. We all know smoking is bad for you (if you are really trying to still rationalize that it isn't, or that you are not a smoker even though you smoke, just stop!). Believe it or not, smoking is linked to back pain. Active and past smokers are three times more likely to develop back pain than non-smokers. Smoking, past or present, impairs the flow of oxygen to your spinal tissues, increasing the intensity and probability of Back Attacks. So just put down the cigs once and for all.

HEELS. It would be embarrassing to tell you how many pairs of high heels I actually have . . . I love them. In fact, I spent the four days before I quit my job at Morgan Stanley secretly taking home over a dozen pairs of shoes from under my desk. The thing is, high heels can cause intense lower back pain. In order to stay balanced as we prance about in our stilettos, our pelvis tilts forward, crimping the muscles and nerves of the lower back and throwing off our natural spinal curves. To avoid Back Attacks from your expensive tall shoes, keep them in your bag or under your desk like I did, putting them on only when you really need to, and opting for supportive flats or one-half-inch heels the rest of the time.

CARS. Did you know that every time you get out of a car you could be planting the seeds for a major Back Attack in the future? Most of us get out of cars one leg at a time, abnormally twisting our lower sacral spine, and then we reach for something still in the car, improperly stretching our thoracic and upper lumbar spines. This combo routinely causes an inexplicable back pain, one that takes longer than most to get better. Try turning your whole body out of the car at once, and then stepping out with both legs at the same time. Once you are out of the car, lean in to get whatever you left behind.

CHAIRS. No surprise that sitting can cause back pain, but it cannot be eliminated from life altogether. Whether you are sitting at your desk, in the car, or on the couch at home, try to make sure your pelvis is in a neutral position and evenly balanced on both sides. Uncross your legs, placing both feet with equal weight on the floor—it's the new sexy. Then, place your hands on your lower back, fingers down, and drag your back up with the heels of your hands. Finally, roll the front of your shoulders back and even out your chin, making sure it is not too far down nor too far up, thus keeping the cervical spine in its neutral position. You can throw in a slight Jalandhara Bandha if you like as well. In addition, choose seats that are relatively firm—soft, squishy seats make you more susceptible to slouching and misaligning your pelvis.

SLEEP. As counterintuitive as it sounds, sleeping on the stomach almost always leads to Back Attacks, so you must change your sleeping position if you're a stomach sleeper. When you sleep on your stomach, you compromise the entire alignment of your spine. It puts pressure on your joints and muscles, which can then irritate nerves of the back and lead to a tingling feeling in the limbs. It also puts intense stress on your cervical spine, creating an overstretching of one side of the muscles of the neck and extreme contraction and thus tightening of the other. Try sleeping on your back as you fall asleep or your side as a second best option, and your back will be much, much happier.

STANCE. Another unavoidable life habit that may be causing you back pain is standing. When you stand, check first that you have even weight on both legs; having more weight on one than the other will lead to the pelvic imbalance discussed earlier. Then make sure your lumbar spine is in a neutral position, and that you are not sticking your stomach out. The best way to do this is to place your hands on your lower/middle back and roll your back muscles into them. Then, check that you are

not hunching over and rounding your upper back. Take a deep breath and imagine someone is pulling the top of your head up with a string. Your back will be relieved and you will probably feel instantly taller, too.

RETOX

There is not one food that will take away your back pain or prevent Back Attacks from ever happening, but a healthy combination of these foods in your daily diet can and will alleviate back pain and help prevent its onset.

CHERRIES. Cherries are packed with nutrients and color. The pigments that make them red are polyphenolic flavonoid compounds known as anthocyanin glycosides. These anthocyanins work as anti-inflammatory agents by blocking cyclooxygenase (COX-1 and COX-2) enzymes, as well as reducing pain. In addition, the high levels of melatonin in cherries can calm the nervous system, which can help abate emotional links to Back Attacks. Start each morning with a big bowl of cherries or snack on them throughout the day.

GINGER. Ginger is an age-old remedy for muscle aches across all cultures. Add it to your morning juice, grate it into cooked meals or salads, or sip on a fresh ginger tea and it will help soothe your Back Attack muscles.

CRANBERRIES. Often back pain results from an irritation in the kidneys, which lie on the back side of your body at your lumbar spine. Cranberries are the most potent foods for kidney health, so try a half cup of simple juice, mixing juice with seltzer water for a cranberry spritzer, or sprinkling some dried cranberries into your salad or sautés.

TURMERIC. Usually reserved for hippy vegan restaurants and Indian curries, turmeric is actually a strong anti-inflammatory spice that can relieve pain and enhance nerve and cellular function. Try sprinkling it into or on whatever you eat.

HOT PEPPERS. Hot peppers contain capsaicin, the active ingredient that makes them spicy. Capsaicin is an analgesic, used to relieve pain topically and internally, as it stimulates nerve endings to a point that they become unable to report pain. With a chronic exposure to capsaicin, which I do not recommend, neurons are actually depleted of the neurotransmitters they need to relay pain signals. However, in moderation, hot peppers are helpful. Try adding a few slices to whatever you cook, and if you are really gung-ho, add a few slices to your sandwich.

ARNICA. The first time I ever used arnica was after I fell down thirty-five steep marble stairs in my new, bright red patent leather heels, but that's another story. Arnica is an herb that sort of looks like a daisy and has incredible anti-inflammatory effects on bruises and wounds. Try boiling arnica in hot water then adding the water to a bath, or rubbing it on your aching back. If that is too much work for you, just buy arnica cream, but the infusion will be much more effective for soothing your Back Attack.

SNACKS

Bowl of cherries
Candied ginger
Dried cranberries

RECIPES

Golden Fish

- 1 tablespoon extra virgin olive oil
- 2 cloves garlic
- 1 large yellow onion, sliced
- 4 (6-ounce) wild caught Alaskan cod (or wild caught fish of choice)
- Juice of 2 lemons
- 1 teaspoon turmeric

Heat oil in a large skillet over medium heat. Add garlic and cook until just starting to turn golden. Add onion and cook until translucent. Squeeze lemon juice over fish and sprinkle with turmeric. Cook fish 5 minutes per side or until it easily flakes with a fork. Serve with a side of rice and vegetables.

Spicy Broccoli

- 4 tablespoons extra virgin olive oil
- 2 hot chili peppers, chopped
- 3 cups broccoli florets

Heat oil in a large skillet over medium heat. Add chili peppers and cook until they start to soften. Add broccoli, stir, and partially cover pan with a lid. Cook until broccoli is tender, about 10 minutes.

77

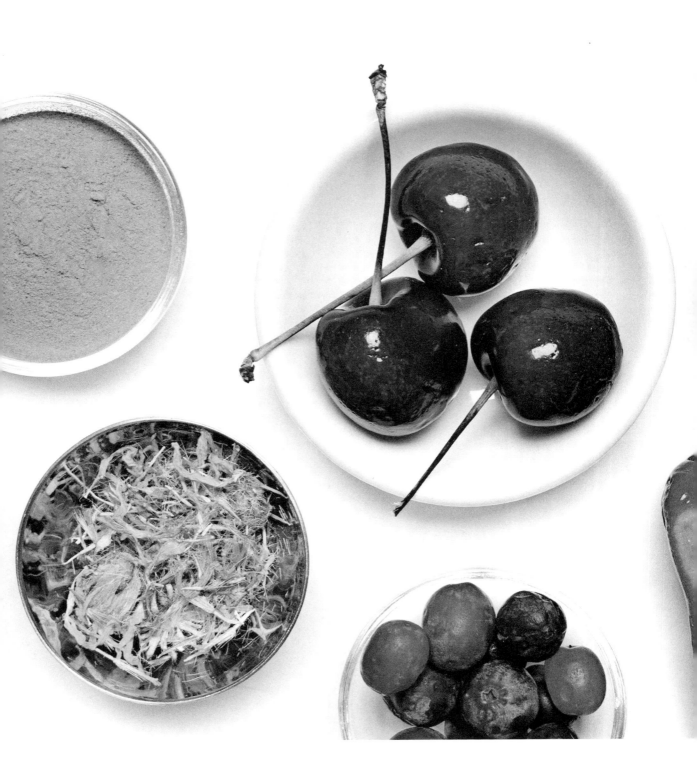

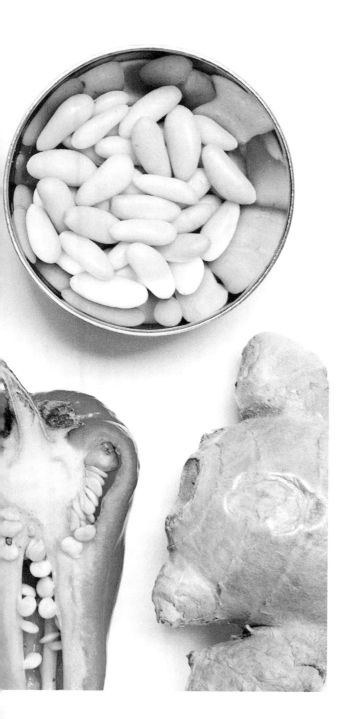

Pain-Free Back Veggies

3 tablespoons extra virgin olive oil, divided

½ cup pine nuts

½ cup dried cranberries

3 cups veggies (spinach, broccoli, cauliflower, zucchini, or a mixture)

Heat 2 tablespoons olive oil in a large skillet over medium heat. Add pine nuts and heat until they just start to turn golden. Add cranberries and stir. Cook 2 to 3 minutes and then add the vegetables. Drizzle with the remaining 1 tablespoon of oil, cover, and cook until the veggies are tender. Makes a great side dish or snack.

MINDSET

What if someone told you they were going to take away your back pain, right here, right now, forever, without you doing anything? It would be pretty back-tastic, wouldn't it? Glad you agree, because that is what you are going to do for someone else.

Tonglen is an ancient Tibetan Buddhist meditation dating back to the 1100s. It is a practice of giving and taking, or sending and receiving. *Tong*, or *jampe* in Tibetan, means "giving," as in giving someone what they want. *Len*, or *nyingje* in Tibetan, means "taking." Specifically it refers to identifying and removing pain and suffering in someone else. This is actually one of my favorite meditations because it is about taking away someone's pain and giving them happiness. What's better than that?

Tonglen is not an esoteric endeavor; it is a pure mind power practice that will transform you from the inside out. It is said to turn pain into compassion, discomfort into ease. When you practice Tonglen, you shift the focal point of pain away from you, allowing your mind, and from there your body, to radiate in a pain-free light.

This mindset practice cannot singlehandedly remove your back pain, but it can help soothe it so that you can begin to heal and prevent Back Attacks. I have taught Tonglen to dozens of people suffering from back pain, even the most skeptical of high-powered CEOs and Hollywood stars, and in all cases, Tonglen has proved an essential ingredient to subsiding their pain. Trust me—it works.

RETOX

Take a comfortable seat in a chair or on the floor, spine long. Gently close your eyes and draw your attention to the tip of your nose. Start to notice your breath, in and out through the nostrils.

Bring your attention to the top of your head. Look down into your body with your mind's eye and see everything that you know to be there—all the muscles, bones, tissues, and organs. Slowly start to clear out everything you see, all your interior contents, until you are totally empty on the inside, but still you on the outside. Almost like a shell of you.

Bring your attention back up to the top of your head, and look down into the clear, vast you. Now fill your body with a radiant, blue light, like the color of the perfect sky or sea. Fill every corner of your body with that light. This is your blue light body.

Now see in front of you someone who is suffering. Maybe it is a family member with back pain, a colleague having a rough time, someone you passed on the street who had a slight grimace on their face. Whoever it is, bring them to your attention. See how they look, what they are wearing, where they are.

Now slowly, imagine drawing out their pain with your breath, like a stream of black smoke exiting their body with your every inhale. See the stream leaving them and forming a cloud right underneath your nose and your blue light body.

On your next inhale, take in that black cloud of pain. See it move up through your nostrils, to the top of your head, then down to the area of your heart. There, see it dissolve into your radiant blue light body, like Disney stardust in the sky.

Sit with this radiant blue light body of yours, and see your friend's body now also totally radiant, bright, clear, and pain free. You may even notice that your pain has dissolved as well.

Retox Soundtrack:
"No, No, No" —EVE

BACK ATTACK

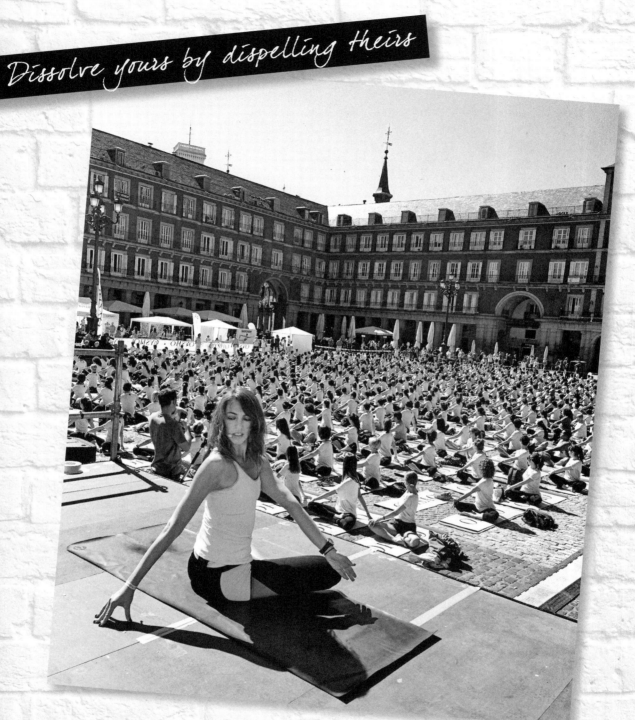

Bringing I.AM.YOU. to my favorite plaza in the world with our resident mixologist DJing. Two thousand people, Madrid.

HANGOVER HELPER

RECOVERING FROM

AND PREVENTING

I take refuge in me

THERE IS YOUR FIRST HANGOVER. Your worst hangover. And the blur in between.

Personally, I arrived late to Hangover-land in comparison to my peers; keg stands in dark California high school driveways hours before morning sports practice never quite appealed to me. But when I arrived, I went big. I was in Madrid for the summer, learning Spanish, working, and, above all, enthralled with the freedom and sense of self-discovery I found in this big city thousands of miles away from home. I became brave enough to shed a layer of my tomboy garb for Zara skirts and slinky tops, and gamboled across the city day and night, speaking with anyone and everyone who was patient enough to decipher my beginner Spanish. I was uncovering layers of my personality and discovering confidence in myself that I hadn't even realized I lacked. I felt like a cool kid.

One of my last evenings in Madrid, I took my new self-assured cool-kid pass and led a pack of globetrotting friends throughout the city. I was showing off my now nearly fluent Spanish and gregarious people skills, while drinking everything in between. I woke up the next morning in pain, my cool-kid pass clearly turned in for a passport to Hangover-land.

I could not eat lunch, which naturally worried Dolores, the housemother where I was living. Her husband, Fernando, on the other hand, took one look at me and escorted me to his study. "Sit," he said. "What did you drink last night?" He opened his bar, filled with slightly dusty bottles and crystal tumblers, and awaited my answer. As I stared at the shelves blankly, not knowing where to start, he handed me a shot glass filled with a clear gasoline-scented liquid. I wondered if he was trying to kill me. He nodded toward my shot of *orujo*, closed the bar, and left me in the room alone to fully experience my own hangover. I got the point.

Let's face it: Hangovers suck. But as I later learned on Wall Street, there are those nights when you know you are going into a full pour, whether you really want to or not. Client dinners, group holiday parties, celebratory cocktails, the list goes on and on. Yes, of course you can decline when offered, but we all know that saying no to a drink can occasionally come with a price tag in business, fair or not. And, besides, a few drinks can make the unbearable work affair bearable.

And then there is your social life. A night out with friends, talking and laughing over cocktails is fun. But sometimes you forget to pace yourself, and that's a sure ticket to Hangover-land. Life is life, and we should live it to the fullest, even if it means getting slightly overpoured from time to time. I have been there, for good reasons and bad, and know from my personal experience, as the hangoveree and the Hangover Helper, how to make it better.

In this chapter, I am going to show you how to prevent getting a hangover, even when in those heavy drinking situations. Then I'll offer you yoga relief and food cures for those inevitable slips.

YOGA

Telling a yoga teacher that you are hung over is pure blasphemy! The first time I went to yoga hung over from a never-ending client dinner the night before, the teacher hovered over me for what felt like the whole class, pontificating on the evils of alcohol, coffee, meat, cheese, capitalism, and leather, for that matter. *Seriously, shut-up-now-please-my-head-is-pounding*, I thought, as I attempted a Tree pose, wavering in the alcoholic winds of my breath.

But as I developed my personal yoga practice and continued my studies, I soon learned that yoga can actually help hangovers, as it is one of the few physical activities that penetrates the deeper layers of the body—namely, the organs. The key to Hangover Helper yoga is to practice specific poses that target and heal the places the alcohol has attacked. (Furthermore, not all ancient yoga traditions ban alcohol, so there is no need to involve guilt of any kind.)

The vast majority of my students have come to me with a hangover at least once. I have treated hundreds of them with my Retox methods. Now, even if a student tries to hide their hangover, I see it. The glossy eyes, the disheveled hair, the faint scent of vodka sweating out their pores, the backward stretchy pants . . . I keep the student after class, not for a talking to, but for some simple tips that will offer relief.

I have put together a combination of poses to eradicate toxins, oxygenate the bloodstream, and wring out the liver, the organ responsible for processing all the booze.

RETOX

DESK FIXES

TWISTING CLEANSING BREATH*

Sit in your seat and place your fingertips on your hips, or on your shoulders. Inhale to a comfortable level. Begin short, sharp breaths out of the nose, where the inhale is simply a reaction to the exhale, as the diaphragm pumps on the abdominal wall. It should feel somewhere between sneezing and blowing your nose. As you pump, on each exhale, twist left and right. Continue pumping the exhales and rotating from side to side for thirty to sixty seconds. End in the center. Relax your arms and breathe normally.

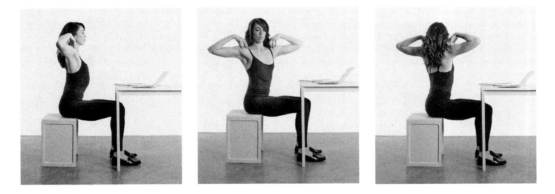

FISTS INTO ABDOMEN FORWARD FOLD*

Make your hands into fists and bring them to your abdomen, below your rib cage, knuckles touching. Inhale fully, then exhale and press your fists into your abdomen. Inhale again, and on your next exhale, fold forward, keeping your fists pressing in and now up into your abdomen.

KIDNEY RELIEF BACKBEND

Place your hands by your sides or on the chair behind you. Inhale, lift your chest. Exhale, find a backbend in your middle and lower back. Breathe into your kidneys and optionally drop your head back. Hold three to ten breaths.

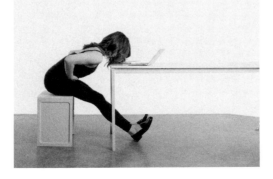

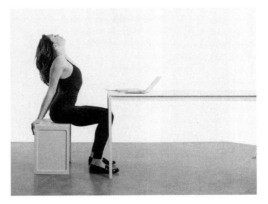

QUICK FIXES

SUN SALUTE A

Start standing with your feet together and your hands touching at your chest. Inhale, reach your arms overhead. Exhale, fold forward, and bring your forehead to your shins. Inhale, extend your spine, look forward. Exhale, Chaturanga or Plank pose. Inhale, Up Dog. Exhale, Down Dog. Close your eyes and hold here five breaths. Then inhale and step or jump your feet between your hands. Exhale, fold forward. Inhale, reach your arms up, look up. Exhale, hands to your heart. Repeat five to ten times.

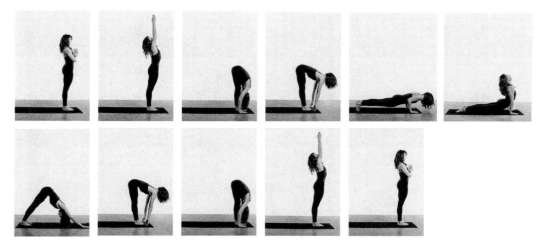

TWISTED CHAIR*

Stand with your feet together. Inhale, bend your knees into Chair pose and lift your arms up. Exhale, twist to the right, bringing your left elbow outside your right knee, palms touching and thumbs to sternum. Look up and hold five to ten breaths, then repeat on the other side.

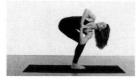

REVERSE BACKBEND LUNGE TWIST

Start in a high lunge, right leg forward. Inhale, and lift your left arm up and back. Exhale, place your right hand on your back thigh. Twist and bend back, looking at the palm of the hand or down at the floor. Breathe five to ten breaths, then repeat on the other side.

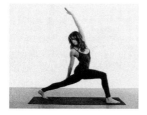

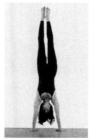

Bonus!

HANDSTAND AT WALL

Place your hands on the floor, a palm's length from the wall. Lift one leg into the air. Jump up onto your hands until your heels reach the wall. Rest your body on the wall, press into your hands, look down, and breathe. Hold for as long as you can to boost your circulation.

87

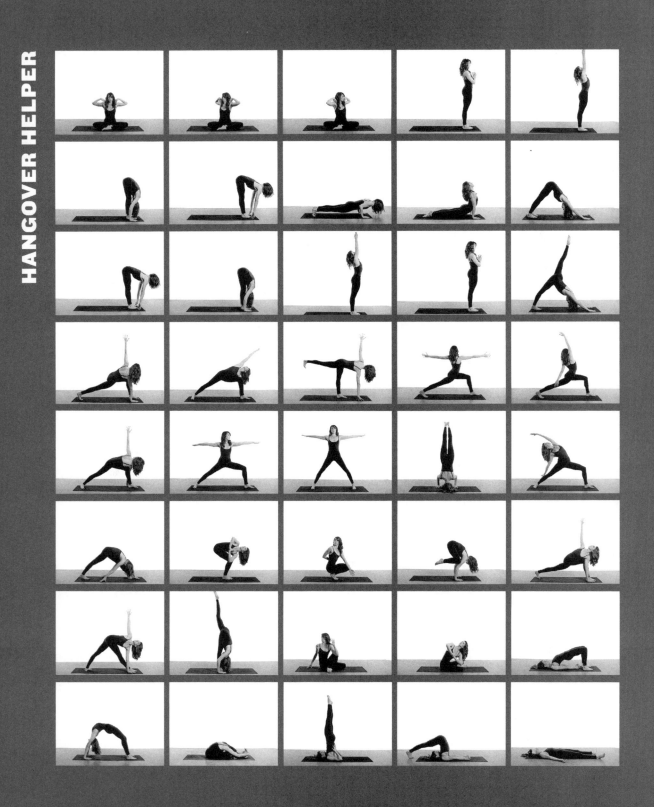

NOURISHMENT

There are three parts to this phase of Hangover Helper: The before—what you do before you go out to prepare your system for the toxins that will invade its bloodstream; the during—how you manage your alcohol intake in the moment; and the after—what you later ingest to make it all go away.

DETOX

When it comes to hangovers, the Detox phase is less about eliminating foods or habits, and more about preparing the body to best handle a night of too much alcohol.

THE BEFORE

MAGIC FOODS. These foods help boost the levels of enzymes in your body necessary to break down the alcohol once it hits your system: broccoli, asparagus, spinach, and tomato. Eat them together in a salad, snack on them as crudités, or cook the broccoli and asparagus and snack on them during the day or at work. If you prefer to juice, juice them together for the pregame.

SKIP THE SKIPPING. It can be tempting, especially for weight-conscious folks, to eat lightly the day you expect to drink. But that is asking for pain! Skipping meals or eating lightly before you drink is actually more of a detriment to your body than the small additional calories would be on your waistline. Without proper food in your system, the alcohol has more of a straight shot to the organs and blood, almost ensuring a hangover. It can also damage the lining of the stomach, likely causing that gross feeling in your tummy the next day. Make sure you eat normally the day you drink, and if possible snack from the Magic Foods list before you head out.

HYDRATION. Alcohol dehydrates your system. Dehydration is actually one of the main causes of headaches and hangovers. Make sure you hydrate with one to two liters of flat, room temperature water before you go out.

THE DURING

1:2. Have one full glass of water for every two drinks you have. I would ideally recommend 1:1, but I know it can be a pain to get to the restroom when you're in a crowded bar.

TOP UP ON TAPAS. Many cultures never offer alcohol without a bite of food at the same time. Spain, Turkey, Italy, Hong Kong, and Colombia are a few of my faves in this camp. If you're at a restaurant, order an appetizer or bar snack for the group. At a party, position yourself close to the snack table. Even nuts or bread will help absorb the alcohol, line your stomach, and brace your system.

MODKA SODAS. The I.AM.YOU. Modka Soda should be the hottest drink in town. Seltzer water with a twist of lemon or lime, it looks exactly like a vodka or gin cocktail. If you are willing and able to abstain, or you have imbibed enough but do not want to appear "lame," order Modka Sodas.

RETOX

After a night of imbibing, you need to get your body back in prime condition. Follow these simple tips and you'll be on your way to beating the hangover blues.

AFTER

HOT WATER AND LEMON. The morning after your epic eve, fill a mug with warm water and squeeze half a lemon into it. This will help you eliminate the toxins from your organs and bloodstream and further help your body produce the bile it needs to remove the toxins from your system entirely.

KEEP DRINKING . . . WATER. Keep yourself hydrated. Plus the water will help clear out the toxins.

BANANAS, POTATOES, AVOCADOS, OH MY! Your body has lost a lot of potassium, so it's a good idea to replenish. Bananas, a boiled or baked potato, or an avocado sprinkled with salt can all do the trick and will be gentle on your upset stomach.

CARBS ARE OKAY. Today is not the day to be on a low-carb diet. To settle a queasy stomach, ingest some carbs to absorb some of the alcohol and mix it with food as it processes in your body. Bread, saltine crackers, pasta, and rice all do a hung-over body good.

ORDER EASY. Back in the day, my friends and I thought there was nothing better after a night out on the town than to go to a diner on the way home. They would order cheeseburgers, fries, sometimes with cheese, and giant stacks of pancakes, all with OJ. I, on the other hand, was the weirdo with a massive chopped salad or vegetable omelet. We each assumed we had the best way to absorb all the alcohol in our systems. Boy, did they learn the hard way! Cheese, hot sauces, sugar, and orange juice are some of the worst choices. The inflammatory agents in each of these will make the feeling of the hangover worse once they enter your system, even though they may taste like a slice of heaven in the moment.

SNACKS

Pear
Banana
Fennel
Honey
Artichoke
Beets

RECIPES

Hangover Helper Salad

3 cups chopped greens (iceberg or romaine lettuce, spinach, or a combination)

¼ bulb of fennel, sliced thin

½ cup cherry or grape tomatoes, cut in half or quarters

½ cup chopped cooked broccoli florets

½ cup chopped beets

1 to 2 tablespoons extra virgin olive oil

Juice of ½ lemon

In a large bowl, mix the greens, fennel, tomatoes, broccoli, and beets. Toss with olive oil and lemon juice.

Hangover Helper Scramble

3 eggs

1 teaspoon olive oil

4 asparagus spears

½ cup cherry or grape tomatoes, cut in half or quarters

Black pepper, to taste

Crack the three eggs in a bowl and scramble. Heat the oil in a small frying pan. Add asparagus and tomatoes and cook until asparagus are soft. Add egg and cook until set. Top with freshly ground black pepper, if desired.

Pasta Toss

1 (16-ounce) package pasta of your choice

1 tablespoon extra virgin olive oil

2 cloves garlic, minced

1 (14-ounce) can artichoke hearts, drained and chopped

1 cup grape or cherry tomatoes, halved

Freshly ground black pepper, to taste

Bring a large pot of water to boil. Add pasta and cook according to package directions. While pasta is cooking, heat oil in a large skillet over medium heat. Add garlic and heat for 1 minute. Add artichokes and tomatoes and cook until soft, about 7 minutes. When pasta is cooked, drain and add directly to skillet. Toss with vegetables and season with black pepper, if desired.

Artichoke Water

2 artichokes

Cut the stems off the artichokes and cut the top inch off of the leaves. Fill a large pot with water and bring to a boil. Add artichokes and boil for 30 minutes, or until you can easily pull off the bottom leaves of the artichoke. Remove artichokes and save for a snack. Let the water cool and then drink a cup of it. This will help your liver detoxify itself and your entire body.

Hangover Helper Juice

1 beet, peeled and chopped

1 cucumber, chopped

1 stalk celery

½ lemon, peel and pith removed

¼-inch piece of ginger, peeled

Handful cilantro

Handful fresh mint

Put everything in a juicer or blender and enjoy.

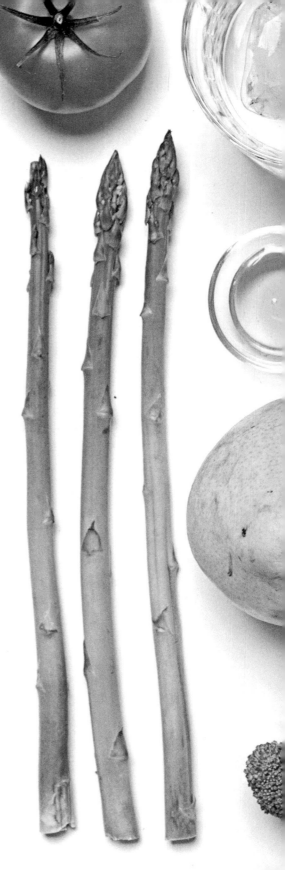

92

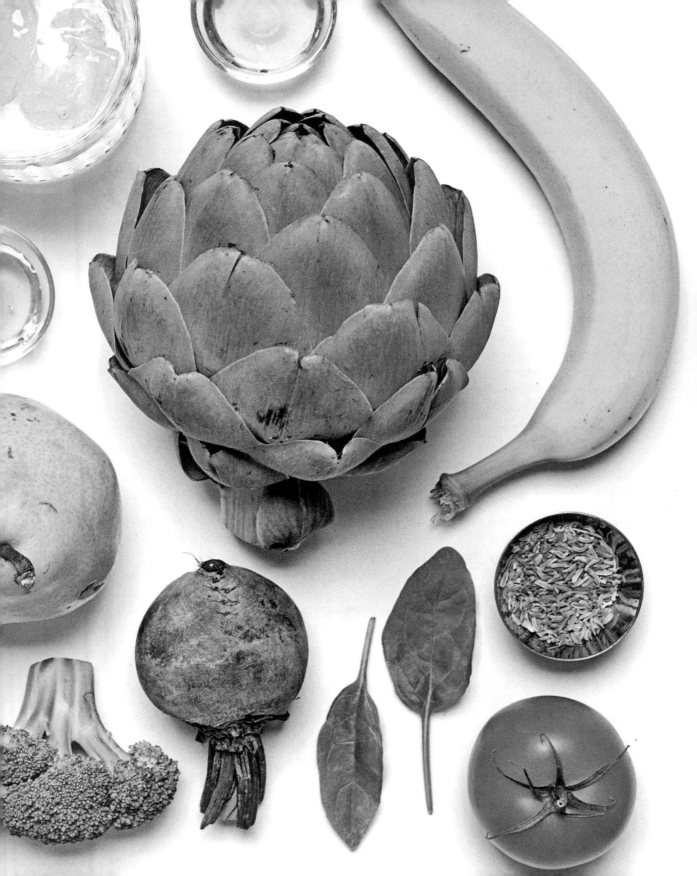

MINDSET

It probably is not something you want to hear from someone like me, but I have woken up plenty of mornings and declared before noon that I need a drink. Straight up. I blame the morning's trials and tribulations, of course. Am I an alcoholic? No. Just an honest, hardworking, modern woman who wears a hundred different hats and juggles as many roles. And sometimes I want quick relief.

My old, default Cali-urban ex–Wall Street reaction on these days of stress is to find a chocolate chip cookie, go sweat it out on the mat, and then grab a drink. In total candor, I have spent those chaotic mornings pondering whether it should be Malbec or Tempranillo that will soothe me that evening. The reality is that neither a fruity nor a leathery blend will actually do the trick, as both are free tickets to Hangover-land.

A hangover is literally defined as a thing that survived from the past. In today's world, the things we are most generally referring to are toxins. As discussed earlier, there are both tangible toxins (such as alcohol, cigarettes, chocolate, cheese, sugar, processed food, chemicals, and smog) and intangible ones (such as stress, anger, worry, anxiety, depression, sadness, and extreme emotions).

Hangovers can thus take on many forms. There are those from two glasses of wine and a full dinner, and those from five tequila shots and no dinner. There are hangovers from a fight with your boyfriend and hangovers from a workaholic day in the office. There are hangovers from screaming kids and from whiny wives. There are hangovers from an overindulgent shopping spree and ones from eating too many gummy bears. They come not solely from alcohol you intake, but rather from an array of toxins that overwhelm your system. These Retox mindset tools help target the hidden cause and prevent it from happening over and over.

Let's look at a bad day. You leave work and what do you do to feel better? Or you put the kids to sleep and where do you head? Where do you turn when things are less than fine? Is it a new pair of shoes or lingerie? Chocolate or a pint of Ben & Jerry's? Back-to-back spin classes? Blasting heavy metal? Whiskey?

In Tibetan yoga philosophy, these are all considered places of refuge. Refuge, or *sangye choe* in Tibetan and *namo* in Sanskrit, is where you flee when you are yearning to feel better. It is what you do to appease yourself or find solace. But at some point, these places of refuge don't work. So then what? It is time to go deeper to find a truer refuge, which is what I am here to help with.

RETOX

The next time you text a friend telling them that your day sucked and you need a drink, pause and remember this: The drink is not going to make the day better. But you have it in your power to create what actually *will* make it, you, and your world better. So go for your drink, but while you wait for them to pour your alcoholic refuge du jour, try this exercise.

Take out a piece of paper and fold it in half, or grab a bar napkin or a new iPhone note if you want.

If there is an emotional focal point at the moment, such as something upsetting you, something to celebrate, or something that

94

makes you want to flee or escape, write it across the top. If you cannot pinpoint anything, just leave the space blank.

On the left side of the page, write down everything you are craving in that moment that will soothe you. Maybe it is crawling into a ball on the couch, sweating for hours in a sauna or gym, crying, running, pigging out, or simply downing that dirty martini you can almost already taste. Remember, I was honest about my cookies, sweat, and red wine refuges, so be honest with yourself.

Now take a moment, even a nanosecond, to close your eyes and breathe.

Open your eyes, and below each item of refuge, write down one negative side effect of it. For example, for the dirty martini you crave, you could write a hangover; for the pizza and ice cream, feeling gross; for the sympathy shopping spree, spending money you don't have.

Take another moment to close your eyes and breathe.

Open your eyes, and now on the right side of the page, write down what makes you truly happy, what makes you truly feel great, like when you are on vacation with no problems. Don't hold back—write it all down.

Take another nanosecond to close your eyes and breathe.

Now mentally text a note to yourself and commit in your mind to fully indulging in a real feel-good activity in the next twenty-four hours. Maybe it is doing yoga or cooking a meal, calling your mom to talk or going to a museum, reading a book or inviting over a friend. Whatever it is, do it. This is your true refuge.

And if it is having a few drinks that makes you feel better, I am willing to bet you will not suffer from the same level of hangover the next day, because instead of drinking to take cover in refuge, you were having a drink because you really wanted to, inside and out.

Retox Soundtrack:
"Shimmy Shimmy Ya" —PRINCE FATTY

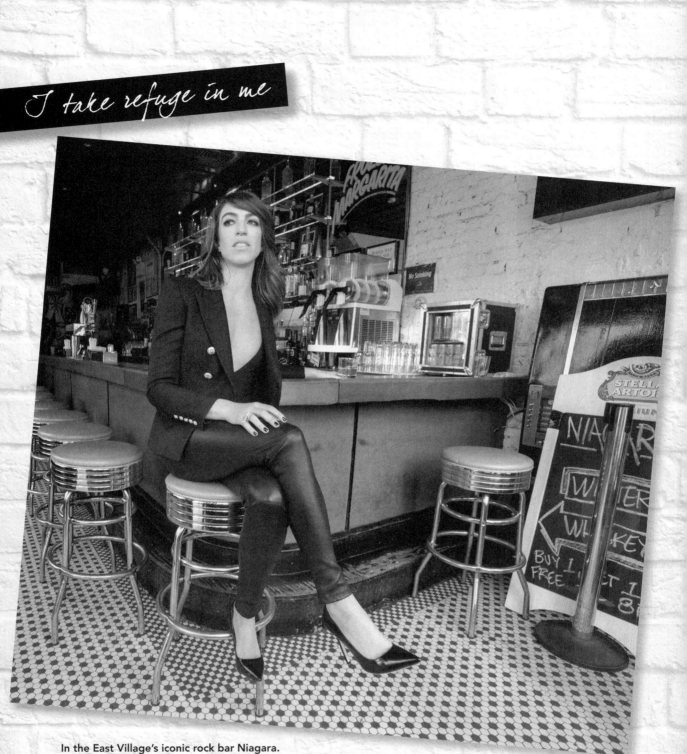

In the East Village's iconic rock bar Niagara.
New York City. Photograph by Mick Rock.

THE NEW
MILE-HIGH CLUB

MAKING TRAVEL A
HEALTHY TIME FOR YOU

Go for a ride inside

THERE ARE CERTAIN DAYS WHEN I look at my bag with utter disgust. I sincerely cannot believe that I have to lug it through another airport or train station; I would rather chuck it out the window. Other days, I see my suitcase glistening with opportunity, begging to be taken on a new journey. In both cases, I rarely have a choice, as travel for work, family, and, sometimes, pleasure beckons.

These days, taking an airplane can be as commonplace as jumping on the bus, train, or subway. But flying has a unique and specific impact on your body. The airplane air is recycled, the security checks and bag carrying are exhausting, and the service often leaves much, if not all, to be desired.

If you are anything like Peter, a digital ad salesman with two round-trip flights weekly, you need a plan to maintain yourself physically and mentally. Peter came to me a haggard mess; he sort of reminded me of a beat-up piece of luggage, lost and waiting to be found. He immediately told me how much he traveled, and proceeded to recount his back pain, headaches, leg cramps, inability to sleep, swollen feet, and digestive issues. I was quick to notice his dry, pale skin, lackluster eyes, and hunched posture. Having personally gone through phases of travel even more intense than Peter's, I immediately indoctrinated him into the new mile-high club, a Retox plan designed specifically to relieve and prevent travel woes.

This chapter provides yoga to help you overcome jet lag, bloating, and all the other unpleasant side effects of flying. It includes tips on how to eat in-flight and at the airport, and a reconstruction plan for your mind to keep you calm and alert throughout it all. Peter and countless other travelers across the globe use these tips before, during, and after their trips, making their experience a true journey to inward, radiant health.

YOGA

I am not that weirdo sprawled on the terminal floor in a Pigeon pose or handstand. That's just gross. I am, however, the over-traveled gal who will make time to do the yoga so that I feel and attempt to look like a billion bucks no matter where I go. Try the Desk Fixes in your seat, the Quick Fixes in the aisle before or after your journey, and the full sequence before or after you take off, or both. The poses reach the muscles and fascia most affected by travel, as well as boost your circulation and metabolic systems so that you feel refreshed, strong, lean, and un-jet-lagged wherever you go.

RETOX

DESK FIXES

ENERGY BREATH*

Lift your arms straight up and open them into a V. Inhale to a comfortable level. Begin short, sharp breaths out of the nose, where the inhale is simply a reaction to the exhale, as the diaphragm pumps on the abdominal wall. It should feel somewhere between sneezing and blowing your nose. (If you are pregnant, skip khapalabhati.) Keep these up for one minute, energizing your body with each pump.

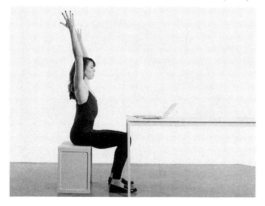

SECRET PRAYER

Bring your arms behind the back and put your hands together as if in prayer. If this is too difficult, grasp your forearms with the opposite hands. Stretch across the front of your chest. Stay there and breathe normally or add the energy breath.

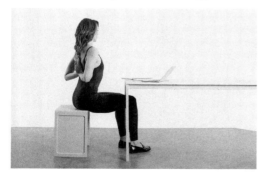

SIDE STRETCH

Lift your arms straight up. Hold your left wrist with your right hand. Inhale, grow long and pull up. Exhale, lean to the right. Make sure both sitz bones are on the chair so the stretch is through your left side. Hold here, then repeat on the other side.

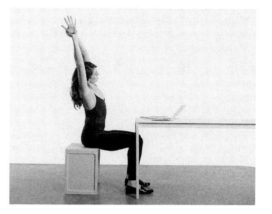

HALF ANKLE TO KNEE

Place your left ankle on your right lower quad, just above the knee. Flex your left foot. Press your left hand down on the inner left thigh or knee. Optionally, fold forward. Hold there, then repeat on the other side.

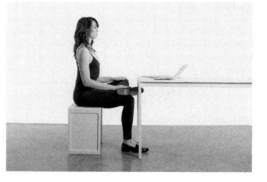

99

QUICK FIXES

WEEPING WILLOW

Start standing. As you inhale, bring your left knee into the chest. Place the sole of the left foot to the inseam of the right leg, above or below the knee but not on it. On your next inhale, lift your arms up. Exhale, drop your left forearm to the top of the left thigh. Inhale, stretch the right arm up. Exhale, lean to the left side, stretching the right side of your body. Stay here five to eight breaths, then repeat on the other side.

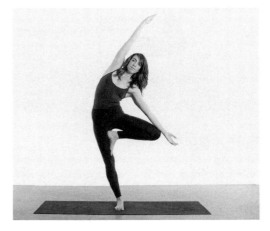

STRADDLE

Sit with your legs wide into a V. Reach your arms in front of you and fold forward. Hold here eight to twenty breaths.

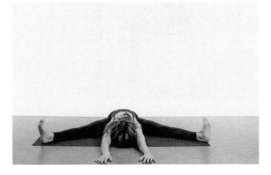

SWIVEL SIDE PLANK

Start in Plank pose with your shoulders over your wrists and body parallel to the floor. Swivel onto your left hand, inner edge of right foot, and outer edge of left foot, with one foot in front of the other. Raise your right arm alongside your ear and look up. Lift your hips and stretch from ankles to middle finger. Hold here five to ten breaths, then repeat on the other side.

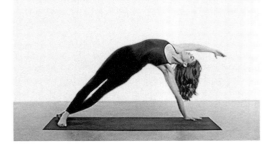

SHOULDER STAND*

Lie on the floor. Lift your feet up and over your head and place your hands on your back. Inhale, lift your legs straight up into the air. Look at your toes or close your eyes and breathe here for ten breaths, or up to five minutes.

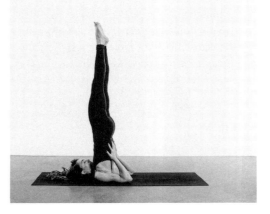

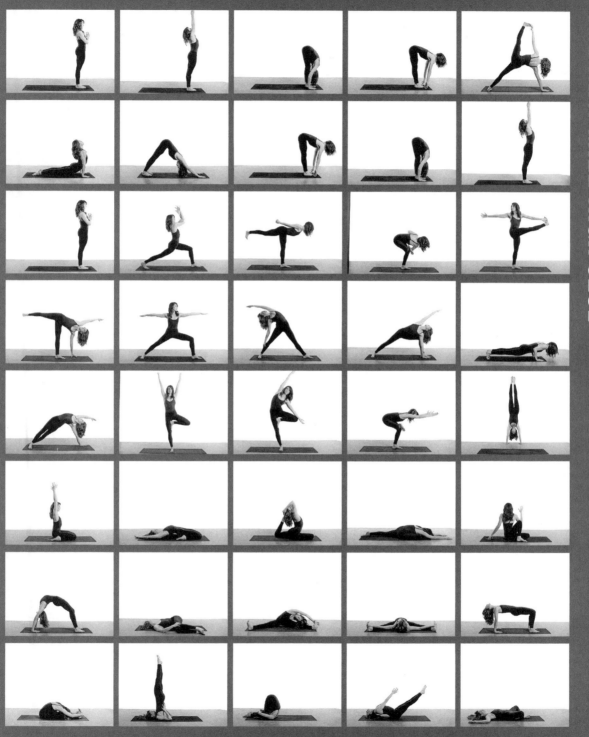

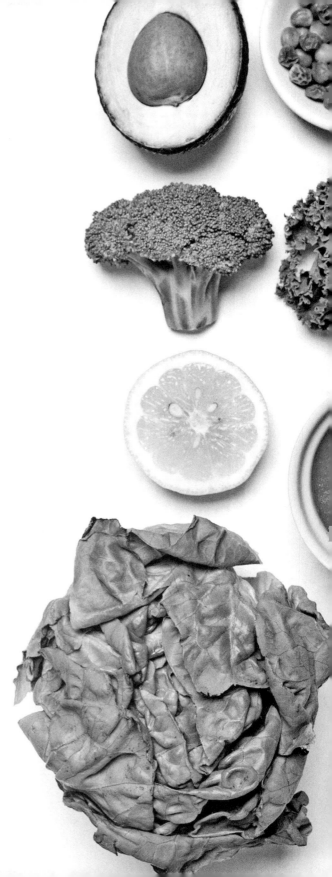

NOURISHMENT

Traveling is not an excuse to eat crap. Travel already demands so much more of your system that giving it, well, poison makes no sense. Sure, pick up a pack of your favorite candy to have while you watch the in-flight flick, but don't try to tell me that McDonald's, Auntie Anne's, or Cinnabon are necessary so you don't get hungry on your journey. You will pay for it when you get there.

Figuring out what to eat can be tricky, but it is not impossible. There are three parts to nourishment for the new mile-high club: the before—what you do before you get to the port of departure; the during—how you manage and select your intake while en route; and the after—what you later ingest to smooth out the ride.

DETOX

THE BEFORE

HYDRATION. Flying and travel dehydrate your system. It is thus imperative to stay extra hydrated. Try doubling your water intake the day before you travel, and taking a liter to drink en route to the airport. You may be sprinting to the restroom before security, but it will be well worth it. Drink another liter before you take off as well, making a quick bathroom stop on the way to the gate, if you need to.

FUEL UP. It can be tempting to avoid eating before a series of sedentary hours, and it's easy to "not have time" to eat as you run around preparing for your journey. Yet maintaining stable blood sugar levels is critical to managing stress and acclimating to the jour-

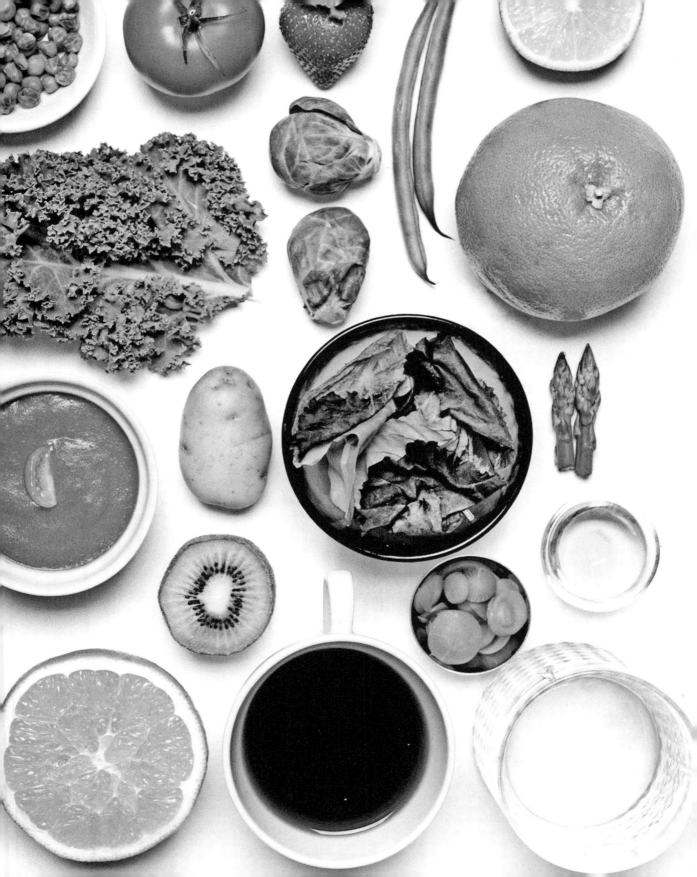

ney and the destination. Make sure you eat normally the day before and the day of travel, focusing on the Golden Ticket Foods.

GOLDEN TICKET FOODS. These foods will help stabilize your metabolic system and boost immunity so that you feel strong and calm as you travel:

- **Cooked Vegetables:** Load up on cooked veggies like broccoli, spinach, string beans, and zucchini. The "green" factor will keep your skin and inner system vibrant, and the fact that they are cooked makes them easy to digest so as to mitigate bloating in-flight.
- **Soup:** Choose a soup as your last meal before takeoff. The warmth will soothe your internal organs, boost immunity, and prevent digestive discomfort in the air.
- **Vitamin C:** Load up on vitamin C–rich foods so that your immune system can protect you as you maneuver through the hundreds of people around you. Focus on broccoli, kiwis, oranges, and other citrus fruits.

THE DURING

CHUG. Admittedly the bathrooms are usually nasty, but even worse is your internal system dehydrated. Buy a liter of water en route to the gate, and then proceed to ask for two glasses of water, no ice, every time the in-flight team passes by. Every time you go to the bathroom, get another one to two glasses of water. Your goal should be to drink at least one liter on a short flight, two to three on a medium- to long-haul flight.

GO VEGAN. Travel is one of the rare times I suggest going vegan. Avoid meats, eggs, and cheeses in-flight, as they will merely inflame your system and disrupt digestion as you are up in the air. Not to mention the quality of these items at the airport is usually subpar, mass produced, and full of hormones and other chemicals you probably would never want to ingest on land. Stick to pasta, crackers, fruit, and vegetables at the airport and during the flight.

PICK SMART OPTIONS. Sure, you can pack your own meals and snacks for the trip, but really, who has time? And if you do sometimes, are you like me and usually forget them all in the fridge at home? I usually pick something healthy at the airport, which, by the way, is easier to find than most people think. I have yet to be at an airport anywhere in the world where I cannot find some or all of the below:

For snacks, keep your eyes on nuts, blueberries, raisins, bananas, apples, quinoa chips, salads, and vegetable sticks. For a larger meal, look for veggie burgers, vegetable sandwiches, steamed vegetables from the Asian places, salads, vegetable platters, and maybe even soup.

AVOID COFFEE AND ALCOHOL. Okay, if it is your honeymoon, totally have the glass of champagne, but for the most part, skip the in-flight booze, coffee, and caffeinated tea. They all dehydrate and inflame your system, which will likely make you even more bloated when you land.

RETOX

THE AFTER

GO GREEN. Greens are your magic potion. Eat them raw, cooked, or in a salad as the focal point of meals and snacks throughout the next twenty-four hours. Focus on lettuces, spinach,broccoli, and avocado. They will all revitalize and hydrate you, as well as keep your circulation in top shape.

FRESH AND WILD. The more fresh, raw food you eat after you land the better. Go for all the vegetables and low-glycemic fruits you can find as snacks and meals. This will help reduce bloating and get your system going again on all levels.

OLIVE OIL. Think of olive oil as a lubricant for your somewhat stagnated digestive system. Have a tablespoon straight up or just include a healthy pour over your salad.

COFFEE. Let yourself sip a warm, black coffee after you land. It will help reduce some bloating and make you more alert for whatever the day brings.

WATER. Obviously. Drink a liter within six hours of landing.

Go cooked before, gluten free and vegan during, and raw and fresh after.

And, yes, I know how many bathroom trips are involved in this Retox plan. Not to worry, you have the time to kill anyway!

MINDSET

You have a choice—you can see travel as a total pain, whining about it out loud and to yourself before, during, and after the trip, or you can shift it into a positive experience you long for, just for you. No, I have not gone crazy. The former will drain you and augment the already challenging aspects of the journey; the latter will energize and relax you in a secret meditative nest. It is up to you, and I will explain why and how.

Tibetan yoga philosophy extols and mandates *pratyahara* as a step on the pathway to success, freedom, and bliss (a word not too commonly associated with travel). Pratyahara is a withdrawal of the senses, a bridge from your outer world to your inner you. In redirecting the senses inward, it gives the five senses that dictate our continual body, mind, and life experience a chance to chill out and just be. In practicing pratyahara, we gain a renewed sensibility with which to perceive our reality, one that expands your perceptual capacity and feeds the true you.

The problem is that there is so much commotion, so much continual external stimulation, that our ability to go inward is obstructed. We are constantly bombarded by emails, phone calls, advertisements, colors, people, smells, errands, stressors, texts, and endless other subliminal and up-front demands, all of which push and pull on our own true nature, leaving us drained, frazzled, and longing for an escape.

In today's world, travel is arguably one of the best and most efficient places to practice pratyahara. Travel is an incubator for you; pratyahara is merely the gateway.

Whether you are up in the sky or barreling across the tracks, travel creates a pure, unobstructed period of time just for you. You can opt out of calls and emails (you can always say the in-flight Internet did not work), you cannot go work out or run an errand. It is just you with time for you, in a perfectly contained and tempered pod. Despite the schlep and hassle, travel is a forced withdrawal of the senses, one that your body is likely starved for. You have undisrupted time to read and watch movies, write and snooze, draw and let your mind wander. No one can bother you, no one can force you to be anywhere else but seat 27B. It is just you and you.

RETOX

This plan has allowed me and dozens of my jet-set clients to uncover the precious, hidden aspect of travel, and turn our journeys into multihour-long meditation and nourishment sessions for the parts of ourselves day-to-day life often forces us to neglect. Try to implement these practices into your regular travel routine, and you will start to relish your journeys in a whole new way.

DAY BEFORE YOU FLY. Get two books, two to three movies, and your favorite binge series. Download your favorite music and charge your devices.

AT THE AIRPORT. Get all the newspapers and magazines you never have time to read.

AS YOU BOARD. Put on your headset and listen to whatever music calls you. Once you sit, keep one book, the newspapers, and half the magazines out on your lap. Flip through the guilty pleasures of *US Weekly* and get the last drops of email and social media as you wait for the doors to close.

AS YOU TAXI. Turn your phone off, let your eyes flutter shut, and let your mind wander. You may even note that with the pressurization of the cabin that you drift into a light slumber. That's good! Stuck on the tarmac? No worries, you literally have nowhere you can go but inward.

IN THE AIR. Enjoy. Read. Watch. Stare into almost space. Doodle. Indulge. Let yourself be free, without feeling guilty about what you should or should not be doing. Going into you is the only thing you can do, and thus the only thing you should do for that matter. So ride whatever wave takes you there.

DEALING WITH THE CHALLENGES. Screaming baby behind you? Turn up the volume on your headset. Turbulence? Fasten the seatbelt, close your eyes, and just follow your breath. Nasty smell? Put up your hoodie or spray a scarf with your favorite perfume and wrap it around your neck. Gross food? No worries. It will be great wherever you land, and you have a plan, above, to get you through the flight.

ONCE YOU LAND. Take off your hoodie, toss everything you read, take a big, deep breath, and do some Retox yoga. You may even feel more calm and revitalized than when you took off.

YOUR PERSONAL SECURITY CHECK. Whatever step of the journey you are on, remember you can always close your eyes and find your breath saying:

Inhale, *Serenity.*
Exhale, *Protect me.*

Inhale, *Serenity.*
Exhale, *Protect me.*

Anytime the travel mumbo jumbo gets to be too much, repeat this Retox saying and transport yourself into the inner you. Use your breath and mind to simply block out the bad and find the good.

Retox Soundtrack:
"East to the West" —MICHAEL FRANTI

RETOX

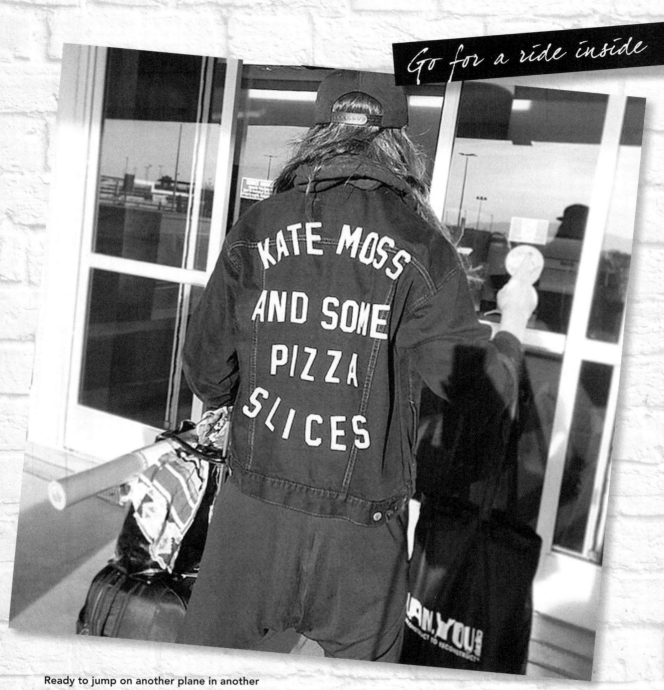

Ready to jump on another plane in another airport, Arizona. Photograph by Emily Nolan.

ALIEN BABY DEBLOAT

GETTING RID OF THAT

ABDOMINAL POOCH

THERE IS DEFINITELY A DON Draper in me. At the very least in my love of the perfect suit and crisp button-down. In fact, I was wearing such a button-down the first time the Alien Baby came to life. I was twenty-four years old and sitting at the trading desk at work when I got tapped on the shoulder. (On Wall Street, this is rarely a good sign.) I looked up, and it was the infamous Ben from London. He had a reputation for being a genius, more akin to the Nutty Professor than Albert Einstein, and was now heading up my group in London and making a killing. "Let's go," he says.

We sat in an office to chat, and before long he says, "I want you to come to London with me. We are starting a business in Turkey and I want you to be a part of it." I could barely believe what I was hearing. Being selected to be a part of a new business for the firm, live abroad again but with a job, and get free regular travel to a country that has always fascinated me? The left lobe of my brain was in. Then he said, "And we want you to start in two weeks." The right lobe of my brain panicked. He explained a bit more about his vision, which the left side loved, and then gave me a week to think about it, which made the right side tremble.

I went back to my desk to work for the rest of the day, noting not only a furious match of mental ping-pong going on in my brain, but also a small bulge starting to push at my button-down. By the end of the day, the ping-pong had tired out, but I had a bump the size of a football pressing against the bottom part of my shirt, so large, in fact, I was almost able to rest a small water bottle upon it. I had never seen this before. And it did not go away. I felt pregnant, *Spaceballs*-style, with an alien ready to pop out of the front of my abdomen and dance. The Alien Baby was born.

All joking aside, this Alien Baby of mine was one of the most uncomfortable physical moments I have ever experienced. I had to wear my work shirts untucked, dig out my loose sweater sets, and make sure my boyfriend did not stand at any angle where the baby was visible.

I went to my yoga teachers, who told me to become a vegetarian, which I already was. I called my mother and grandmother daily for home remedies. Ultimately, I went to the two best GI specialists in NYC, which naturally resulted in tests and more expensive tests, all of which came out normal, and IBS being the general, vague, and unhelpful diagnosis. I ended up moving to London four weeks after

Ben sat me down, about half a dozen doctors' visits later, and looking roughly four or five months pregnant. Needless to say, my Alien Baby came with me.

Unsatisfied with the various doctors' diagnoses, prescribed pills, and suggested remedies, I decided to take the matter into my own hands and experiment with new natural ways to get rid of the painful pooch and bloat at the bottom of my belly. After months and months of experimentation and study, I discovered there are acute food and mental triggers for the Alien Baby, as well as certain yoga poses that can reduce the pain and size of the baby very quickly.

Once I figured out the key to my own divine anticonception, I started to use the same tools on my girlfriends and colleagues, who were also "conceiving" their own Alien Babies. Word quickly got out that I was some sort of Alien shamanic doula, and from those initial ladies to the current I.AM.YOU.ers across the globe, I get weekly requests for Retox solutions for Alien Baby debloat—or as I like to say, getting that sh*t flat and gone.

Some people come to me knowing exactly what the problem is, while others describe an unidentified discomfort and bloating, too shy to share details. Yet all seem to find a comfort in my lighthearted name for this annoying, prevalent, and sometimes embarrassing condition, not to mention relief in the Retox cocktails I serve them up.

Take Desiree, a pretty chill thirty-year-old gal from Boston. She and I crossed paths at a birthday party in the park for a mutual friend. Every time she reached for a bite of the snacks, she winced a bit. I asked what was wrong, but she was too timid to share despite my desire to help. Thankfully, someone passed a platter of crudités, and the opportunity to delve into her discomfort appeared. I politely declined the raw veggies, saying I am careful with them so as to avoid my Alien Baby, looking at Desiree specifically when I answered. A few minutes later, she asked what I meant, I told her what I have just told you, and she immediately lifted her shirt to show me how much she was suffering. I told her to put the carrot down, not to stress, and to let me help her. Thankfully, she did.

By the end of the party, I had given Desiree (and a few other party guests) the tools to make her Alien Baby go away, and to prevent it from coming back in the future. We discussed what she had eaten in the past few days, allowing me to quickly identify a few culprits for her to eliminate, all of which she had mistakenly thought were remedies. Then I got her on the lawn with some yoga poses, and ultimately on the mat with a longer sequence devoted to the inner anatomy of Alien Baby eradication.

Within twenty-four hours of putting down the carrot and sharing her problem, Desiree's Alien Baby had abated. Within a few days, it was gone entirely. Now she finally knows what causes her Alien Baby, as well as how to reconstruct a pain-free, deflated abdomen. Here is how she did it.

YOGA

The point of the yoga poses in the Alien Baby debloat cocktail is aimed at soothing symptoms, decreasing inflammation, and quelling discomfort. Think of it as getting you moving, and your Alien Baby grooving its way away.

RETOX

DESK FIXES

FISTS INTO ABDOMEN*

Make your hands into fists and bring them to your abdomen below your rib cage, knuckles touching. Inhale fully, and as you exhale, press your fists into your abdomen. Inhale again, and on your next exhale, fold forward keeping your fists pressing in and up. If you want to extend your legs and fully fold forward reaching your forehead to your thighs, you can do that as well.

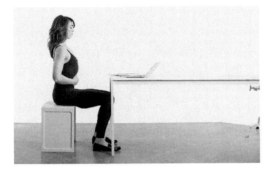 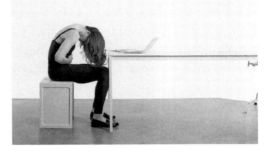

STOMACH RUBS

In Traditional Chinese Medicine, bloating and digestive issues mean that the qi, or energy, in the stomach and spleen are blocked. I have adapted one of their techniques to your daily desk life. Sit in a comfortable seat. Warm your hands if they are cold by rubbing them together. Begin rubbing your stomach in concentric circles to the left around the belly button. Then repeat to the right. Ideally you would do one hundred on each side, but if you are pressed for time, then just do as many as you can. Repeat as you can and desire.

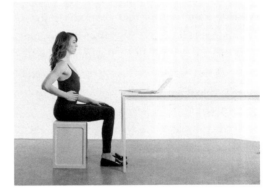

CHAIR TWISTS*

Sit up tall in your chair, feet even on the floor. Inhale, grow long; exhale, twist to one side, making sure both sitz bones stay on the seat. Stay here five to ten breaths, then repeat on the other side.

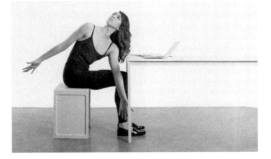

QUICK FIXES

STRONG CLEANSING BREATH*

Stand tall, feet wide apart. Inhale through your nose and lift your arms up. Exhale out of your mouth as you fold forward, bending your knees. Place your hands on your thighs, and when you are totally empty of breath, close your lips and straighten your elbows. Hold here, bringing your abdomen toward your spine. Remain empty. If you are doing it well, you almost feel as if your stomach is up in your throat. Now pump your stomach against the abdominal wall, either straight out or in circles. This is something you need to experience and get via trial and error. When you have to inhale, stop the pumps, inhale through your nose, lifting your arms alongside your ears and straightening your legs. Exhale, bringing your hands to your heart.

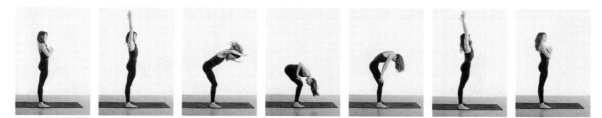

CHAIR WITH TWIST*

Stand with your feet together. Inhale, bend your knees into Chair pose and lift your arms up. Exhale, twist to the right, bringing your left elbow outside your right knee, palms touching and thumbs to sternum. Look up and hold five to ten breaths, then repeat on the other side.

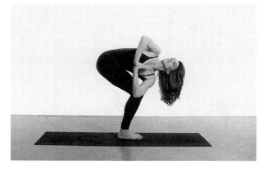

SQUAT TWIST*

Start by standing with your feet together. Bend your knees and come to the balls of your feet bringing the thigh bones parallel to the floor. Place the back of your left hand on the outside of your right leg and lift your right arm up. Hold here five to ten breaths, then repeat on the other side.

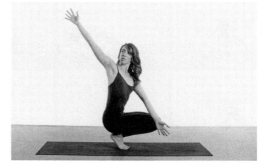

Bonus!

BELLY ROLL*

Roll up a blanket or towel into a neat ball. Come to lie on top of it facedown, with the roll pressing between your pelvis and your lowest ribs. Bring your forehead to the floor or one cheek to the side and breathe for one to five minutes.

ALIEN BABY DEBLOAT

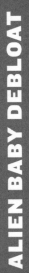

ALIEN BABY DEBLOAT

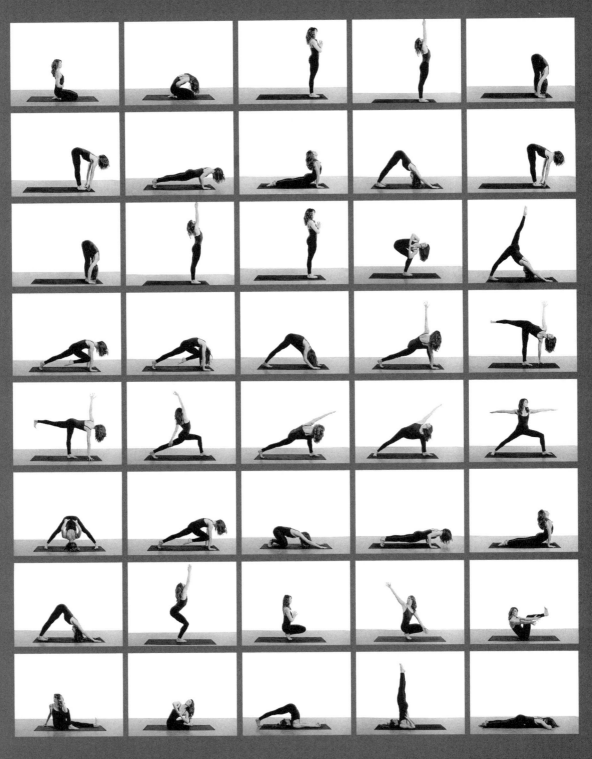

NOURISHMENT

Embarrassing tidbit: You know when you go to a spa and they put slices of cucumbers on your eyes to de-puff them? Back when I was twenty-four I thought that logic could apply to my belly. So I started to eat one to two cucumbers a day and drink cucumber juice in attempt to de-puff my abdomen and get rid of the Alien Baby. You know what? It did *not* work! In fact, it made it way worse, as did all the light salads I was eating to try to "get my system going." Now after years of experimentation and study, I have figured out why.

When you are bloated and have stomachaches, abdominal pain, and/or diarrhea, the insides of your intestines are irritated and, quite frankly, pissed off at you. Specifically, the villi, or tiny hairs that line your intestinal walls, get inflamed. Because your intestines are over twenty feet long, one microscopic inflammation can become one giant abdominal bloat.

The key to nourishment in the Alien Baby debloat cocktail is actually simple: You have to avoid foods that your system biochemically protests. Each of us is slightly different, but luckily there are many foods that are common denominator Alien Baby triggers for almost all of us. Just eliminating these can make a big difference.

DETOX

Avoid these foods:

EGGPLANT. The seeds get stuck in the intestines and inflame them.

CUCUMBER. Same as eggplant.

NUTS. Like seeds, the broken-down nuts get stuck in the intestinal hairs.

CHIA. Like the small bits of nuts, they get stuck in the hairs, and worse, they expand.

SOY SAUCE. Soy sauce has one of the highest gluten contents of anything out there. The gluten in the soy sauce, even sodium-free kinds, will trigger inflammation across your body, especially your gut.

SOY PRODUCTS. Many people have a slight soy allergy without realizing it. Notice if you bloat after eating tofu, soy milk, or other soy products and then remove them from your diet.

SPICY SAUCES. Spice inflames your body inside and out, and when ingested can lead to all sorts of Alien Baby symptoms.

RAW FOODS. Raw foods are jam-packed with nutrients, yes, but they are also incredibly hard for your digestive system to break down. Raw foods often travel through your intestines only half processed, especially if you ate rushed or stressed, aggravating your intestines further.

PROCESSED FOODS. All processed foods include additives and chemicals, and many contain gluten or one of its derivatives to enhance texture, consistency, and taste. This gluten is very different from natural gluten in fresh wheat, and has a direct effect on the Alien Baby. The same goes for MSG, soy derivatives, and xantham gum, a common ingredient in gluten-free foods.

115

RETOX

INSTA DEBLOATERS

WARM WATER. Drink a glass of plain warm water three times a day, at least thirty minutes before you eat. This will help pacify your villi and get your internal system moving.

RICE. Rice is your friend. A bowl of steamed white rice will help absorb excess acidity in your stomach and sooth your Alien Baby like a little blanket.

COOKED FOODS. When a food is cooked, your stomach and digestive system have to work less to break it down. When it works less, it can recover and do its job with less aggravation (aka inflammation). If you are at the height of Alien Baby pregnancy, cut out raw foods entirely until you normalize. As general prevention, have one meal a day that is all cooked, perhaps even two in the cold winter months when your body needs warmth to be able to function smoothly.

TEA. Chamomile, mint, or dandelion teas are instant tummy soothers.

SNACKS

Crackers, especially the old-school
    saltines
Small cup of rice
Baked potato with the skin
Licorice root
Candied ginger

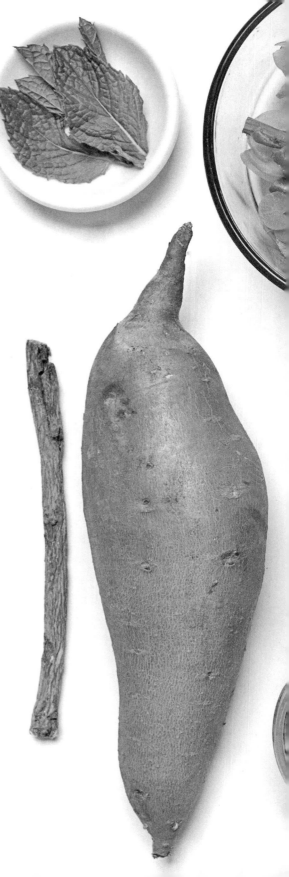

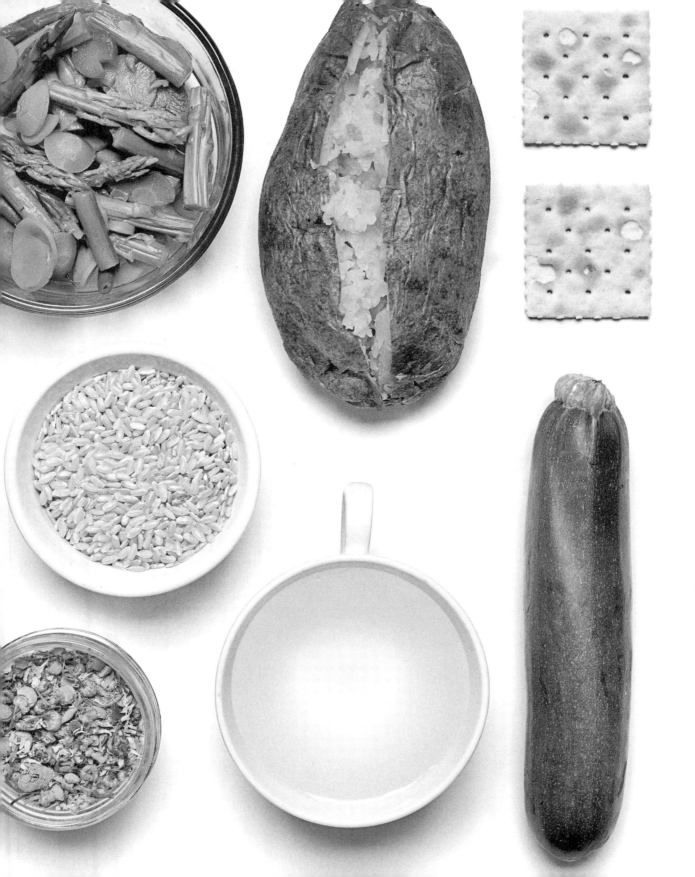

RECIPES

Chata's Vegetable Soup

1 tablespoon olive oil

1 yellow onion, diced

1 (6-ounce) can of tomato paste

2 teaspoons salt

1 carrot, chopped

2 stalks celery, chopped

1 zucchini, chopped

1 potato, diced

Fill a large pot two-thirds full with water and bring to a boil. As you wait for the water to boil, heat oil in a small sauté pan. Add onion. When the onion is soft, add the tomato paste and salt. Add carrot, celery, zucchini, and potato to the boiling water. When the tomato/onion combo starts to look a little orange, add it all to the pot of water and vegetables. Stir and cover with a lid. Let cook until all vegetables are soft, about 20 minutes. Enjoy!

Zucchini and Rice

1 cup rice, uncooked

3 tablespoons olive oil

2 gloves garlic, minced

3 large zucchini, chopped

Sour cream for garnish (optional)

Cook your favorite type of rice according to the package directions or just buy it precooked. In a large frying pan, heat the oil and garlic over medium heat. Add the chopped zucchini to the pan. Stir a couple times and let cook until the zucchini is soft. Serve the rice with the zucchini on top. Add a dollop of sour cream, if desired.

Sautéed Spinach

1 tablespoon olive oil
2 cloves garlic, sliced thinly

2 (9-ounce) bags baby spinach

Heat oil in a large sauté pan. Add garlic and let cook until it just begins to turn golden. Add spinach to pan and stir. Cover and let cook until spinach is completely wilted, about 5 minutes. Serve as a side dish or a snack.

Alien Potato Mash

4 sweet potatoes, peeled and chopped

1 tablespoon butter
Salt, to taste

Put potatoes in a large pot and fill with water. Bring to a boil, then reduce heat and let simmer until the potatoes are soft, 8 to 10 minutes. Drain potatoes well and transfer to a large bowl. Add butter and salt and either smash them with a fork or whip them with an electric hand mixer.

MINDSET

Remember earlier when I told you my left and right brains started fighting over Ben's proposal to move to London? One side really wanted it, knowing it would be killer for my career and personal growth, while the other side was scared to move so far away and leave my life, family, and loved ones behind. The point between the two sides, the vagus nerve, was torn.

As we have all heard, the gut is often referred to as your second brain. What this specifically means is that the vagus nerve connects the stem of the brain with the abdomen. It is a cranial (that is, brain) nerve that connects to the nerves for the colon and intestines (that is, Alien Baby nerves), and transports messages to and from your brain to your gut. What does that mean? Your gut has a direct line to your mind, and your mind to your gut.

This connection between the mind and the body is what makes mindset such a powerful ingredient in the Alien Baby debloat cocktail. If you can learn to manage your intangible mind, you can learn to manage your quite tangible Alien Baby. I do not at all mean to ignore your mind or stop it from thinking, as many common yoga philosophies encourage by "letting go," but rather to guide it in a better direction. In doing so, you can prevent and control the unappealing, anatomical babies that result when unpleasant messages are sent down there, and you can feel fantastically free.

The key to this lies in the concept of water. The Tibetan philosophers say *Chula chu chapka*, or in English, "Water poured into water."

If you pour a glass of water into a pool of water, you will not be able to distinguish between the two. The water from the glass will dissolve or get lost in the large pool, as if nothing had happened. On the other hand, if you pour a glass of oil into the water, the oil gets stuck on the top, does not dissolve, and creates pollutions of various kinds. The pool water with the cup of oil is visibly and forever changed.

Thoughts and emotions are poured into your body every second of every day. Some are like water poured into water and go unnoticed. Others enhance your life, making the water sweeter and more soothing. And some act like oil in water, getting stuck in your system and agitating it, tangibly and intangibly. Because of the vagus nerve, these thoughts transport themselves directly into your intestines and digestive system and get stuck there, almost like the coating from an oil spill. The "oil slick" externally manifests itself as abdominal bloating and discomfort, also known as the Alien Baby.

The goal for Alien Baby debloat is to Retox your mind in a way that it can perceive and process the events and emotions around you, just as smoothly as if you were pouring water into water. It is about transforming the gook into a smooth, continuous flow. My clients, such as Desiree and Kendra, have found that not only does this abate the Alien Baby, but also makes them more aware of all the thoughts they are inviting into their system.

Kendra is an entrepreneur and stay-at-home mom in her midthirties. She quit her corporate job after she had her baby and started her own consulting business so she could work at home. But Kendra had completely underestimated the demands of working for oneself, let alone with a little one. She had big goals, for her career and family, no support staff, and a whole lotta stress. She spent most of her days running around like a crazy woman multitasking, but ultimately felt like neither her business or her baby were getting the best of her. The only thing that seemed to be thriving was her Alien Baby.

She initially came to I.AM.YOU. to lose a few pounds, but soon we started focusing on the Alien Baby, and determined that hers was due almost entirely to emotional stress. She used this mindset exercise to eradicate her Alien Baby, and keep it away throughout all her future baby bumps as well.

RETOX

Grab a piece of paper and write down anything and everything that has been unpleasant, or less that pleasant, in the past couple of days. Write down everything that happened, that is stressing you, worrying you, or keeping you anything but super smiley and happy. You can write one word, or you can write a full paragraph. Whatever comes naturally. When you are done put the paper to the side.

Now sit up tall, find a comfortable position, and close your eyes. Bring the attention to the top of your head. See everything you know to be there, the bones, ligaments, tendons, intestines, stomach, blood, muscles. See it all, then slowly start to clear it all out as in LSP (page 26).

Use your mind's eye to clear out all the interior contents until you see yourself empty on the inside, and just a shell of you on the outside. Take as long as you need to do this.

Then bring your attention to the crown of your head, and fill yourself with a clear blue stream of light, like the color of the perfect sea or sky. Fill every corner of your body with that light.

Sit here in your blue light body for ten breaths. If a thought comes up that is stressful, unpleasant, or agitating, envision more clear blue light pouring into your body. See the stress or whatever comes up, then see the light pouring over it and dissolving it completely.

Take as long as you need, and when you are done, continue your day in this fluid blue-lit body.

Retox Soundtrack:
"Confusion" —NEW ORDER

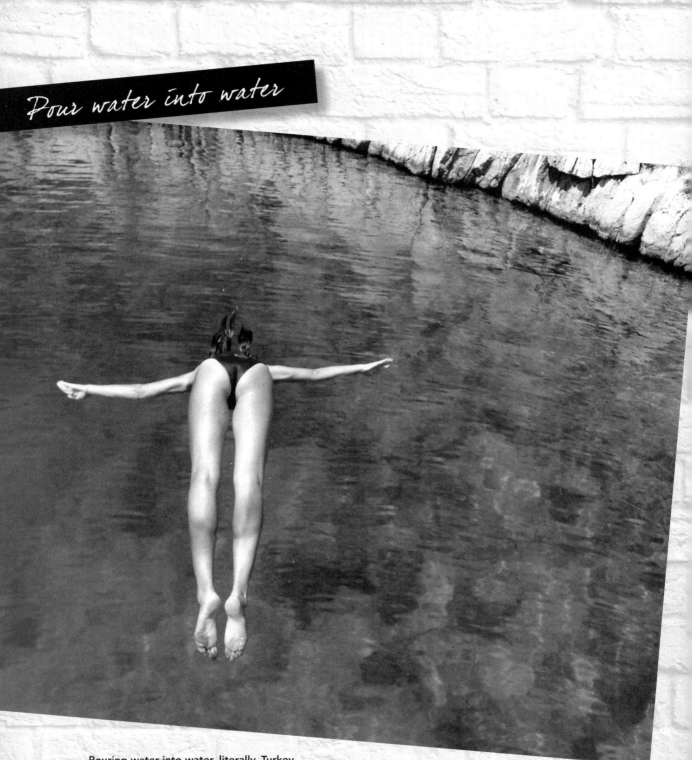

Pouring water into water, literally. Turkey.

RAGE AGAINST THE FEMALE MACHINE

HANDLING PMS AND

THE VICIOUS CYCLE

It's coming from me

THE HORROR SHOW USUALLY GOES something like this . . .

I walk to my closet to get dressed. Despite dozens of items in front of me, I have nothing to wear. Top after top, pant after pant, skirt after skirt, nothing fits or looks right, and it all just feels gross. A small pile starts to grow in the middle of the room, items I have disgustedly torn off myself in search of something, anything. Lack of time ultimately forces me to throw "whatever" on and head out into the world . . . with a beautiful pimple on my chin.

Over the course of the next few hours, I get angry about the line at my coffee place. I snap at my mom on the phone and engage in a pointless, borderline mean text exchange with my man. My back starts to hurt and I am tired, even though I just had my coffee. My waistline feels tight, so I get salad for lunch. Then I am hungry and craving pizza, hamburgers, and candy to the umpteenth degree. I am supremely anxious, worrying about things months into the future, and everyone is annoying me, especially the lady doing my nails who refuses to paint the entire nail. I proceed to engage in an all-out war with the mobile phone carrier on how they repeatedly sneak charges into my bill, screaming like a lunatic but telling myself I am logically debating, at which point I decide that chocolate is the only answer. I head out to the bakery, already feeling the soothing effects that first bite will engender

throughout my system, but when I get there, they are all out of chocolate chip cookies. I start to cry.

When I realize I'm crying over cookies, that's when I understand. It is PMS.

Without running the risk of sounding like a Midol ad, I will just say that being a woman is full of often unpleasant physical issues, ones I generally categorize as Rage Against the Female Machine. Between our monthly period, PMS, possible challenges with fertility, the trials of pregnancy, post-pregnancy, perimenopause, and finally, menopause, we ladies have a whole other dimension to our body and life, one my husband often says should come with an instruction manual and warning label.

This chapter gets to the core of female issues, hormone fluctuations and imbalances, and uses yoga poses, easily accessible foods, and a quick meditation to help us ladies balance it all out. We will focus on PMS and periods, because it is something we all suffer from, and where Retoxing has an incredible track record.

Take Cristina, a thirty-six-year-old I.AM .YOU.er originally from Minnesota. When I met her, she was miserable ten days a month. And when I say miserable, I mean *miserable*. Cristina had been suffering from acute PMS since she was a teenager. PMS would hit her so hard that many times she could not get out of bed. She had intense cramps, nausea, and back pain, none of which were remedied by the various medicines her doctors had prescribed over the years. When the height of PMS would pass and Cristina would be able to drag herself into work, her performance was lackluster and clouded by a "bad attitude," according to bosses. She did not make social or exercise plans during those days, and would just go home and curl up into a ball in the baggiest clothes she could find. This was the regular routine for a third of the month, every month, for twenty-plus years.

Like many, Cristina came to me desperate for help, yet only half believing that I could offer something all the specialists and pills had not. I asked her to trust me, which she did, and we embarked on a full PMS Retox cocktail program, starting with yoga.

YOGA

I get that when you are PMSing or have your period the thought of exercise seems miserable and, in all honesty, usually loses to a manicure with a back massage followed by ice cream on the couch, but yoga is imperative to your female well-being. When done in the I.AM.YOU. Retox methodology, yoga serves as an essential tool to abate PMS and period discomforts. It also works to balance your hormones the rest of the month so that your monthly cycles become less painful, and eventually maybe not even noticed.

RETOX

DESK FIXES

ANTI-RAGE BREATH

Sit up tall and rest your hands where they feel comfortable, maybe even on the abdomen. Inhale, counting to five. Exhale, softly out of the mouth, counting to five. Repeat five to ten cycles.

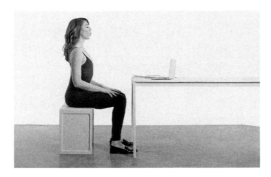

DESK GARLAND

Slide to the edge of your seat. Place your feet on the floor touching each other. Drop your knees out to the sides. Inhale, sit up tall. Exhale, fold in between your legs and let your head hang. Breathe here as long as you can.

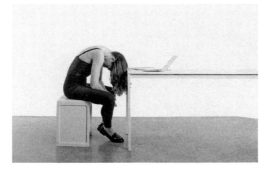

GENTLE TWIST*

Inhale, sit up tall. Exhale, twist to the right. Look over your right shoulder. Hold here five breaths, then repeat on the other side.

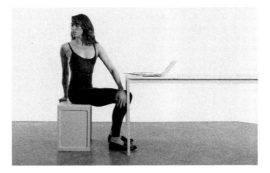

CHAIR FORWARD FOLD

Come to the edge of your chair. Separate your feet hip distance apart. Extend your legs forward and flex your feet so the heels press into the floor. Inhale, sit up tall. Exhale, fold forward, reaching your hands toward your ankles or shins. Let your head hang here and hold for five to fifteen breaths.

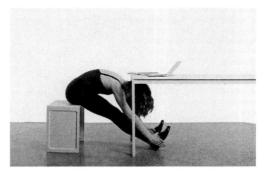

QUICK FIXES

GARLAND

Stand with your feet together. Come to your tip-toes, bend your knees, and open your knees wide. Drop your forearms to the floor between your knees, drop your head, and relax your neck. Hold here, breathing.

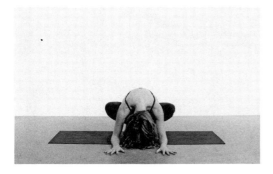

LEGS UP THE WALL

Lie on the floor, bringing your butt to the wall. Lift your legs up the wall, either feet touching or letting them flop out to the sides. Open your arms wide or place one hand on your abdomen and one on your heart, and breathe here as long as comfortable.

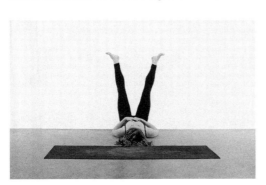

V-SHAPE CHILD'S POSE

Kneel with your shins in a wide V shape, knees apart, feet together. Bring your butt to your heels and your forehead to the floor, letting your chest fall between your legs. Extend your arms alongside your body. Hold here, breathing.

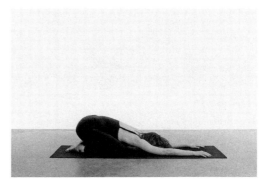

RECLINING DIAMOND

Lie on your back with your knees bent. Bring your heels together and drop your knees to the sides. Place one hand on your abdomen and the other hand on your heart. Optionally, put a heavy blanket on top of your abdomen. Close your eyes and breathe thirty breaths.

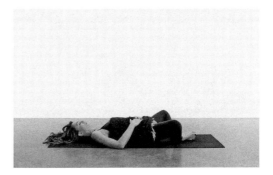

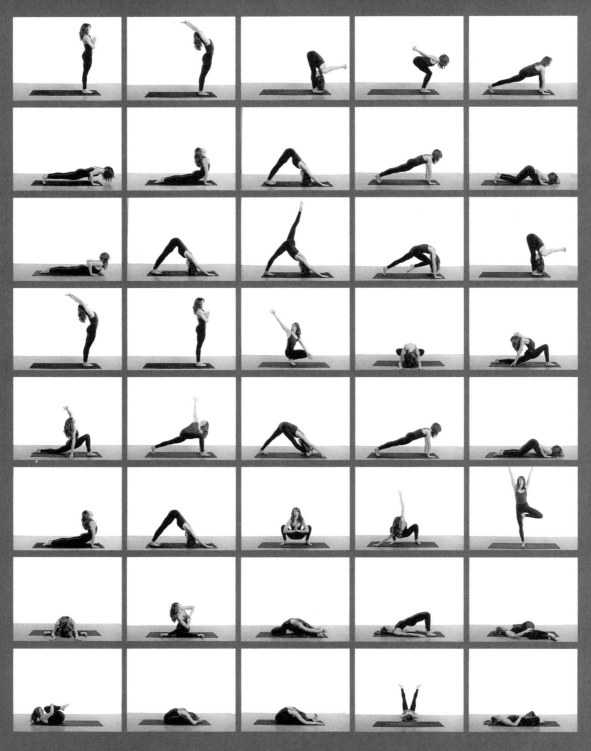

NOURISHMENT

Cartagena, Colombia. January 1, 2004. I had just enjoyed three magical days in this old colonial city on the Caribbean Sea, basking in its vibrant colors, smells, tastes, sounds, and magical realism that has made the town so well known. But my vacation had come to an end, and I was at the airport patiently waiting to board my flight back to the gray urban jungle of New York City. As I started to climb the stairs to the door of the airplane, a flight attendant stopped me. "I am sorry, you cannot board the plane," she said. "Why?" I asked, perplexed and worried. "Because you are pregnant!" she exclaimed with a look of abhorrence on her perfectly made-up face. I am pretty sure the look on my not-made-up face was one of confusion. Nonetheless, she proceeded to ask me to go back to the gate, collect my luggage, and refund my ticket, telling me that per the airline's rules, I could not fly if over six months pregnant. But I was not pregnant, I told her, first calmly, and then more agitated. Let's face it—she was basically calling me fat!

The conversation went on and on, causing me to feel worse about my body every second. Finally my boyfriend convinced them of the truth—I was not pregnant; I was merely a very bloated, mid-period, American.

As we finally boarded, I resolved right then and there to figure out why my PMS symptoms were so severe, and how to manage my bloating and cramps so that this embarrassing scene would never happen again. Back in New York, I started studying my diet and how it affected my PMS, coming up with the Retox plan I shared with Cristina and am about to share with you.

DETOX

Avoid these foods to quell the rage:

DAIRY. Despite many Western studies saying that dairy helps PMS, Traditional Chinese Medicine and more recent functional medicine studies have found that dairy actually intensifies the effects of PMS, making the cycle itself and symptoms more severe. Dairy inflames the body, and during that time of the month, it can lead to worse bloating and cramps. Try cutting out dairy for a month and you will likely notice how much smoother and pain free your period is the next time around.

SUGAR. No matter how much your brain may tell you it wants that candy or brownie, it will just make you more miserable, as more ups and downs are the last thing your already manic body needs. Try reducing both natural and processed sugar leading up to and during your period, trading in the fruit and candy for some nuts or veggies.

SOY. Soy products can cause bloating. Soy milk has also been shown to change hormonal levels. Although you may think that replacing regular dairy with soy will benefit your system, soy products actually add more turmoil to your body's hormonal balance and instigate painful cramping and bloat. Just skip the soy.

CAFFEINE. I love my coffee, believe you me, but while PMSing or during my period, I just swap the regular for decaf. Caffeine can increase levels of anxiety and stress, making us more moody (or even intolerable) than we need to be. When you do have the coffee, have it black or with almond milk.

129

RETOX

BROCCOLI AND CAULIFLOWER. I know this can sound counterintuitive given the bloating factor that many people feel from these two veggies, but broccoli and cauliflower are powerful cleansing agents for extra estrogen floating around your body. When you have your period, estrogen increases and progesterone decreases, creating a hormonal imbalance. Adding broccoli and cauliflower can help even it out. Just make sure it is cooked to make it easier on the digestive system.

FENNEL AND FENNEL SEEDS. Both contain volatile oil and aliphatic acid, shown to eliminate abdominal pains associated with menstrual periods. They also help regulate the motion of the stomach to prevent gas produced in the digestive system. Slice some up and munch on it during the day, or cook with fennel seeds at night.

CARBS. They are not the enemy! Complex carbs have been shown to soothe PMS systems, especially those related to mood swings. Go for natural grains like rice, potato, and oats.

SAFFLOWER AND SAFFRON. These vibrantly colored spices are used in Eastern medicine to strengthen the blood and circulation. They have been shown to ease pain caused by blood stagnation such as menstrual pain, and help you stay strong as you bleed. Try adding a drop of their oils to a glass of water or cooking with them.

BEEF. It should be what's for dinner. When you have your period, you lose blood and, with it, iron. Have organic red meat a few times through your cycle and you will feel stronger and more stable.

CHAMOMILE TEA. Chamomile soothes your body, muscles, and mind. Sip a cup and you will feel calmer almost instantly, not to mention you'll have less bloating, cramping, and back pain.

SNACKS

Cooked broccoli and cauliflower florets
Corn tortilla chips and mild salsa
Oatmeal
Fennel and Green Bean Salad (see recipe on page 132)

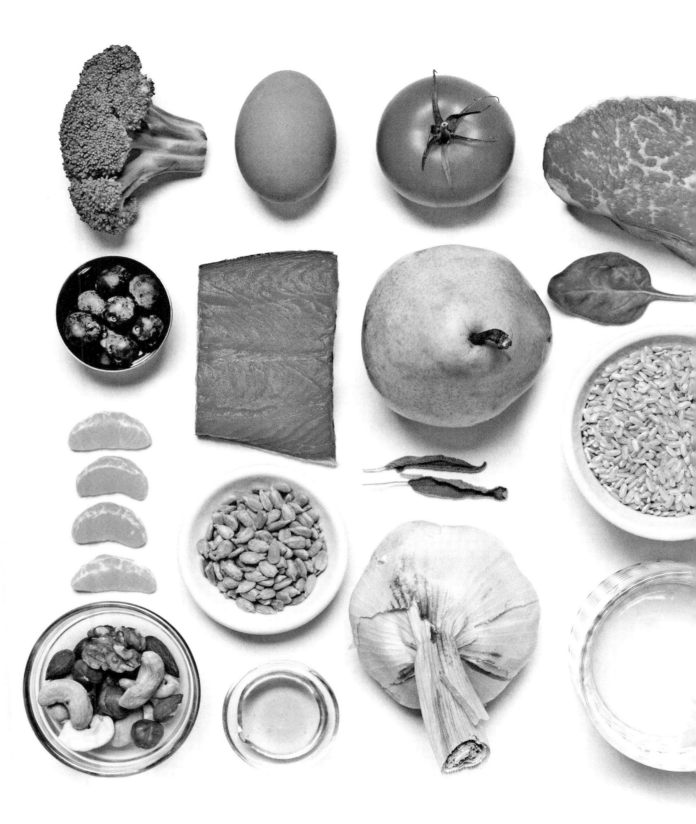

Anti-Rage Paella

1 tablespoon extra virgin olive oil

1 clove garlic, minced

1 onion, diced

4 tomatoes, chopped

1 cup chopped kale or spinach

1 zucchini, chopped

1 cup peas, fresh or frozen

1 pinch salt

2 pinches saffron

3 cups cooked rice or quinoa

Heat oil in a large pot. Add garlic and onion and cook until onion is translucent. Add tomatoes and stir. Cook covered for 15 minutes. Add kale and zucchini. Stir and cover with lid. When zucchini is tender, about 5 minutes, add peas, salt, and saffron. Stir. Add rice or quinoa. Stir and cover with lid. When quinoa has absorbed the color of the rest of the veggies, it is ready to serve!

Fennel and Green Bean Salad

1 pound green beans, trimmed

1 bulb fennel

3 tablespoons extra virgin olive oil

1 tablespoon balsamic vinegar

½ teaspoon oregano

Salt and pepper, to taste

Steam green beans in a pot or steamer or sauté them in a pan. While they are cooking, slice fennel and place in a salad bowl. Add green beans, oil, vinegar, oregano, salt, and pepper, and toss.

Broccoli Soup

1 tablespoon extra virgin olive oil

4 cloves garlic, minced

2 heads broccoli or 2 (16-ounce) bags frozen broccoli, chopped

2 cups vegetable broth (or chicken broth or water)

Salt and pepper, to taste

Heat oil in a large pot over medium heat. Add garlic and cook until it turns golden. Add broccoli, broth, and salt and pepper, to taste. Bring to a boil, then reduce heat and cover, letting simmer for 20 minutes, or until broccoli is soft. Remove pot from heat and use an immersion blender to puree. You could also puree the soup in a blender in batches.

Beef, "It's What's for Dinner"

We all know what the period implies. Iron out means we need to put iron in. Go buy your favorite cut of beef, ideally grass-fed organic. If it is a steak, literally just put it in the pan or on the grill and cook to your liking. For me, that means well done and 20-ish minutes if a steak. (I know, but not even the French have been able to sway me.) For you, it may mean rare and just a couple of minutes a side. Or, if you want something softer, buy some ground beef and make into patties. Place in the pan, cook to your liking, and serve with a side of veggies.

133

MINDSET

If you are reading this chapter, chances are you are highly irritable, moody, and anxious as is, so I am just going to give it to you straight, quick, and dirty. And men, if you are reading this for your ladies, please hand the book over to them and let me deliver the message, not you . . . (you've been warned).

It's not them. It's you.

I am serious.

It's coming from you, not at you.

The heinous woman who stole your place in line. Your evil boss who asked you to do a new project. Your bitchy friend who pushed back dinner. The annoying fitness instructor who would not stop prattling in her high-pitched voice during class. Your mother who keeps calling to say hi. The call center agent who will not pick up no matter how many times you press 0. Your evil man who purposely leaves stuff all over the home. All of this is coming from you, and only you.

Chances are, these people have no idea that they are driving you crazy, because it is the farthest thing from their intention. So your desire to impale them, or wail upon them, is straight-up coming from your mind. It is your problem, not theirs. Granted, the problem is propagated by an intense mishmash of strong hormones that you are just starting to manage with Retox yoga and nourishment . . . but even when you master the physical movements and diet, your mind and moods will remain.

The fact that it is coming from you, not at you, is one of the most powerful tenets of the Tibetan yoga philosophy I.AM.YOU. is based on. It implies that you, yourself, create every experience of every moment of every day. That's pretty intense, and cool.

Let's take the boss. She gives you a new project. You can be furious that she is so rudely adding more to your already intense workload, get upset, mutter to yourself for hours, complain to your friends via text to the point of a thumb ache, then hash it out even further over a glass of Malbec. Or you can see the same boss, and the same new project she gives you, and be excited that she is entrusting you with it, proud of yourself for being a go-to within the company, and psyched to get to use your energy and capacity to its fullest, and maybe even learn something while you are at it. Same boss, same new project—two totally different perceptions and reactions, and from there life experiences.

Believe me, I know it can be really tough to swallow this on already PMS-filled days, but it is the key to managing mood swings during the female cycle. It is, to be blunt, the key to keeping your job, friends, and loved ones.

You not only have the power to control your experiences, but you *are* that power. Simply because none of it is coming at you, and all of it is coming from you. That's the magical reality of it all.

To help you cultivate that power, I have created a quick and easy meditation that you can do wherever you are, no matter who is driving you nuts and how irrationally (or rationally) upset you feel.

RETOX

This Retox mindset plan is a straight shooter.

Every time someone says or does something that bothers you, respond with sweet, positive kindness.

If the woman across the street shoots you a bitchy look, smile back. If the repair man is unsuccessful and you have to buy a new refrigerator, genuinely thank him for his effort. If the deli guy messes up your lunch order, say that it's okay, you know he is overwhelmed, and you are lucky to have a proper meal. If your kid is nagging you, tell her how much you love her. If your partner is being aloof, thank him for being present in your life.

For each and every negative thing coming your way, send out a happy, compassionate one. You may not want to initially, but within a few hours you will notice a massive shift in your outlook, mood, and life.

Retox Soundtrack:
"Take the Power Back" —RAGE AGAINST THE MACHINE

RAGE AGAINST THE FEMALE MACHINE

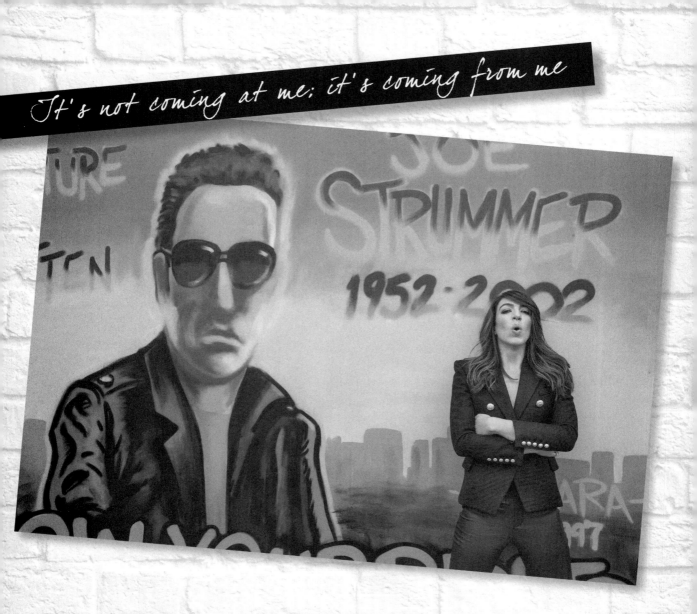

Rocking through the rage. New York City. Photograph by Mick Rock.

S&M...
AND THE GIANT F

STABILITY, MOBILITY,

AND FLEXIBILITY

I trust me

DON'T WORRY. THIS CHAPTER IS RATED PG.

S&M in Retox terms stands for *stability* and *mobility*. At the crux of it lies flexibility, something I never used to care about, in large part because I am not naturally flexible, and I prefer to focus on strength and endurance. In fact, I used to arrogantly look down upon those flexible people, aka show-offs, like they were weirdos, all while secretly jealous of how graceful and pain free they appeared. This nonflexible superiority complex of mine really reached a pinnacle in that first yoga class I told you about earlier. I mean, really, who has time to spend stretching when you could be burning calories? I used to think flexibility was overrated.

Yet, as I started longer hours on Wall Street and clocking more miles after work to sweat out the stress and alcohol, everything slowly but surely started to hurt. My lower back and knees wailed at me every day. My hips, especially the left, were an overall disaster that no amount of cortisone shots, foam rolling, or rest could appease. My shoulders twinged every time I moved my arms, so I pathetically tried to soothe them with massages at the nail salon (it was time efficient, after all), and I was often unable to turn my neck to one side or the other at least a couple times a month. And the biggest crisis of all was that leaning over to put on my stilettos or tie my kicks was, well, less than elegant. It was pathetic. And I was twenty-two.

The thing is, flexibility matters. It leads to mobility. Flexibility and mobility combined stabilize the body and from there the mind. Flex-

ibility is most definitely not solely for dancers, yogis, and little kids; it is for all human beings, of all ages, and imperative for good health.

The catch is, as we age and become more sedentary, our bodies tighten and our tissues lose moisture content, making us less supple, more stiff, and more prone to injury. Just imagine what happens to a grape in the sun: It starts round, soft, and juicy, but over time it shrinks, loses its moisture, and dries into the firm shape and size of a raisin. That's what's happening to your body, especially if you do not pay heed to its need to be flexible and mobile.

Before you start scoffing at me, I want you to give yourself a test run. Reach down and touch your toes. Go ahead, just do it. And now stand tall, balancing on your tippy toes, and lift your right foot off the ground and count to ten. How did it go? I am guessing the first was mildly painful, and the second was not perfectly graceful. Don't worry, you are in the same camp I was in, along with the majority of people over twenty these days.

As much as you may think S&M isn't for you, and that as a result you really do not care about flexibility . . . it is, and you do. Or at the very least, your physical, tangible machine of a body does. It is vital for injury prevention, sleep, and general getting around.

In this chapter, I have crafted a three-part plan to get you strong and flexible, so that you can be stable and mobile. I have based the yoga on physics and straight-up anatomy, nourishment on the biochemical properties of foods to make you more agile, and mindset on how to find your comfort zone. Let's get down and dirty.

YOGA

Yoga is as much a science as it is a philosophy. As with all science, data is necessary, so it's time to get geeky. The root of flexibility lies in the body's connective tissues, or the tissues that bind us together into a whole. Ligaments, tendons, and fascia are the most important of these. Almost all well-taught yoga nourishes these tissues, bringing them new blood and oxygen to aid in cellular regeneration, lubrication, and other healing agents.

However, you need to be cognizant of the difference between tendons, ligaments, and fascia, and take care to treat each in the appropriate way. Tendons connect muscle to bones. They are relatively stiff and should not be stretched. Ligaments connect bone to bone inside the joint capsules (think rotator cuff). They

are a bit more supple, but should only be stretched a minor amount. Their role is to limit flexibility and keep you safe. Fascia bundles up muscle fibers into distinct working units. Imagine stuffing balls of socks into panty hose. The socks are the muscles, the nylon panty hose is the fascia. Fascia makes up about a third of the body's total mass and is responsible for about 40 percent of what we call *flexibility*. It is the only connective tissue that you can safely stretch.

Injuries and frustrations in yoga and flexibility most commonly occur for three reasons:

- **Poor Instruction.** Poses and anatomy are incorrectly taught, and poses are incorrectly focused upon the tendons and ligaments, which should rarely be stretched.
- **Ignoring the Fascia.** The fascia is completely overlooked in the importance of flexibility, stability, and mobility, leading to a lack of progress despite a student's repeated efforts.
- **Disregard for Physics.** Of the many things that enthralls me about physics is the Newtonian concept that for every force there is an equal and opposite opposing force. For every up there is a down, every in, an out. For every action, a reaction. Turns out Newton was actually a yogi, because this is actually a fundamental cornerstone to both the tangible and intangible practices of yoga.

In every yoga pose (that is properly aligned), there is a muscle that is strengthening, and one that is lengthening. There is a grounding action and a lifting action. There is a forward reach and a backward pull. In every yoga pose assist (that is performed safely), there is a grounding action and a lengthening action. A stabilizing force and a mobilizing one. You can see these most obviously in the front thigh of Warrior 2, where the quad strengthens and the hamstring lengthens; in a handstand, where your hands press down but your torso lifts up out of the shoulders; in a seated forward fold assist, where you ground the pelvis and lengthen the spine. In anatomy, they refer to this as reciprocal inhibition, or when one set of muscles contracts, the automatic nervous system causes the opposing muscles to release. If you do not contract one, the other will not stretch. Or if it does, it may stretch in the wrong way causing an injury there or somewhere else. It is as simple as that.

Given our newfound love of physics and opposing forces, I am going to share with you two opposing Retox S&M wonder stories. The first involves Mark, a thirty-three-year-old digital geek, also more professionally referred to as Internet coding genius. He came to me only because his boss and close friend forced him to, after he complained about chronic, crippling back and wrist pain and headaches They were worried he was really sick and had sent him to a doctor who just wanted to prescribe painkillers and a trendy yoga class that offered no help. Then they found me. I instantly noticed that Mark's problems were firmly rooted in a desperate need for S&M . . . and some good ol' F.

Before finding his true coding calling, Mark had been a very high-level collegiate athlete in Michigan. His body was used to intense training and accomplishing superhuman feats on football fields on a regular basis. Now he coded, CrossFitted, lifted, coded some more, and ran.

His body was hating him. Mark was so stiff that he could not even bend forward, and his circulation was stagnated as a result. He had a myriad of random injuries, ones that a thirty-three-year-old should not have, and felt he was underperforming on his runs, CrossFit challenges, and in the gym. He thought he needed a good stretch, which he did, but the Retox way.

After the first hour of working together, Mark was already a transformed person. He could bend over, could almost touch the middle of his quads, and said he felt "light and free." We continued to work together using the longer sequences you will find in this chapter, and I had him do the Desk Fixes once a day. He now can touch his toes, do a split, and is running and lifting at his college times and weights. All with Retox yoga.

Charlotte, on the other hand, was a gymnast her entire life. Once she graduated college in Ohio, she turned that passion into a professional dancing career in Miami. She was the opposite of Mark in that she could put her leg behind her head without blinking, but similar to him, was suffering from a litany of injuries that her thirty-five-year-old body should not have had. She also needed some S&M Retox relief, but one that would focus her innate flexibility more on the S than the M, or on the stability more than the mobility.

Because Retox yoga is firmly based in anatomy, I was able to use the exact same poses for Charlotte that I used for Mark; we just slightly shifted the focus and purpose behind each pose. Within a few weeks, Charlotte was as bendy as always, but infinitely stronger and pain free.

So whether you are more like Mark, Charlotte, or me . . . it is time to get down and dirty.

RETOX

DESK FIXES

SIDE STRETCH

Lift your arms straight up. Cross your left wrist behind your right wrist. Inhale, grow long and pull up. Exhale, lean to the left. Make sure both sitz bones are on the chair so the stretch is coming from the right place. Hold here, then repeat on the other side.

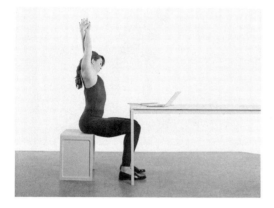

WIDE CHAIR SQUAT

Place your feet wider than your chair, toes forward or out to the side. Open your legs wide and place your elbows on your inner thighs. Inhale, lengthen your spine. Exhale, press your arms straight and back into your legs. Stay here and breathe as long as feels comfortable.

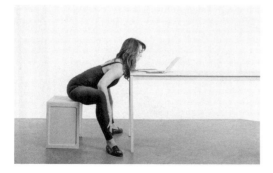

SHOULDER AND CHEST STRETCH

Sitting or standing, clasp your hands behind your back. Try to bring your palms to touch. Inhale fully, grow your spine tall, and straighten your elbows. Exhale, reach your hands back and down, whichever direction feels best. Hold five to ten breaths, then repeat as needed.

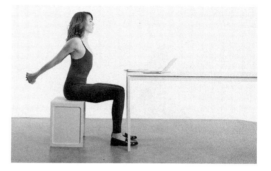

HALF ANKLE TO KNEE

Place your left ankle on your right lower quad, just above the knee. Flex your left foot. Press your left hand down on the inner left thigh or knee. Optionally, fold forward. Hold there, then repeat on the other side.

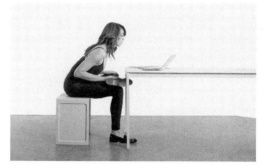

QUICK FIXES

BENT-KNEE DOWN DOG SPLIT

Start in Down Dog. Inhale, lift your left leg in the air. Exhale, bend your left knee and open the pelvis. Bring your left heel toward your butt and look under your left armpit. Reach your right heel to the floor. Hold here five to ten breaths, then repeat on the other side.

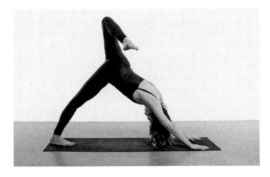

PYRAMID

Start standing with your hands clasped behind your back. Step your left leg about two to three feet behind you. Place the heel down with your toes pointed at a 45-degree angle. Straighten your right leg in front of you. Inhale, lengthen your spine. Exhale, fold forward over the front leg. Engage the quads and pull the right hip backward. Hold here five to ten breaths, then repeat on the other side.

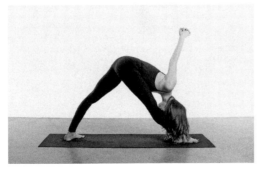

EXTENDED HALF MOON

Stand with your feet hip distance apart, then shift your weight to your right leg. Take your left leg behind you in the air. Place your right hand on the floor under your right shoulder. Inhale, lift your left arm up and open the pelvis to the side. Exhale, reach your left arm alongside your ear. Point your right toes. Hold here five to ten breaths, then repeat on the other side.

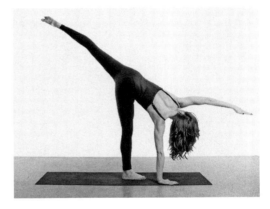

REACHING HALF DIAMOND

Start sitting on the floor. Bring your right knee into your chest. Place the heel of the foot as close to the groin as possible and drop the knee out to the side. Frame your chest over your left leg. Inhale, sit up tall. Exhale, fold forward over your left leg, trying to reach your right rib cage to the knee cap. Inhale, lift your right arm up. Exhale, reach the foot with both hands. Stay here five to fifteen breaths, then repeat on the other side.

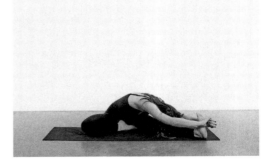

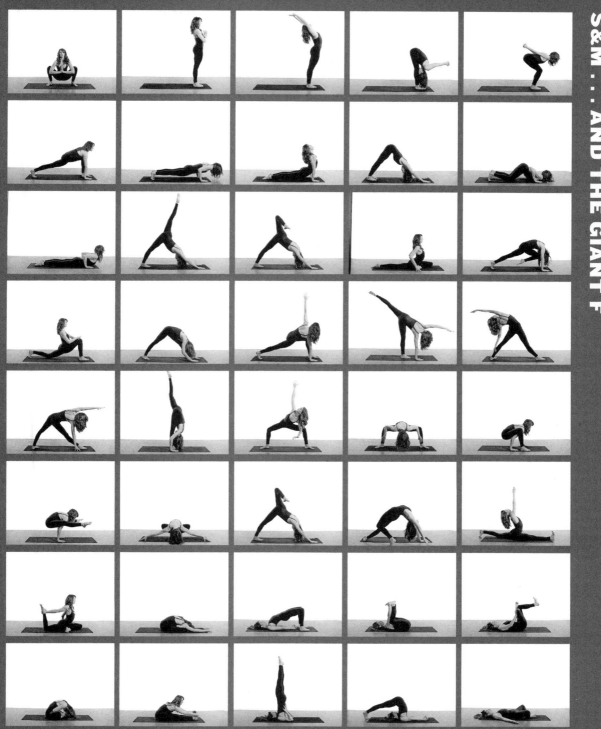

NOURISHMENT

Flexibility is something you can feed, stability something you can nourish. In fact, there are many foods that directly hinder your mobility, making you more rigid with every bite, and others that enhance your flexibility and inner stability, from the fascia to the muscles, energy to the mind. It is easy to think that because you do not have time or that you are trapped in an office that working on S&M is impossible, but with these nourishment Retox tips, you can eat yourself into a more open, mobile, supple, and sexy body, one bite at a time.

DETOX

pH BALANCE MATTERS

Very simply, a neutral to high body pH leads to increased stability, mobility, and flexibility. A lower pH level means there is higher acidity in the body. Higher acidity leads to increased inflammation. Increased inflammation leads to a more rigid, less flexible, and less mobile body.

> pH down = acidity up = inflammation
> up = rigidity up
> pH up = alkalinity up = inflammation
> down = rigidity down
> healthy S&M = higher pH

The most obvious example of this is someone with arthritis, like Gloria. Gloria is an overall healthy, strong individual, and an ex-dancer, yet she has been suffering from arthritis for some time, which puts a spotlight on the effects of acidity on S&M in the body. Every time she eats highly acidic foods, her hands and knuckles become stiff, she can barely bend over let alone get up out of bed, her body hurts, and she is somewhat immobilized. The acid increases inflammation in the joints already suffering from arthritis, often within the hour. When Gloria keeps a high-alkaline diet, she is able to run, jump, and dance just like she did when she was a kid. We worked together to limit acidic food in her daily diet and added the alkaline foods discussed below so that she could eat her way to flexibility.

Avoid these highly acidic foods: raw tomatoes, cranberries, cheese, milk, shellfish, soy beans, soy products, soy milk, peanuts, corn, pineapple, and black coffee.

RETOX

Add these alkaline foods to your diet: garlic, dark leafy greens, seaweed, broccoli, avocado, apple, peach, cucumber, beets, lettuce, peas, cantaloupe, lemon, blueberries, almonds, eggs, seeds, honey, and spirulina.

ELECTROLYTES RULE

As much as I love lemon-lime Gatorade, there are much better, and more natural, sources of electrolytes, which are necessary for our muscles and tissues to activate, contract, relax, and move. The primary ions of electrolytes—sodium, potassium, calcium, magnesium, hydrogen phosphate, and hydrogen carbonate—ionize in water and other solvents, and are responsible for muscle and nerve function, as well as hydration and pH blood balance. If you do not have sufficient electrolytes, your muscles will be weak, immobile, or even severely contracted, which we conventionally call a cramp.

Potassium is one of the most important electrolytes as it helps regulate fluids in the body. Try adding bananas, avocado, oranges, sweet potato, watermelon, carrots, avocado, ground organic beef, and lentils to your diet. Other electrolyte-rich foods include spinach, artichokes, and cooked green veggies.

SULFUR AND MICRONUTRIENTS, THE OTHER S&M LAYER

These tiny little particles influence the creation and health of your connective tissues, respectively:

SULFUR. Sulfur is needed to make glucosamine sulfate and chondroitin sulfate, both of which facilitate the formation of connective tissues in your body, especially the fascia. Add these sulfur-rich foods to your daily diet: broccoli, Brussels sprouts, cabbage, cauliflower, garlic, leeks, parsley, chives, onion, and radishes.

MANGANESE, COPPER, AND ZINC. These three micronutrients are imperative for fascial health. Add these micronutrient-rich foods to your diet to feed your fascia, the most important aspect of flexibility: cacao, sesame seeds, oysters, nuts, pumpkin seeds, beef, bran, and flax.

In addition to including the above in your diet, here are two other tips to Retox your way to flexibility:

COOKED FOODS. Warm, cooked foods help your body process and retain electrolytes and micronutrients better than raw foods. Instead of going all raw, try sautéing or steaming your veggies. Instead of grabbing a juice on the run, go for the soup. Try to have at least one warm, cooked meal a day, ideally one using foods from these pH or micronutrient lists.

WATER. This should be pretty obvious, although easily forgotten about when we are busy and stressed. Moisture implies supple mobility, and your body needs water to stay moist. Just imagine a fresh, wet stick or leaf versus a dry one—one moves as you touch it, the other splinters and breaks. Shoot for three liters of water a day, four if you are highly active.

SNACKS

Figs
Raisins
Watermelon slices
Chilled cooked asparagus
Almonds
Orange wedges
Radishes

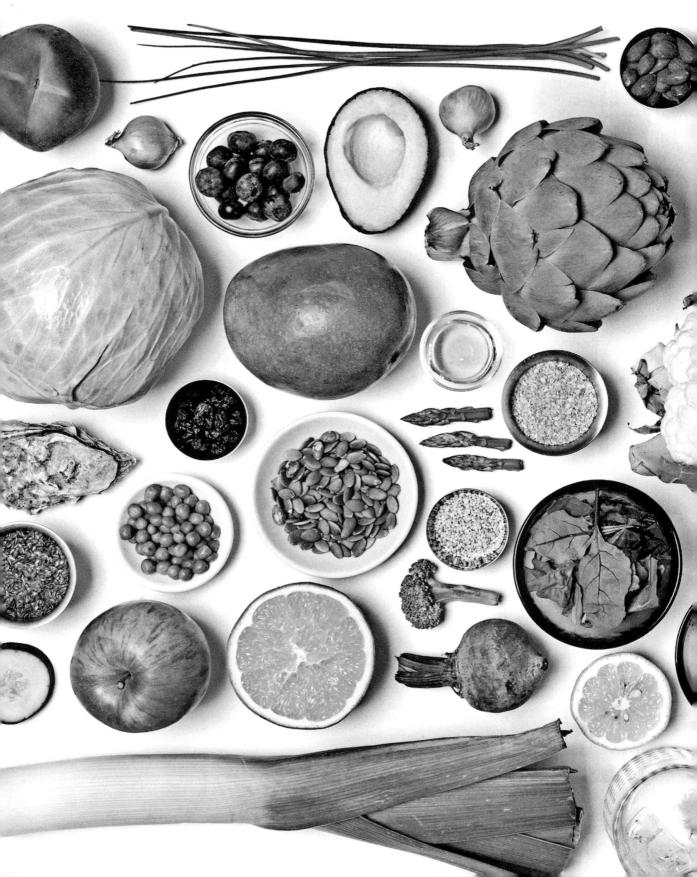

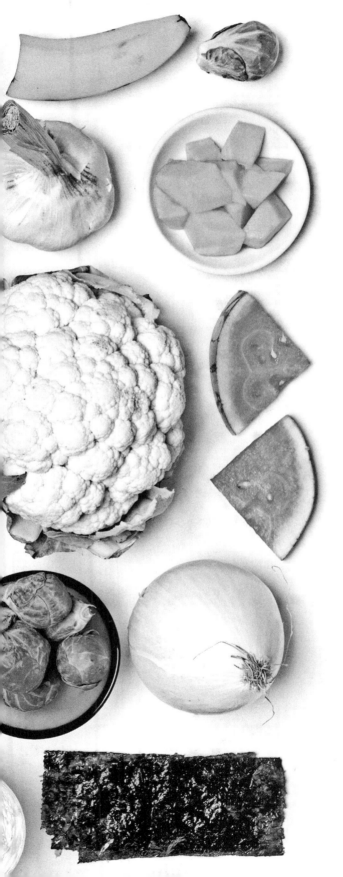

S&M Breakfast Bowl

- 1 banana, sliced
- 1 cup cherries, pitted and sliced
- ½ apple, sliced
- 1 orange, peeled and separated
- 1 teaspoon honey
- Juice of ½ lemon
- 1 tablespoon ground flaxseed and/or 2 tablespoons slivered almonds

In a bowl, mix together all the fruit. Drizzle with honey and lemon juice and stir. Sprinkle with flaxseed and/or almond slivers, stir, and enjoy.

S&M Juice

- 2 cups spinach
- 1 stalk celery
- 1 orange, peeled
- 1 cup papaya
- ½ lemon, peel and pith removed

Place all ingredients in a juicer or high-speed blender and enjoy!

S&M Lentil Salad

1 cup dry lentils

1 tablespoon olive oil

½ yellow onion

1 head broccoli, chopped

1 head cauliflower, chopped

2 zucchini, chopped

½ tablespoon chili powder (optional)

½ cup toasted sesame seeds

Chopped chives, for garnish

Place lentils in a pot and fill with water. Bring to a boil and cook until lentils are cooked, 20 to 30 minutes. (You could also buy them premade.) While lentils cook, heat oil in a skillet over medium heat. Add onion and cook until translucent. Add broccoli and cauliflower and cover. Let cook for 5 minutes and then stir in zucchini. Replace cover and cook until all veggies are soft, about 10 minutes. When lentils are cooked, drain and add to skillet. Stir in chili powder, if desired, and cook until everything is heated through. Right before serving, sprinkle in sesame seeds. Stir and top with chives.

FlexiBurger

This burger combats inflammation and boosts alkalinity, autoimmune function, and overall health.

1 tablespoon extra virgin olive oil

2 cloves garlic, minced

2 cups kale, trimmed and washed

2 cups baby spinach

2 cups chopped broccoli, steamed

½ cup raw cashews

½ cup raw walnuts

In a large pan, heat oil and garlic over medium heat until garlic just starts to turn golden. Add kale, spinach, and broccoli. Cover and cook until veggies are soft, about 10 minutes. Add to a food processor with nuts. You can just do one type of nut, if you prefer. Blend until slightly soft and mushy. Make burger patties with your hands and place them again in the skillet, adding a drizzle of oil if needed. Cook until crisp on each side. Serve on your favorite bread with your favorite toppings (such as sliced red onion, tomato, and avocado) and enjoy!

Sesame Thai Stir-Fry

1 tablespoon extra virgin olive oil

1 white onion, chopped

2 Thai chilies, sliced (optional)

3 tomatoes, chopped

1 zucchini, chopped

1 cup asparagus tips

1 cup chopped broccoli

1 cup snap peas

2 cups chopped spinach or kale

2 cups cooked quinoa or brown rice

¼ cup toasted sesame seeds

Fried eggs for serving (optional)

½ avocado for serving (optional)

Heat oil in a large pan. Add onion and chilies, if using, and cook until onions turn translucent. Stir in tomatoes, zucchini, asparagus tips, broccoli, and snap peas. Stir and cover with a lid. Cook until all veggies are soft, about 15 minutes. Stir in spinach or kale and cook until completely wilted, 3 to 5 minutes. When the greens are soft, add in the quinoa or rice. Stir in sesame seeds. Serve with a fried egg on top or with avocado slices.

MINDSET

Let's take a step back to the old yoga texts before we get all hot and bothered. The connection between stability and mobility stretches back to the first-ever book written on yoga, the *Yoga Sutras of Patanjali*. There in the second chapter he writes, *Sthira Sukham Asanam*.

Sthira means "stability" in Sanskrit; it also translates into "trustworthy." *Sukham* means "mobility" in Sanskrit; it also translates into "flowing and ease filled." You cannot have stability in your mind or body without having mobility. And you cannot have mobility without having stability. Patanjali is telling us that with stability and mobility together you can succeed; with strength and ease you will find success and harmony. The crux of the message? Flexibility and trust.

Without creating a stable foundation you believe in, you cannot move forward and evolve. And without allowing yourself to evolve and ride the waves of life, you will not be able to become grounded and stable. Trust is the lubricant that makes strength and motion possible.

Trust is a belief that it will all work out. It is a sign that you know you can bend without breaking. It allows you to be susceptible to adapt, able to yield. Flexibility is trust itself, a trust that it all evens out, and you will be okay.

The question becomes, how do you foster it? First, you listen. Listen to your body, listen to your mind, listen to the inner you. Then you allow it to grow with ease, knowing that wherever life takes you, you have S&M to fall back on. In a word, you become flexible in mind, allowing you to trust yourself, thus becoming flexible, and through that both stable and mobile in life.

Once you implement this pattern, S&M will become second nature, and you will be radiating from the inside out.

RETOX

This one is so simple and pure.

Take a comfortable seat, on a chair, the bus, or in the car. If you are at home or in a quiet place, close your eyes. If you are driving, please keep them open.

Inhale, saying to yourself, *Here I am.*
Exhale, saying to yourself, *I trust you.*

Inhale, *Here I am.*
Exhale, *I trust you.*

Repeat this for as long as you can, and at least once a day. It will stretch your mind, body, and life to new incredible levels.

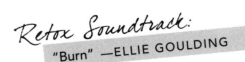

Retox Soundtrack:
"Burn" —ELLIE GOULDING

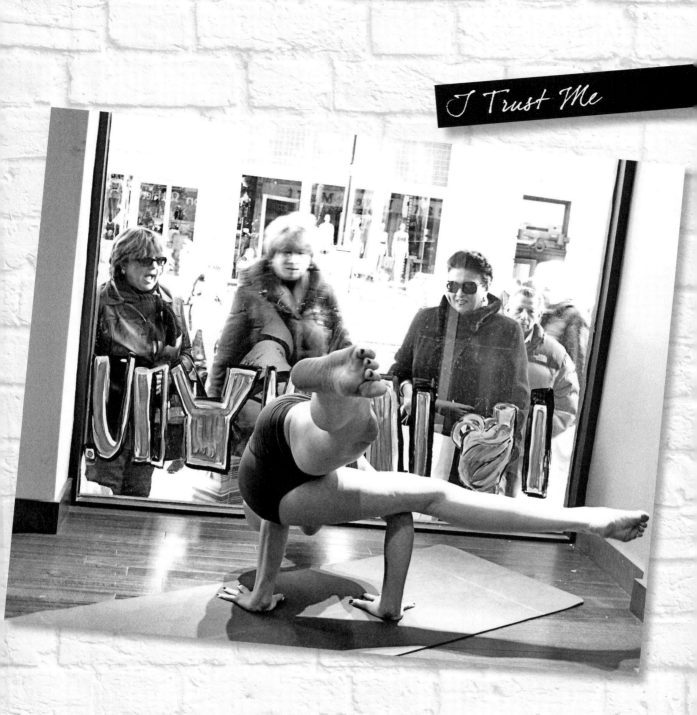

Entertaining the streets. New York City.

DREAMING OF SLEEP

NATURAL SLEEPING AIDS

Make the space for it to come

KENTUCKY, THE BLUEGRASS STATE, HOME of the Kentucky Derby, champion race-horses, and rich tobacco. Bordered on the north by the Ohio River and the west by the Mississippi, Kentucky became a state in 1792 and shares borders with seven other states. Kentucky fought for the Union during the Civil War, but thousands of its citizens joined the Confederate forces. In fact, both Abraham Lincoln and Jefferson Davis, opposing presidents during the war, were born in Kentucky, less than a hundred miles apart from each other. Fascinating, right?

My somewhat random obsession with Kentucky started when I first experienced trouble sleeping. Stressed and unable to relax into a smooth slumber, I would toss and turn, wide eyed, annoyed, and ultimately utterly upset about still being awake. I tried counting sheep, cows, pigs, and birds; I paced the halls, watched boring television, and stared at the ceiling. Then I found Kentucky, nestled in the middle of the 1990 World Book Encyclopedia, volume 11, J–K. That's a paper edition, if you are wondering. For whatever reason, reading about Kentucky was the only thing that soothed me to sleep.

Drifting easily into a soft slumber at the end of a day and waking up to the sound of chirping birds is a luxury that often only a holiday or innocent youth can provide. As we age, the difference between night and day is less, with workdays continuing long after the sun sets and mornings with kids, bosses, workouts, and chores often starting before the sun rises. Technology further obfuscates the haze making it more challenging for our bodies to fall into each of its naturally intended states. Most of the time, we try to squeeze in a few hours of sleep, during which we fidget and wake up multiple time. We may even succumb to using sleeping aids to get us some shut-eye. Between fifty and seventy million Americans suffer from sleep deprivation. Over 43 percent of Americans between the ages of thirteen and sixty-four say they rarely get a good night's sleep on weeknights. More than 60 percent say they experience a sleep problem every night, and over 63 percent say their sleep needs are not met. Over 15 percent say they sleep less than six hours a night, but my experience leads me to think that number is much higher.

The thing is, insomnia is not an illness. It is a condition all too often caused by modern

154

life. Part of the challenge of getting proper shut-eye is identifying what stands in its way. The problem is, usually those with trouble sleeping are too tired to figure out the root cause, choosing instead to suffer through it or go the pill-popping route. Sleeping pills are a gold mine for the pharmaceutical industry—in 2011, sales of generic Ambien were over $2.8 billion and Lunesta $912 million. That is almost $4 *billion* of prescribed, non-authentic sleep.

The problem with popping sleeping pills is that they mask the reason your body is keeping you up. Sleep is natural; your body wants it and knows to do it. The challenge is quelling the unnatural hindrances to it so that the natural sleep can arise. Sometimes the problem relates to poor food choices, other times it's a decrease in melatonin or adrenal fatigue. You could be awake due to jet lag, bad bedtime habits—such as electronics, social media, and pets in bed—or the dreaded and infamous Mental STDs. It could also be an imbalance in your internal energetic systems, which we will discuss later, or the all-too-common modern-life late-to-bed, early-to-rise pattern. I could actually bore you to sleep with how many things could be causing your lack of ideal slumber, but I would rather just help you, like I helped Valerie and countless others.

When I met Valerie, she was thirty-three and hiding behind layers of concealer caking the bags under her beautiful but exhausted blue eyes. She averaged about three and a half hours of sleep a night, usually interrupted, routinely took Ambien, and said the word "tired" close to every other sentence. I am fairly certain she called me up secretly hoping that I would turn our session into an hour-long *shav-*

asana, aka naptime. Despite her busy schedule, we began working together, on two conditions: (1) no sleeping pills and (2) only Retox cocktails. The night after our first session, Valerie fell asleep in less than half an hour after going to bed. A week later, she slept six hours for the first time in two years. And now, a year later, she sleeps six hours a night during the week, seven to eight on weekends, and only wakes up once in a while. She has not taken one sleeping pill since we started and has traded in the dark circles for a radiant glow.

If you are reading this, I am guessing that, like Valerie, you are either having trouble falling asleep, staying asleep, or getting any sleep at all. That's okay—this chapter serves as a 100 percent natural sleeping pill of yoga, which prepares your body to sleep and allows you to rest undisrupted, recipes and nutritional tips to help your system wind down, and a breathing meditative practice to help clear your mind and body for the peaceful shut-eye it needs. Shall we get the Z's on the way?

YOGA

Retox yoga for catching some Z's is all about your internal sleeping mechanism. It focuses your hormones and internal energy, much like Traditional Chinese Medicine. When you are up at night, there is an imbalance in your system, one that Traditional Chinese Medicine addresses with needles, and Retox addresses with postures and breath.

Traditional Chinese Medicine has what they call the organ clock, a system that helps pinpoint where there may be challenges. In the organ clock theory, certain hours of the day correspond to specific organs of the body. There are fourteen major flows of energy (qi), or as yoga would call them, energy channels, each linked to a two-hour period. Each relates to an organ, its functionality, thoughts, and emotions. If you are waking up every night at the same time, or having difficulty going to sleep before a certain time, it likely has to do with an imbalance linked to the corresponding channel. For example, if you are waking up between 1 and 3 a.m., the liver hours, you may be upset, angry, harboring stress, or need to give your chocolate, cheese, avocado, meat, wine-loving liver a break.

The Retox yoga I prescribe here is meant to re-create your natural equilibrium, helping the energy flow freely so that your body can both easily drift into sleep and sleep through the night. Try the Desk Fixes as tune-ups during the day, and the Quick Fixes or the full sequence in the evening, either right before a light dinner or a couple hours before bed, so that your body is most balanced as you head off to a sweet sleep.

RETOX

DESK FIXES

DESK UTTANASANA

Stand in front of your desk. Separate your feet hip-distance apart. Fold forward and reach your hands toward your ankles or shins. Hold here five to ten breaths.

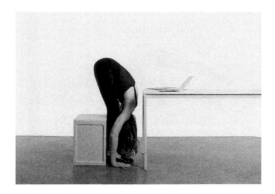

DESK SLEEPING

Exhale all the air out of your nose or mouth. With lips closed, inhale a third of the way. Pause. Inhale another third. Pause. Inhale the final third. Pause. Exhale all the air out. Repeat ten times.

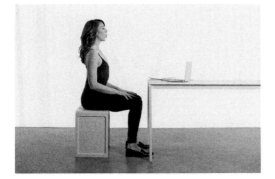

CHIN-DOWN STRETCH

Drop your chin toward your chest. Inhale fully, stretching across the front of your chest. If you would like to place your hands behind your head to enhance the stretch, do so. Exhale, relax your arms and your hands behind you or on your lap.

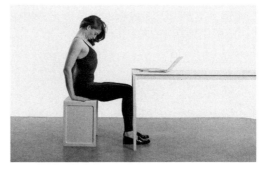

TEMPLE MASSAGE

Place your thumbs on the sides of your forehead. Let your fingers rest on your skull where it feels natural. Start to move your thumbs in a circular motion, using as much pressure as feels good. Massage your skull for three to twenty breaths, maybe while you are on the phone, staring at the screen, waiting in line, watching TV, or sitting in traffic, and at least once before bed.

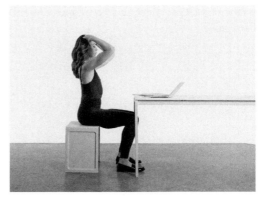

QUICK FIXES

LENGTHENING STANDING FOLD

Separate your feet a bit more than hip distance apart. Inhale, stand up tall. Exhale, fold forward. If it feels good, wrap your arms behind your legs, holding the inner calves or even reaching through toward your head. Close your eyes and breathe here five to ten breaths.

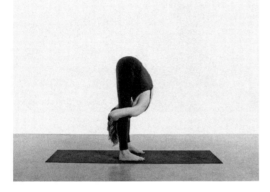

FORWARD BEND WITH BLOCK

Sit on the floor with your legs extended in front of you. Place a block, pillow, or stacked books on your thighs. Inhale, sit up tall. Exhale, fold forward and rest your forehead, right above your brow line, on the block. Let your arms drop by your legs and hold here.

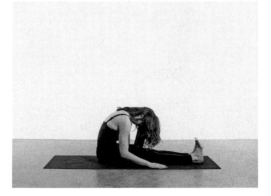

PLOW

Lie on the floor. Lift your feet up and over your head to the floor. Flex your feet, straighten your legs, and interlace your hands behind your back. Bring hips over shoulders and hold here five to twenty breaths.

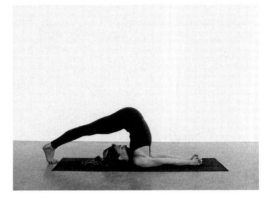

LEGS UP THE WALL

Lie on the floor, bringing your butt to the wall. Lift your legs up the wall, either feet touching or letting them flop out to the sides. Open your arms wide or place one hand on your abdomen and one on your heart, and breathe here as long as comfortable. You can also come to a full Shoulder Stand (page 100).

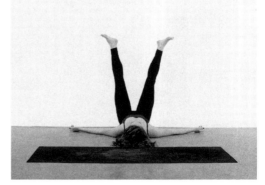

158

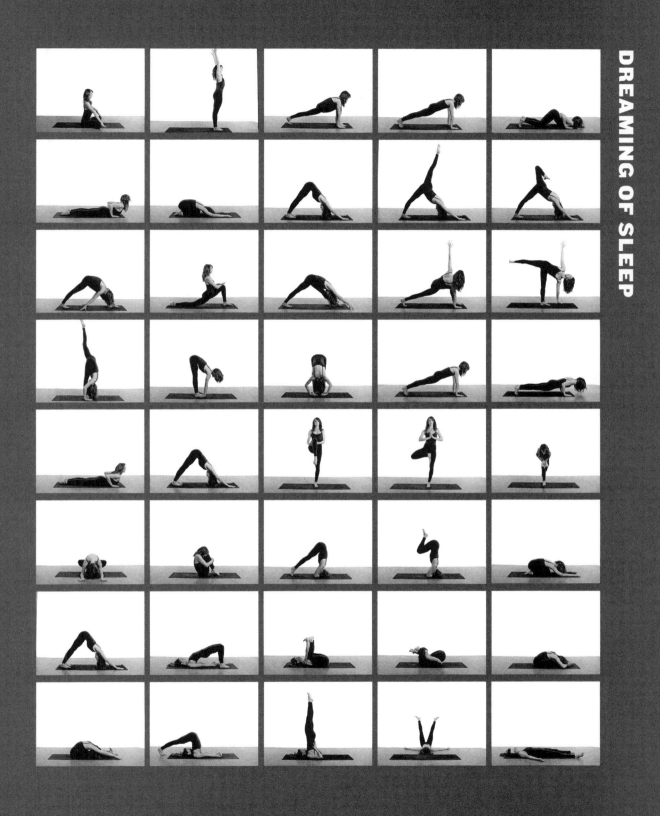

NOURISHMENT

Food stimulates the body, both in a waking, energizing direction and in a pacifying, sleep-inducing one. Oftentimes, insomnia and/or an inability to sleep through the night are connected directly to the diet, something that pill-prescribing doctors rarely mention. Valerie insisted that she was eating well, but when I finally inspected what she ate and drank with a fine-tooth Retox comb, I realized that she was unknowingly disturbing her sleep patterns. I gave her the following guidelines, which had her snoozing better within days. Here are some of the most sleep-divesting foods followed by sleep-inducing foods and recipes.

DETOX

These are nourishing nightmares if you are having a tough time drifting into slumber:

CAFFEINE. First and foremost, if you are having trouble sleeping, do not have caffeine before bed. This includes the obvious coffee, but also chocolate, teas, and sodas. After 2 p.m., put aside your simmering cups of green, black, and white teas and swap them for non-caffeinated versions. While many teas have caffeine and keep you up, chamomile tea has been shown to relax your system and help you drift off to sleep. Sip it throughout the afternoon and have a cup right before bed. Keep the chocolate, coffee, and other caffeinated products only in the pre-lunch routine as well.

RAW VEGETABLES. Raw vegetables are extremely hard to digest, let alone before entering a horizontal position. Eating them at dinner or before bed can exacerbate indigestion and keep you up longer than desired. Swap raw veggies for cooked ones in the eve, saving big salads for lunch.

SPICY FOOD. Smoking hot dreams can be tantalizing, but spicy foods have been shown to change sleep patterns by reducing the time spent in the deep-sleep stages, thus causing less sleep overall. In addition, elevated body temperatures after eating spicy food make it harder to actually a fall asleep. Keep the spice to the daytime and go mild at night.

RED MEAT. Red meat contains tyrosine, which stimulates the production of cortisol, the "stress" hormone that counteracts sleep. It is also high in protein, which makes it difficult for your body to digest while you are falling asleep. Either move the meat to lunch, or save it for nights you know you are willing to toss and turn a bit more.

RETOX

These foods will help you to some sweet dreaming:

CARBS. Carbs are your sleepy friend. Carbohydrates such as rice, bread, and other grains stimulate the release of insulin. Insulin clears out amino acids that compete with tryptophan, thus allowing more of the sleep-inducing tryptophan to circulate throughout your body and making it easier for you to fall asleep. Try having rice, tortillas, pasta, or bread with dinner. Yes, another reason to eat your carbs.

CHEESE AND DAIRY. The calcium in dairy helps tryptophan produce sleep-inducing melatonin. Try some melted cheese or some bites of yogurt before bed to help your body get on the sleep train.

Note: The combination of carbohydrates and dairy has been shown to make tryptophan more available to the brain and promote sleep. Good news for pizza and quesadilla lovers everywhere!

VITAMIN B6. B6 converts tryptophan to niacin and serotonin, which in turn regulates sleep patterns. Decreased levels of B6 can prevent a good night's sleep by disturbing the metabolism of tryptophan and thus limiting the levels of serotonin in the body. Try adding more B6 foods to your diet such as pistachios, tuna, salmon, sunflower seeds, and lean beef.

MAGNESIUM. Chronic insomnia is a main symptom of magnesium deficiency. Loading your diet with magnesium-rich foods such as whole grains, spinach, banana, nuts, seeds, and fish will help your slumber.

SNACKS
Pistachios
Sunflower seeds
Banana
Chamomile tea

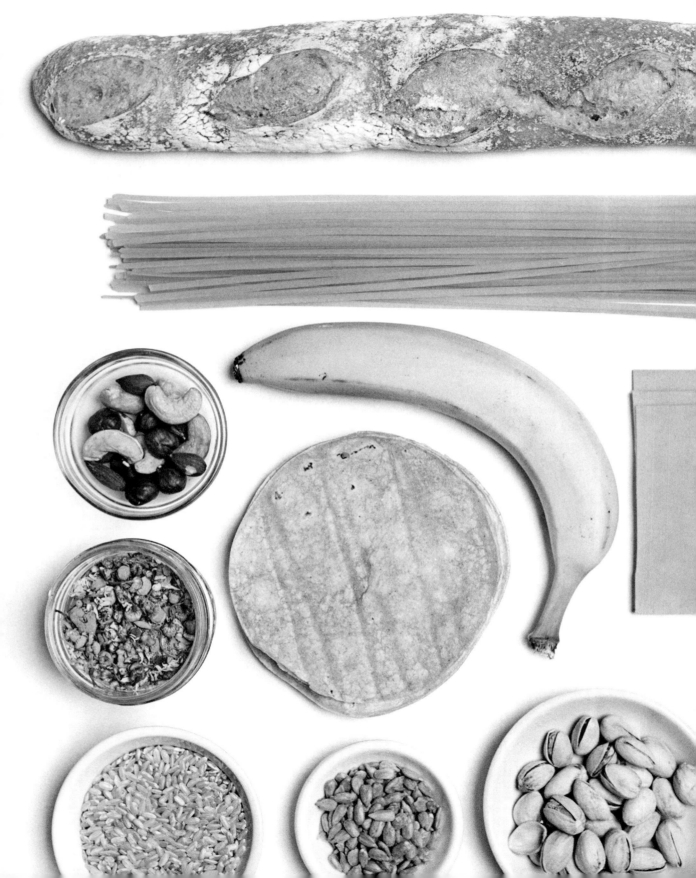

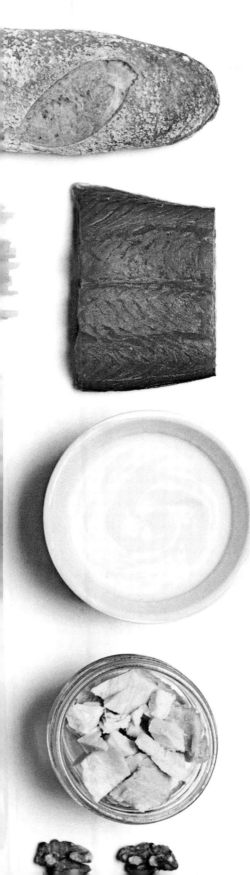

Retox Milk

This is a Retox take on the old wives' glass of warm milk—tastier and more effective.

Warm up a glass of almond milk in a steamer, pot, or microwave. Serve in a mug and enjoy. You can add a dash of cinnamon if you choose. The warmth will soothe your system while the magnesium and tryptophan in the almonds will naturally reduce and relax nerve and muscle function so you can drift into soft slumber.

Quesadillas

1 teaspoon extra virgin olive oil

2 corn tortillas

¼ cup shredded cheese (cheddar, Monterey Jack, or your choice)

Heat oil in a pan over medium heat. Place two corn tortillas in the pan to warm up, about 1 minute. Place cheese on half of each tortilla and fold the other half over it. Cook on each side until cheese is melted. Have for dinner or before bed.

Slumbery Smoothie

This is the perfect afternoon snack.

2 cups baby spinach

1 cup almond milk

1 banana, peeled and sliced

1 teaspoon honey

Place all ingredients in a blender and puree.

ZZZ Pasta

1 (16-ounce) package of pasta of your choice

¼ cup grated pecorino cheese

¼ cup grated Parmesan cheese

Fill a large pot with water and heat until boiling. Cook pasta according to package directions. When pasta is cooked, remove ½ cup of the cooking water and set aside. Drain pasta and place into a large bowl. Add cheeses and mix. If too dry, add a bit of the reserved pasta water, a little at a time until pasta is smooth and creamy.

MINDSET

Let's be honest, counting sheep has never worked for any of us, not when we were in one-piece rompers and not now. Yet I realized one insomniac night a few years ago that there in the green, sheep-filled pastures lay an effective solution for getting to sleep, and that maybe whoever invented this farm-centric practice was not so crazy after all. I have since extrapolated counting sheep into a pure, Retox yoga solution based on visualization and breath.

Pranayama is the science of the breath. The word for "breath" in Sanskrit is *prana. Ayama* means "length and expansion." *Pranayama* thus means "the control and broadening of the breath." A smooth, rhythmic breath pattern is essential for getting to sleep as it soothes the nervous system, relaxes the muscles, and releases the mind from its stressed-out circles of endless thought. If your breath is spastic, your body is spastic. If your breath is calm, your body is calm, and thus able to do what it knows how to do—go to sleep.

I asked Valerie to do this every night. At first she thought it was a load of hogwash, but once she tried it and slept without pills, she was hooked. The plan worked so well that she has gone on to teach it to her husband, colleagues, friends, and family members. Now it is your turn.

RETOX

Find a comfortable position in bed, on your back or side. Let your eyes gently close. Relax the muscles of your face and take a long, slow exhale out of the mouth. Now bring to mind your favorite serene place, such as a beach or huge field, and start to count with me, breathing through your nose:

> Inhale to the count of three—inhale one, two, three.
> Exhale to the count of three—exhale one, two, three.
>
> Inhale to the count of three—inhale one, two, three.
> Exhale to the count of three—exhale one, two, three.

When you feel comfortable there, go up to four.

> Inhale to the count of four—inhale one, two, three, four.
> Exhale to the count of four—exhale one, two, three, four.
> Inhale to the count of four—inhale one, two, three, four.
> Exhale to the count of four—exhale one, two, three, four.

When you feel comfortable there, go up to five.

> Inhale to the count of five—inhale one, two, three, four, five.
> Exhale to the count of five—exhale one, two, three, four, five.
> Inhale to the count of five—inhale one, two, three, four, five.
> Exhale to the count of five—exhale one, two, three, four, five.

Keep breathing like this, inhaling and exhaling through the nose, calmly and rhythmically as long as feels good, then just let your body fall into a peaceful slumber.

Retox Soundtrack:
"Today was a Good Day" —ICE CUBE

Letting the sleep come from within. Lolë White Tour for Peace. Two thousand people, Barcelona.

RETOX

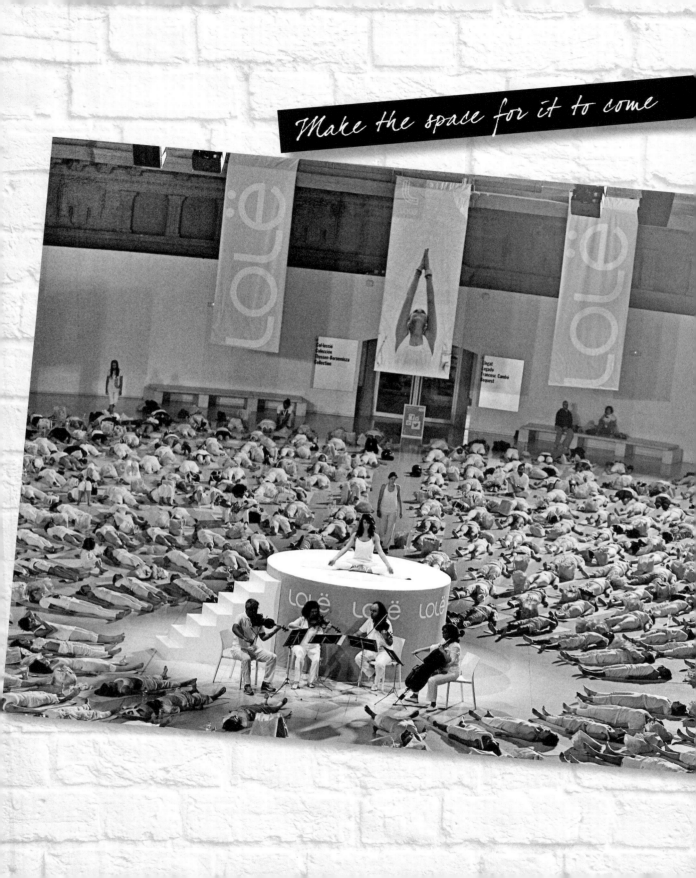

Make the space for it to come

LUMPS ON MODERN LOGS

MITIGATING CONSTANT

SITTING

Create your mental beach

YOU'VE LIKELY NEVER HEARD ANYONE say that they are suffering from being chained to their poolside chaise longue, have you? Yeah, neither have I. Being chained to a desk, driver's seat, or workstation, though? That's another story.

You know why? Because human beings are not meant to sit and stare for hours on end. Our bodies were created to run, hike, gather, hunt, walk, climb, sleep, lie down, lounge, and yes, occasionally sit, but never, ever in hard chairs, even the fanciest, most ergonomically correct ones. Our bodies were built to undergo duress and work hard, but to work with the physical muscles, not solely the mind.

Now, as we all know, sitting in a chair eight hours a day hunched over a keyboard has become the norm. Sitting in a car in traffic or ferrying kids back and forth sucks up a huge chunk of our day. And when we're not doing either of those things, chances are we're sitting, head down, gadget in hand, scrolling through email, updating social media, watching a video, reading an article, or listening to a podcast . . . I, for one, feel like a lump on a log. When you add it all up, I estimate that the average human these days sits for ten or more hours a day. That is three to four times more than the human body was created to sit, and more than the average person sleeps! Our bodies were simply not built for this way of life. In fact, sitting more than six hours a day has been shown to make you up to 40 percent more likely to die before someone who sits less than three hours a day, even if you exercise.

Even with the best posture, the mere act of sitting for more than a few minutes lowers the active digestive enzymes that break down fat by 90 percent, and sitting for more than two hours has been shown to cause a drop in good cholesterol by 20 percent. The activity of sitting lowers your base caloric rate to one calorie an hour and decreases insulin by 24 percent. Those who sit more than four and a half hours a day increase their probability of depression and obesity, and those with jobs that are sedentary have twice the rate of cardiovascular disease as those who do not.

This is just part of what happens to your internal functions; what happens to your muscular-skeletal system is just as bad, if not worse. The hunching forward, rounding of the spine, increased pressure on your sacrum, possible imbalances to your pelvis, and extended head and arms add a whole other dimension that actually lays the foundation for countless back, shoulder, and knee problems.

Society has advanced to get us here, but our bodies have not, and we cannot evolve fast enough to support this lifestyle, and perhaps we never will. This conundrum between how the physical body was built versus what it is required to do is the core of the lump on a log challenge.

If your lower back or hips are sore and hurting, and you let out a low groan when you get out of bed in the morning, sit down in a low chair, or climb in a car, you have definitely become a modern lump. You may have noticed a pooch in your lower belly that no amount of dieting or crunches is taking away. And every now and then, even though you do not tell anyone, you go lie down because of a Back Attack.

John is a perfect example. He came to me in October of 2014, a young, very high-level executive at a multinational media company with a drive to succeed at all costs. Yet the office was making him miserable. He had never done yoga, but he went to a trainer once a week, lifted weights, and ran outside two days a week. A girl he was interested in suggested he try yoga. Eager to win her over, he committed to a private session with me. Hey, I'll take it.

The day after we first met, I received an email from him asking to schedule yoga three times a week, claiming he already felt better than he had since graduating from college more than a decade before. After two weeks of yoga, mindset, and nourishment homework, that feeling we were engendering together and working toward became the norm. A few weeks after that, his aches and pains com-

pletely disappeared. Soon afterward, he had to get his suits taken in, and after a year, he had to have entirely new suits made because the tailor had already taken them in three times. All the work we did together had relieved his pains to the point that he was finally optimizing his workouts and boosting his metabolism as well.

These days, John can touch his toes and almost do a split. He did not change his life; he did not have to. He is at the same job with even more responsibility that keeps him at the office longer than before, but now he has resources that keep his pain at bay and his weight down.

YOGA

Anatomically speaking, sitting and hunching, even slightly, at a desk, table, bar, in the car, or in any seat, tightens the muscles on the front of the body and weakens the corresponding muscles on the back—a fact that most people aren't even aware of. Usually people think back pain must be a "back" issue and thus try to treat it with back exercises or back-centric yoga, but because sitting affects both the front and back of your body, these efforts are likely only working 50 percent of the problem, which is why you are still suffering.

The real problem is not necessarily where you think you are hurting, rather in the muscles supporting your front and your back sides. Sitting causes the muscles alongside your spine (erector spinae) to stretch due to how you have been slouching, sinking in your seat, and reaching forward to the keyboard, steering wheel, phone, iPad, or desk. At the same time, the "six-pack" muscles of your abdominal wall (rectus abdominis) become shortened, pulled back by the lengthening of the muscles alongside your spine, and the hip flexors have simultaneously tightened, making you feel stiffer than you actually are.

Judy approached me fearing she may have morphed into a modern lump. As a stay-at-home mom, she was endlessly running around managing the kids and the house, yet between driving them around, making phone calls, paying bills, helping with homework, and waiting for tutors, piano lessons, and dentist appointments to finish, she actually sat for the majority of the day and was routinely exhausted at the end of it. And all that sitting showed, from the classic shoulder hunch to the abdominal pooch, from slowed metabolism to random aches and pains. Mamma lump for sure.

I knew there was little flexibility in the structure of her day—she was at the mercy of her kids' schedules—so I created a two-part plan. The first was using her legs for standing and walking. No, I didn't tell her to walk for miles a day or to walk instead of driving the kids to school, but I did want her to add standing and walking into her day whenever she could. Instead of sitting at the kitchen table while on the phone, I had her walk up and down the hallway. Rather than sitting in the car waiting for practice to be over, I had her stand outside and lean against it. Instead of driving from one side of the mall to the other, I had her walk it. And as an alternative to scrolling her screen in the lounge chair for a momentary break, I had her implement Retox yoga.

RETOX

DESK FIXES

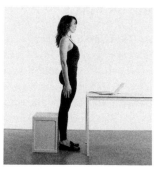

STAND

Literally, just stand up. No one will think anything weirder than that you are about to head to the bathroom. Stand every hour for at least a minute, if not longer. Standing is the perfect time to make and take calls, talk with colleagues, or just think.

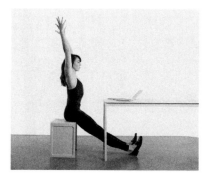

STAFF

When standing is not possible, sit upright in whatever chair you have. Place your hands by your hips. Press down into your hands and lift your sternum up. Lengthen the back of your neck by dropping your chin slightly. Spread wide across the collarbones and bring your abdomen to your spine. Lift your arms up if you can. Hold for five to ten breaths, multiple times a day. No one will ever notice.

SHOULDER-OPENING BREATH*

Clasp your hands behind your back, elbows straight. Inhale to a comfortable level. Begin short, sharp breaths out of the nose, where the inhale is simply a reaction to the exhale, as the diaphragm pumps on the abdominal wall. It should feel somewhere between sneezing and blowing your nose. (If you are pregnant, skip khapalabhati and breathe normally in this pose.)

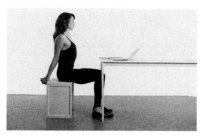

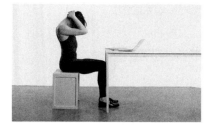

NECK AND SKULL RELEASE

Place your hands behind your head. Let your thumbs rest on the base of your skull. Inhale, lift your skull, stretching the back of your neck. Exhale, use your hands to gently pull your chin toward your chest. Hold five to ten breaths, eyes opened or closed.

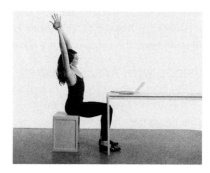

SIDE STRETCH

Lift your arms straight up. Hold your left wrist with your right hand. Inhale, grow long and pull up. Exhale, lean to the right. Make sure both sitz bones are on the chair so the stretch is through your left side. Hold here, then repeat on the other side.

LUMPS ON MODERN LOGS

QUICK FIXES

ANTI-LUMP SALUTE

Start standing with your feet together and your hands touching at your chest. Inhale, extend your arms overhead. Exhale, fold forward and bring your forehead to your shins. Inhale, extend your spine, look forward. Exhale, Chaturanga or Plank pose. Inhale, Up Dog. Exhale, Down Dog. Inhale, put your left foot between your hands, then lift your arms into a high lunge. Exhale, Chaturanga. Inhale, Plank. Exhale, Down Dog. Inhale, put your right foot between your hands, then lift your arms into a high lunge. Exhale, Chaturanga. Inhale, Plank. Exhale, Down Dog. Close your eyes and hold here five breaths. Then inhale and step or jump your feet between your hands. Exhale, fold forward. Inhale, reach your arms up, look up. Exhale, hands to your heart. Repeat five to ten times.

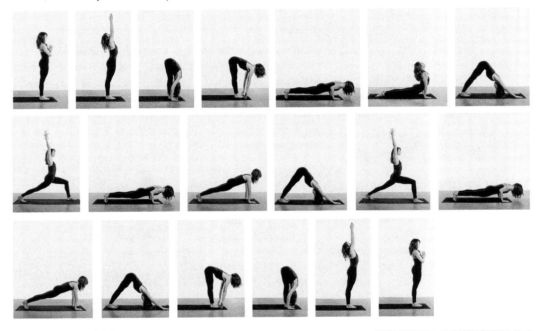

CRESCENT MOON

Start in a low lunge with your left foot between your hands, right leg behind you. Place your back knee on the floor. Inhale, lift your arms up. Exhale, soften your back quad and hip flexor toward the floor. Optionally, place your hands on your front thigh or on the floor behind you for a backbend. Make sure your front knee is directly over your ankle. Breathe here, then repeat on the other side.

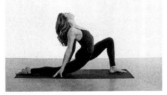

BRIDGE WITH HANDS CLASPED

Lie on the floor and place your feet flat, hip distance apart. Inhale, lift your butt and lower back off the floor into Bridge pose. Exhale, clasp your hands underneath you and pull your fists toward your heels. Reach your sternum toward your chin. Stay here and breathe five to ten breaths, then release your arms and stay there as long as feels good.

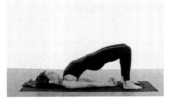

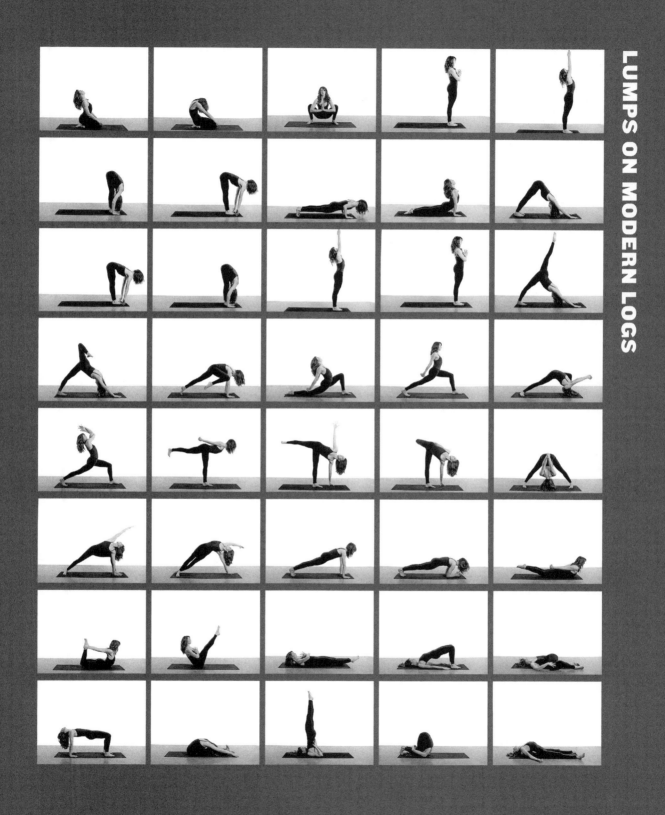

NOURISHMENT

I get it: Making time for a good meal in the middle of your busy day is tough. It's especially hard if you're stuck working at your desk through lunch. But it is not impossible! You just need to learn some tricks for giving your unavoidably sedentary body what it needs to function without getting bogged down. Here are three things to remember:

THE EXPERIENCE IS IMPORTANT

The experience of eating is as important as the food itself. We can probably all agree that eating at your desk is nowhere near as pleasant as sitting outside at a French café with a glass of rosé, but just because you have to eat a boring, sad desk lunch does not mean it has to be bad, or bad for you. If you can make the experience of eating better, the food you eat will taste better and satiate you. Here are some tips to make desk dining more glam:

- Create a placemat out of some sheets of printer paper. Or if you have a private office, keep a placemat in your desk drawer. This simple, thin physical divide between your meal and your work will help your mind separate from the work momentarily so you can focus on the food.
- If you must work while eating, try to keep it to reading, rather than typing or answering emails. It's much less disruptive.
- Keep a bottle or two of your favorite hot sauce, olive oil, or vinegar in a desk drawer. This little dash of you can help convert the taste of the food from something you have to take in to something you actually enjoy.
- Take a moment after you finish to go wash your hands or simply stand up, a subtle way to bookmark eating.

TIMING IS EVERYTHING

You have your own digestive rhythm. Learn to tune in to your body and only eat when your body tells you it needs food. Eating just because it's a certain time or because everyone else is eating can throw off your internal metabolism, actually making you eat more than you need, aka gain weight. Here are some tips on how to avoid it:

- Break the cycle of eating a snack as soon as you sit at your desk in the morning or after an afternoon meeting (a common work avoidance habit). Try to do at least an hour of work before you eat. It will help you get off some habitual schedule and start paying attention to your body. Stop eating by the clock and eat when you're actually hungry.
- Unless it is completely out of your control (for instance, at a company conference with fixed breaks for meals), don't feel you have to eat whenever your colleagues do. And don't feel bullied into eating what they are eating. Have input on what, when, and where you eat.
- When you do decide to order in with your colleagues, take a second to look at the menu. There is always something healthy available; order it with confidence.

- Take your time when you eat. Chew slowly and savor each bite, thus not only enjoying your food, but enhancing the first steps of digestion, which take place in the mouth.

NATURAL IS NOT ALWAYS GOOD

Are natural foods good for you? Yes, but some natural foods are not the best choices when you are sedentary. There are many foods that could be healthy and good snacks, but when ingested while sedentary actually slow the metabolism and help pack on pounds. Here are some common desk foods to look out for.

DETOX

SUGARY FRUITS. Fruits are undoubtedly better for you than chocolate, but be careful with fruits high in sugar such as mango, pears, honeydew melon, and peaches. If you don't burn off the fructose, it will ferment in your system, slow down your digestion, potentially cause some Alien Baby bloat, and pack on waistline pounds.

YOGURT. Yogurt is high in carbohydrates and sugar, which, if you are not moving around, will stick to your system and slow your digestion. If you eat yogurt for the probiotics, make certain the ingredients are pure and that you eat it first thing in the morning. Avoid eating probiotics and all other yogurts as snacks or after meals because it slows the metabolism.

HUMMUS. All natural? Sometimes, yes. Packed with fat and carbs your seated bum will not necessarily burn off? Double yes. Keep the hummus to a minimum, and when you do eat it, mix it with crudités like celery and broccoli to keep your system light and efficient. Furthermore, look for hummus that just has chickpeas, olive oil, tahini, and maybe salt and garlic, but without canola oil or other acids.

NUT BUTTERS. Like hummus, nut butters are packed with energy and fat that if not burned off will stick to your body.

FAT-FREE CHIPS AND SNACKS. They may be fat free, but they are also full of MSG and additives necessary to give them some semblance of flavor. The chemicals in the additives have been shown to lead directly to weight gain and often obesity, not to mention headaches.

RETOX

SNACKS

Almonds, raw or roasted
Berries, preferably blueberries and
    raspberries
Banana
Salad
Popcorn, all natural, without fake
    cheese, and air-popped without
    extra fat
Crudités: string beans, broccoli, or
    carrots
Decaf coffee with almond milk
Lemon water (juice of ½ lemon in 1 cup
    hot water)

Tomato Soup

I always like to have some cans of an organic, natural tomato soup around. Look for ones that have less than five ingredients, such as Amy's. But when I have the time, I like to make a big pot of this homemade soup and keep it in the fridge for a quick snack or meal any day of the week.

  3 tablespoons extra virgin olive oil
  4 cloves garlic, minced
  ½ yellow onion, diced
  2 pounds tomatoes, chopped
  Salt and pepper, to taste

Heat oil in a large heavy pot over medium heat. Add garlic and onion, and let cook until garlic just starts to turn golden. Add tomatoes, two pinches of salt, and pepper, to taste. Cover with a lid and let cook until the tomatoes are completely soft. Turn off the stove and either throw it all into the blender to puree, or use an immersion blender right there in the pot. If the tomatoes are not particularly juicy, you may need to add ½ cup to 1 cup of water while blending. When the soup is smooth, you are done.

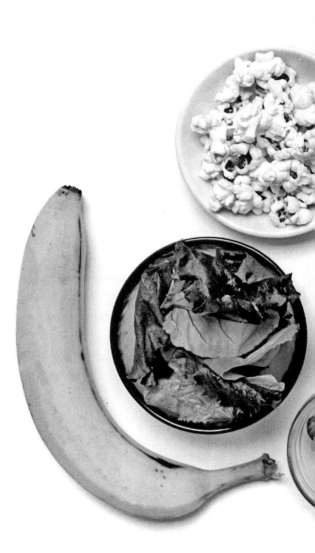

178

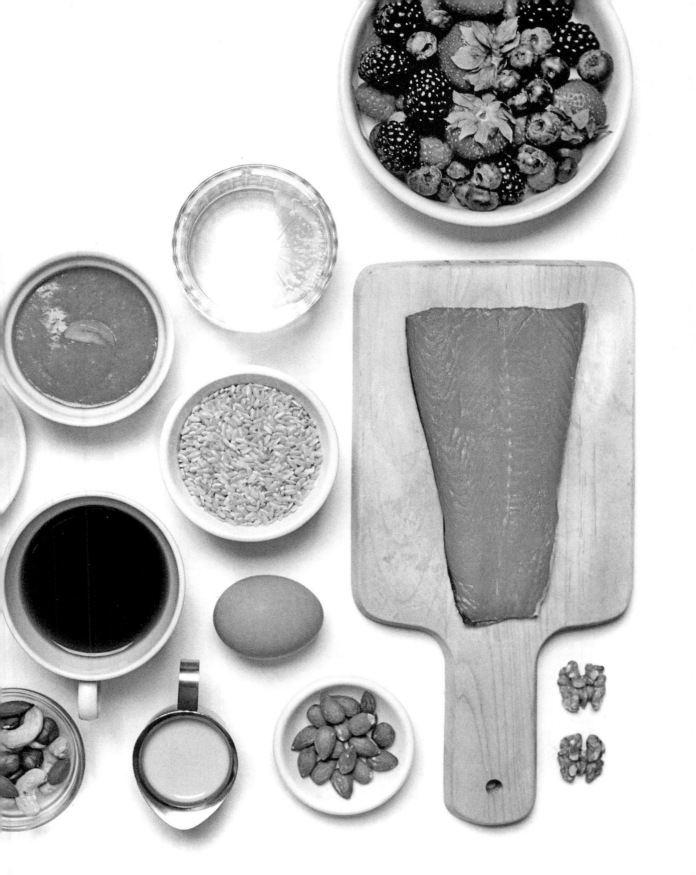

Avocado Boom

Keep an avocado or two at your desk or just toss one in your purse in the morning. Their skin is quite thick so they last, do not get messy, and do not need refrigeration.

Cut open the avocado and scoop it onto crackers or bread, whatever you like and is accessible. If you have to have it, add a dash of salt on top. If you do not have bread or crackers, slice the avocado the typical way and eat it directly from the shell with a spoon.

Quinoa Tabouli

I use this as a snack or lunch, and often double the quantities and make as one batch for the week, even using it as garnish on a larger salad or meal.

½ cup cooked quinoa

2 bunches parsley, finely chopped

½ white onion, diced

1 tomato, diced

1 tablespoon extra virgin olive oil

Juice of 1 lemon

Mix the quinoa, parsley, onion, and tomato in a bowl. Dress with olive oil and lemon juice. Stir and enjoy.

Tortilla

A Spanish staple, done an easy Retox way.

2 teaspoons extra virgin olive oil

1 yellow onion, chopped

2 zucchinis, chopped

8 eggs (or 6 egg whites and 3 whole eggs)

Dash of salt

Heat oil in a large pan over medium heat. Add onion and let cook until soft. Add zucchini and stir, lower heat, and cover. While the vegetables are cooking, beat the eggs in a large bowl. Add salt. Once the zucchini is completely cooked, pour in eggs and cover again. Cook until the top is set, or if you are the adventurous type, place a dinner plate on top of the pan and flip the tortilla onto the plate. Slide it back in the pan and cook 3 more minutes, or until the bottom is cooked. Eat as breakfast or as dinner with a side salad, or take it to work as a snack or in the car as a slice on the run.

Green Machine

Make this once a week and have it for the rest of the week.

1 pound broccoli florets, fresh or frozen

2 zucchini, sliced

1 (10-ounce) box of mushrooms, sliced

1 red bell pepper, sliced

1 hot pepper, sliced (optional)

2 cups baby spinach

2 cups kale (optional)

Place ¼ inch water in a large pan, and add broccoli. Cover it with a lid and let it cook while you prepare the rest of the vegetables. When the broccoli is bright green, add zucchinis to the pan and stir. Next add mushrooms, red bell pepper, and hot pepper, if using. When the vegetables are soft, add the spinach and kale. Stir well, and cook until the greens are wilted. You can eat it warm, cold, or room temperature; toss it with a vinaigrette, or add it to a grain or pasta base. The options are endless.

MINDSET

I had tons of jobs growing up: waitress in Menlo Park, editorial intern at a magazine in New York City, dishwasher at a café in Palo Alto, business development intern in Madrid, trading assistant in Silicon Valley. And of course, my annual summer lemonade stand for petty cash. Given all that, starting my job on the Morgan Stanley trading floors should have been a breeze.

It reality, it could not have been more harsh of a transition. Waking up at 5 a.m. to sit chained to my desk, often for late nights of financial modeling until 9 or 10 p.m depending on what my boss wanted me to do. Having to ask to go to the restroom, and even if granted permission, given no more than a couple of minutes to scurry there and back in the middle of the trading day. Incessant ringing of telephones, the shouting of trades and prices over computers and desks, and the inevitable mean boss and bitchy colleague.

Don't get me wrong—I loved my job. I was hooked by the mayhem and all the accompanying adrenaline. It was a kind of high. But it was so hard to sit there all day long with all the commotion, demands, complaints, and stresses to manage.

I started to notice all the problems my colleagues suffered from and started to experience some myself: back pain, weird uncontrollable weight gain, "blah" moods, and above all, stress. I called my mom exhausted after work one night and she told me, "Just pretend you are on a boat looking out at the sea." Yeah right, Mom.

The next week I felt desperate. Half the group had been fired (one of the many rounds of layoffs I witnessed while on Wall Street), everyone was stressed and panicked, taking out their fury on us young bucks, and there was a low, dark cloud hanging over the floor. I decided to try this whole "pretend I am looking out at the sea" thing. It worked, sort of, except the sea was stormy, and I was getting seasick.

Fast-forward a few years when I was taking a night course on Tibetan yoga philosophy. Not coincidentally, the class was just weeks after Lehman Brothers fell and the tangential market crash and further rounds of layoffs took place at my firm. I hoped the ancient wisdom might provide a new perspective or some skills for survival.

The class began with a talk on Nirvana. *Oh god, here we go*, I thought. How was I supposed to find "inner peace" while sitting on the hardwood floor trying not to wrinkle my suit before having to go back to the warzone of the trading floor for the Asian-hour nightshift? But hey, I came to try to make myself better. So I decided to listen.

Nirvana has many connotations in Western society—from the headbanging of "Smells Like Teen Spirit" to the transcendent state of lotus-seated Buddhas hovering above the earth. What I learned that evening and in subsequent studies was that Nirvana actually means "to transcend something bad." The ancient root *nir* means "to transcend," *va* means "to conquer or to win," and *ana* means "the one who does those things." In traditional Tibetan, the word is *Nanyalemdepa*; *nanyen* is "grief or a negative thing," and *lemdepa* means "to transcend it."

To experience Nirvana is to transcend all the commotion around you so that you can be you. It is like putting yourself in a bubble, a protective force field so that you respond differently when confronted by a disturbing issue or person. It is not just letting things go. That is fake yoga philosophy. Rather, Nirvana is about seeing things and floating past them, or as my mom said, like you are looking out at the sea. It doesn't take *om shanti*s or peace signs, but rather, letting your eyes focus inward on your own world, a world where you can envision yourself producing, thinking, and acting the way you want, rather than in reaction to others. This is the state you want to achieve.

You cannot control the demands of your day: Your boss will insist on that report, your three-year-old will throw that tantrum when she doesn't get what she wants, and you can't obliterate the seemingly inevitable traffic jam you get stuck in when you're already late to your appointment. But you can transcend these moments without letting them dictate your actions and feelings, and without letting them define you. If you transcend where you are, you can always be you.

RETOX

Close your eyes, wherever you are. Bring to mind your favorite place. It can be a forest, a beach, a couch at home, the kitchen table where you grew up, the top of a mountain, your favorite park . . . Let whatever sticks to your mind first be the one. In your mind, hear the sounds of the leaves rustling, waves lapping, wind blowing . . . smell the air, see the details. Take yourself there.

See what you would be wearing, what your skin would look like, how your hair would be. Imagine who would be with you, or if you would be alone. Let your mind fill with any and all details about the place. Literally, *be there*.

Stay with this place in your mind, eyes closed and breathing, for as long as you can, or would like to. When you open your eyes, decide to carry this vision with you.

Do this regularly enough so that the image becomes crystal clear in your mind. When the shit hits the fan the next day at home or at work, or you just can't deal anymore, you can take yourself to that place in your mind. You may start to notice that this becomes your mental chaise longue on the beach.

Retox Soundtrack:
"Smells Like Teen Spirit" —NIRVANA

LUMPS ON MODERN LOGS

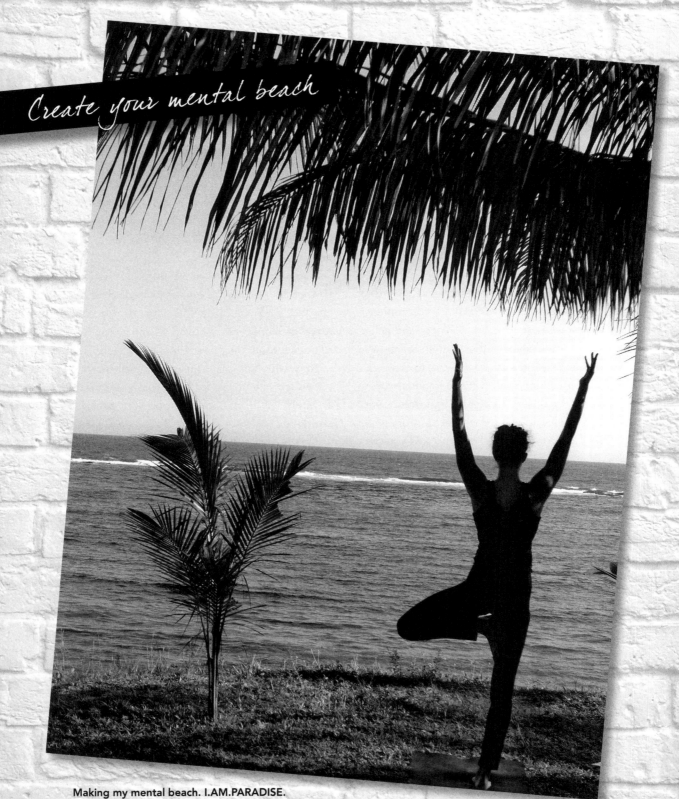

Create your mental beach

Making my mental beach. I.AM.PARADISE.
ESCAPE. Colombia.

iADDICT

Tangible happiness >
intangible scrolling

MY NAME IS LAUREN IMPARATO and I am an addict. To my iPhone. In fact, I am an iAddict.

There is rarely a point in time when my phone, laptop, or iPad is not near me. Sometimes I have all three with me, one in my pocket, one in my hand, and one in my bag at my hip. I would be surprised if it were not similar for you, perhaps even mixed in with a BlackBerry or a Kindle. The brand of device is irrelevant; if it has a screen and information, and you have it within arm's reach the majority of the day, it is time for an intervention.

iAddiction has become the modern-life norm. Although it can be difficult for us to self-discern, there are some obvious signs of gadget dependency. Perhaps you can identify with some of these:

The Morning
When I wake up, I roll to the edge of the bed, take a long stretch . . . to reach for my phone, and immediately check email, Facebook, and Instagram, all while still blurry eyed and under the covers.

I answer five or so emails before I officially start my workday, and I often have a quick call in between.

The Evening
I pick up my phone at least once during dinner to check email and social media.

I check them both again one last time as I head to bed, claiming that I am merely using the light of the phone to guide me so that I do not trip in the dark.

My evening prayer is clearing out my inbox.

The In Between
I refresh my email a minimum of once every half hour.

I have thousands of pictures on my phone—of outdoor scenes, funny moments, and plates of food—and sometimes obsess over the angle of light I am catching in the photo.

The first thing I do in line at the pharmacy or store is load a news website so that I can read while I wait, claiming to be erudite as a result, but usually just scroll through dozen of Instapics.

I view car rides (as a passenger) as a chance to catch up on email and phone calls.

I hold my breath and age a few months when my phone falls, silently praying it has not cracked, and squeal like a kid in a candy shop when it has not.

I rarely turn my phone off. If I do while in-flight, I turn it back on before they have taken off the fasten seatbelt sign.

I use my phone as an escape: an escape from work, my boss, the commuters around me, the kids, life.

I check how many people have liked my latest social media post.

I email, text, and messenger more with my friends than I talk to them on the phone or live.

I have an app for everything, even one that helps me be less digitally connected.

And above all . . .

My legs are splattered with bruises from my walking smack-dab into poles and furniture merely because my face is buried in my phone. I am secretly thankful all I have is these bruises, as I have caught myself walking for five to thirty minutes ensconced in my device, only to arrive at my destination without remembering once crossing the street. I have not been run over (thankfully), but I have run into people . . .

I could go on and on, but then we would have to rename this chapter #confessions.

iAddiction is a problem, as it affects every part our body and life, from sleep to sex, self-confidence to weight gain, relationships to family, back pain to headaches, career to friends. Over a third of divorces are linked to iAddict circumstances, from lack of live communication to arguments over putting the phone down to Facebook trysts. One out of three fights between friends or couples starts over something digital. Personally, I want to impale my husband every time he buries his head in his phone for "one minute" during a conversation, and admittedly I have had intense urges to chuck my dinner companions'

phones out the window before our appetizers even arrive.

Over 50 percent of acute work stress is related to digital overload, specifically emails received when out of the office or on weekends. The leading cause of depression is iAddiction, specifically social media. Over 25 percent of car accidents are related to texting or being on the phone while driving, with texting while driving making a crash twenty-three times more likely. Ten percent of pedestrian visits to emergency rooms result from accidents involving walking and being on the phone (note to self).

To top it off, the most prevalent health issue across the globe—sleep deprivation, including poor sleep quality and insomnia—is rooted in the very screen of your gadget. The short wavelength "blue" light the screens emit has been proven to reduce the production of melatonin, the hormone secreted by the pineal gland that controls sleep and wake cycles. As your eyes absorb the frequency of the light, your body produces less melatonin, and you biochemically cannot sleep as well. In addition, decreased melatonin production increases your risks of cancer, weakens your immune function, and disturbs your metabolic function (that is, causes weight gain).

So we have to ask ourselves—why are we so addicted? Are we endlessly hunting for digital gratification or simply evading the present moment? Whose news do we think can outdo the beautiful real life moments passing us by? Are we living for likes or liking to live?

Often we do not realize we are, in fact, iAddicts. Other times we can sense our digital dependence, but do not know what to do about it. The challenge lies in iAddiction's complexity; there is not one part of your body, mind, and life that iAddiction does not affect, making a 360-degree Retox cocktail imperative and effective, as my student Edward discovered. With a killer position at an investment company, Edward epitomized an iAddict. He would literally fall asleep every night with his phone in hand. He had three laptops, one desktop, one iPad, and a solid couple pounds of charging devices and cables for them all. If he was not on his gadgets for work, he was scrolling through Fantasy Football and sports stats, glancing through an online journal, or playing around with a music app. His friends would try to get him to engage with them, but Edward just couldn't stay away from his screens. Part was work, sure, but most was personal addiction, one that he realized may be a problem when his umpteenth girlfriend dumped him for "not connecting or communicating." With a life of blank, screen solidarity in front of him, I knew it was time for a Retox intervention.

The Retox cocktail for being an iAddict uses yoga to address the physical, tangible results on our musculoskeletal system from grasping our gadget hours a day, as well as to help boost mood and aid sleep. The nourishment section focuses on increasing our awareness and enlivening our stagnant systems, while the mindset part dissects the real reasons we just cannot put that phone down, and why, starting now, we have to.

YOGA

Perhaps you can commiserate with some of the physical ramifications of iAddition: tense fingers, wrists, and palms of the hand from grasping the gadget tight and typing. Tight shoulders and neck from rounding our spine to stare at the screen. Foggy mind from receiving endless information and attention deficit from always being able to quickly scroll to the next thing. Blurry eyesight from staring at a brightly lit small screen. Insomnia or difficulty falling asleep from the reduced melatonin our body produces. And the general malaise that arises from living life through an intangible, digital lens.

Edward suffered from all of these symptoms and used Retox yoga to soothe them as well as to begin to soften his addiction. As a bona fide iAddict myself, I have fine-tuned the yoga tools needed to combat the physical effects of addiction. Some of these are obvious, others more subtle; some you may actively feel, others you may not associate with iAddiction at all.

RETOX

DESK FIXES

EAGLE ARMS BACKBEND STRETCH

Open your arms wide out to the sides. Bring your arms toward each other and cross your right arm under your left arm. Bend your elbows, and if you can, wrap your wrists so your palms touch. Push your elbows and forearms into each other to stretch the upper back and neck. Inhale, arch backward, lifting your forearms up. Exhale, stay there in a backbend, but drop your head, bringing your chin to your chest. Hold here, then repeat with your left arm crossed under the right.

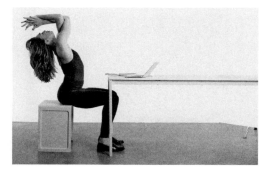

HEAD SHAKE

Take a deep inhale. Exhale strongly out of your mouth, sticking your tongue out, shaking your head left and right wildly. Repeat one to three times.

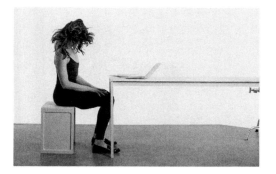

UPSIDE-DOWN PRAYER

Bring the backs of your hands to touch in front of you, fingers pointing down. Press the backs of your hands together and stretch your wrists and forearms out in front of you. Hold here five to twenty breaths. Optionally, begin a Dynamic Breath (page 351) by inhaling and exhaling forcefully and evenly. Eyes open or closed, whatever works wherever you are. Inhale, exhale, inhale, exhale, inhale, exhale. Be careful not to hyperventilate; instead, actively use your muscles to control the forceful inhales and exhales.

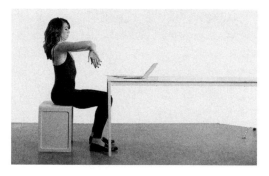

WRIST STRETCHES

Stretch your right arm out in front of you. Drop your fingertips down, and use your left hand to press your right hand down toward your body. Then lift your right hand and use your left hand to press your right palm and fingers toward your body. Hold each for five breaths, then repeat on the other side.

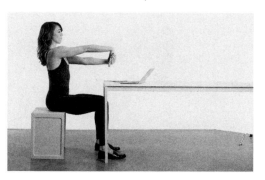

iADDICT

QUICK FIXES

COBRA UNDULATIONS*

Start lying on your stomach. Place your fingertips down on either side of your chest quite wide. Spread your fingers. Inhale and lift your upper body off the floor, letting your head dangle. Stay here for several breaths. On your next inhale, press further into your fingertips and lift your chest and head higher. Exhale and slowly lower your upper body, leading with your chest, letting your head follow. Repeat these slow undulations three to eight times.

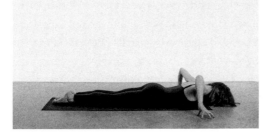

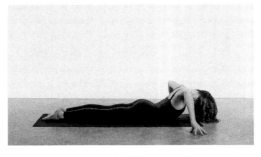

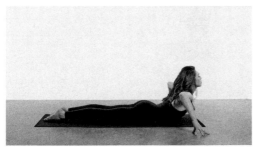

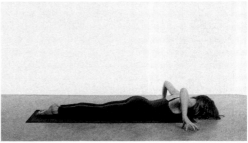

CAMEL

Start sitting on your knees. Place your hands on your hips. Inhale, lift your sternum up. Exhale, arch backward, keeping your hands on your hips or dropping them to your calves or feet. Drop your head back only if it feels good. Hold here five to ten breaths.

INTENSE WRIST STRETCH

Come to your hands and knees. Make sure your hips are over your knees and your shoulders are over your wrists. Turn your hands so the middle fingers are pointing toward the knees. Inhale here. Exhale, lean backward as much as feels comfortable. Hold here five to ten breaths.

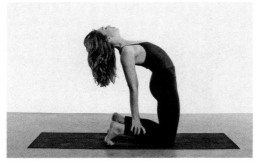

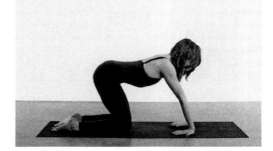

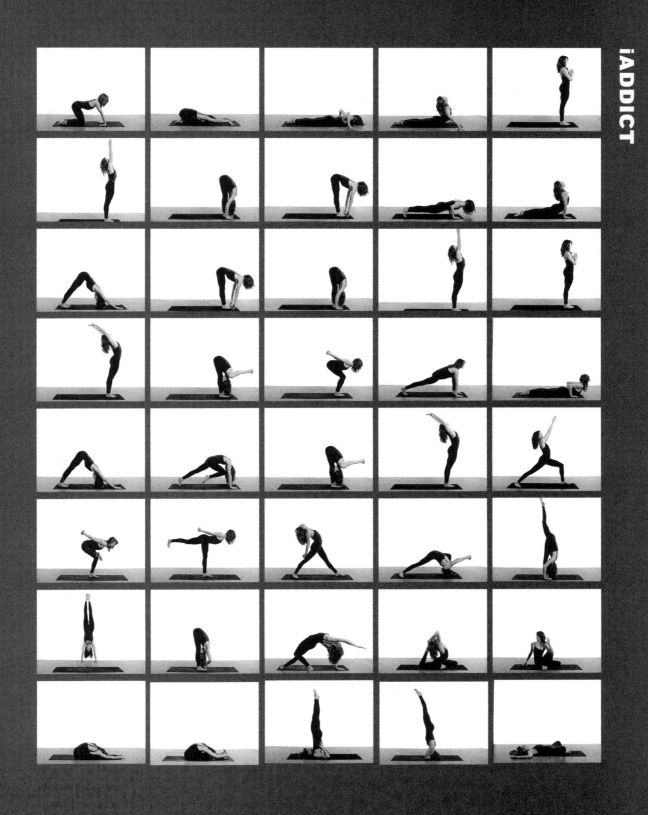

NOURISHMENT

My dining date usually wears tight black pleather . . . in the form of an iPhone case. Sad but true. I spend at least one, if not two, meals a day eating with a gadget. Not just with it near me, but with me actively using it, be it reading, scrolling, emailing, or social media-ing. I used to call it "efficient," given how much there is to do in a day and how much I want, and need, to accomplish in my waking hours, but I have realized through my own personal study as well as that of my nutritional coaching clients that all it does is make me eat more, taste less, and feel blech. In fact, when I have my nutritional coaching clients put their phones away while they eat (which always comes with a protest), they start meeting their weight loss and health goals within two weeks.

Take Amanda, a mother of two who is highly active, energetic, and involved in every aspect of her kids' lives. She had a pesky ten pounds she had been unable to lose after her last child, and she had tried every fad diet and trendy weight-loss program. She came to me hoping that I would be able to work some magic, which we did.

Overall, Amanda's diet was quite healthy. She knew fast food was bad, vegetables were good, and balanced meals were a must. She cooked for her kids and husband every night, avoiding processed ingredients, and exercised three times a week. I quickly realized that her health and weight goals had to do more with how she was eating her food, rather than what she was eating.

As a mother highly pressed for time, Amanda had gotten in the habit of eating while on her iPhone. She would either read something to feel connected and like herself, buy items online for the house, research something for the family, or simply escape into social media. She, like me, thought she was being efficient and relieving stress while also fleeing into her own world for just a few minutes, but she was actually slowing down her metabolism and thwarting her weight loss. I decided to make her go cold turkey and banned phone use from all meals. Within a week, the weight started to come off.

DETOX

Above all, put the phone away. It may seem efficient or pleasurable to eat and stare at a screen at the same time, but it can make you gain weight. As mentioned before, the short wavelength blue light emitted from screens reduces levels of melatonin. In addition to inducing sleep, melatonin helps control weight gain by stimulating the production of "beige fat," a type of fat cell that burns calories in the moment instead of storing them. Beige fat, also known as "thinning fat" or "good fat," helps regulate body weight control, hence its metabolic benefits.

More screens = less melatonin = less beige good fat = more yucky fat
Less screens = more melatonin = more beige good fat = more svelte, fit body

Put the phone or iPad down when you eat. If you are at your desk at work, glance at the paper or talk to a colleague next to you, even if just for a moment.

Paying attention to a screen rather than to the process of eating actually causes people to forget to chew. It's easy to mindlessly shovel food into your mouth when you're engrossed in answering emails or trying to get a report done. But chewing is actually the first stage of digestion. The less you chew the harder your stomach and the rest of your digestive system has to work. And improper digestion can cause a load of health problems. Consciously chew five to ten times per bite. It is totally realistic, totally doable, and much better for your system.

If you are looking at the screen and eating, you are most likely not looking at what is going into your mouth. Take a moment to glance at each forkful and bite before you take it in, even just a nanosecond. This will help you slow down the pace of eating, chew, and be more present in the real life moments outside your digital world.

RETOX

Here are some nutrients that are beneficial to iAddicts:

LUTEIN. With so much attention focused on a screen, it becomes imperative to take extra good care of the eyes. Lutein is a carotenoid concentrated in the macula, or area of the eye essential for central vision. It protects the eyes from stress and the high-energy photons of blue light, so it's a good idea to eat more of it if you are an iAddict, recovering or current. Try adding lutein-rich foods such as eggs with the yolk, spinach, kale, broccoli, peas, carrots, and kiwi to your diet on a regular basis.

MELATONIN. Eating foods with melatonin will help boost the reserve your iAddiction is draining. Try snacking on goji berries, almonds, and sliced fennel. Add coriander to your salads and cooked dishes, and always have a bowl of cherries around.

SPICE. Add some kick to your food to wake you up and get you out of your iAddiction while you eat. Chop up some hot peppers, add a dash of hot sauce, throw in some curry powder . . . whatever you fancy. A little bit of hot spice will force you to pay attention to what you are eating.

TEXTURES. Include various textures to your meals so you become aware of what you are eating. Mix lettuces with crunchy bits like nuts or ground-up tortilla chips. Add green beans as a side to soup, peas to the mac and cheese, or almonds mixed with raisins as a snack. The variety of textures will send a message through your discerning palate to your brain to focus on the interesting things going on in your mouth as opposed to the screen.

SNACKS
Hardboiled egg
Carrots
Kiwi
Chocolate-covered goji berries
Almonds

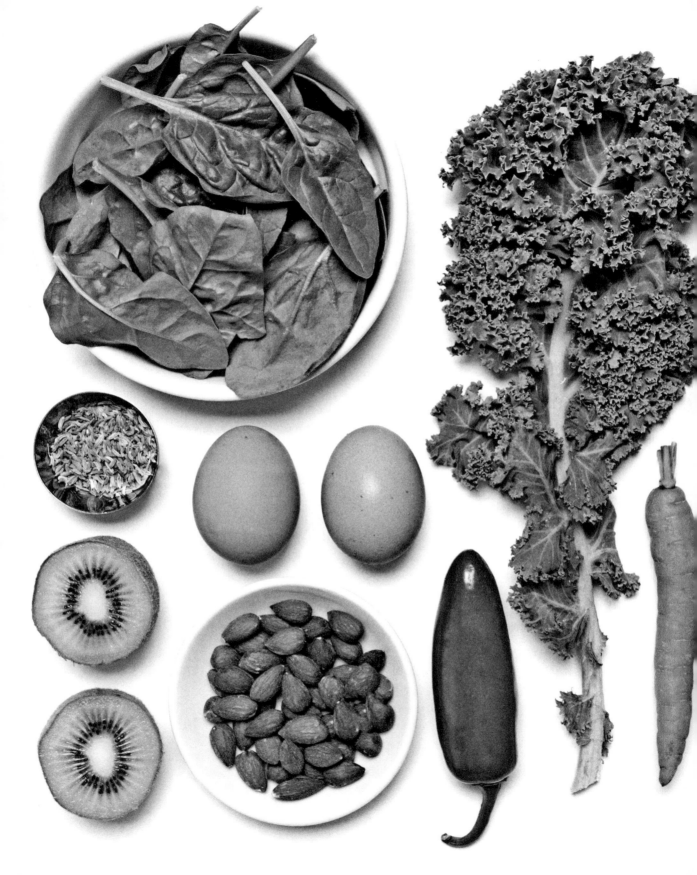

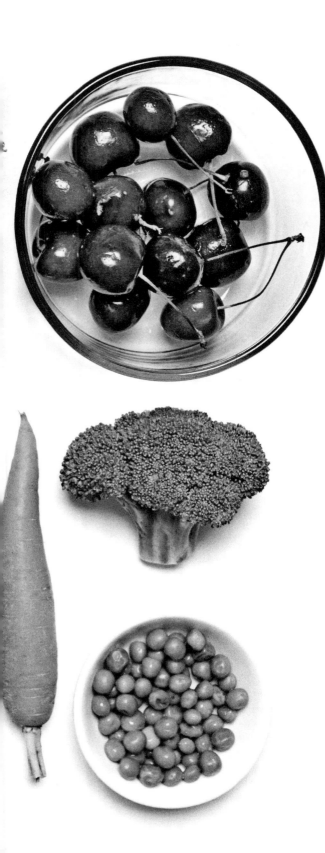

Spicy Scrambled Eggs

- **1 teaspoon butter or nonstick spray/vegetable oil**
- **1 fresh hot pepper of your choice**
- **2 eggs**

Heat butter in a small frying pan. Chop a fresh hot pepper—jalapeño, habanero, chili pepper, whatever you like or have available—and add it to pan. Stir it around so that its juice touches every corner. Let it simmer there while you crack and whisk your eggs. Remove the pieces of hot pepper from the pan and add the eggs. Cook like normal scrambled eggs. If you want to leave the slices of hot peppers to cook in the eggs, do so, just know that it is hard on your digestion. When the eggs are done, enjoy with added spice or as is.

iAddict Juice

- **1 handful kale**
- **2 handfuls baby spinach**
- **1 mango, peeled and diced**
- **1 tangerine, peeled and separated**
- **1 kiwi, peeled and diced**

Blend or juice kale, spinach, mango, tangerine, and kiwi together for a snack or breakfast.

iAddict Mix

1 cup chopped cooked broccoli

½ cup peas, raw or cooked

1 carrot, diced

1 teaspoon extra virgin olive oil

1 teaspoon freshly squeezed
lemon juice

Salt and pepper, to taste

Fresh cilantro, chopped (optional)

Put all the vegetables in a bowl. Dress with olive oil, lemon juice, and salt and pepper. Sprinkle some cilantro on top, if you like, and enjoy as a fresh, crispy side salad.

iDip

1 cup cooked quinoa

½ cup black beans

1 red bell pepper, chopped

1 white onion, chopped

Hot sauce of your choice

Cilantro (optional)

Cook the quinoa according to package directions or buy it premade. Mix together the black beans, bell pepper, and onion and add to the quinoa. Stir in your favorite hot sauce, such as Sriracha, buffalo, chipotle, or plain old Tabasco. If you do not like spice, use olive oil and lemon juice. Optionally, top with cilantro. Use as a dip with celery, green bell pepper sticks, or corn tortilla chips.

Ultimate iSalad

1 cup kale, roughly chopped
without the stems

Juice of ½ lemon

4 tablespoons extra virgin olive
oil, divided

2 to 3 cups baby spinach

1 cup chopped romaine

½ cup chopped broccoli, steamed

¼ cup corn, fresh or frozen
(defrosted)

1 carrot, chopped

1 yellow bell pepper, chopped

¼ cup chopped almonds

1 tablespoon balsamic vinegar

Massage the kale in lemon juice and 2 tablespoons olive oil until soft. Add in spinach and romaine. Add broccoli, corn, carrots, yellow bell pepper, and almonds. Dress with remaining olive oil and vinegar and toss well.

MINDSET

Circling back to the #confessions . . .

I get excited when someone likes my posts and (secretly) feel let down when no one does. I know pointless facts about random people on Facebook. I refresh my email inbox endlessly, hoping for news of any kind. In addition to email, I have at least one other platform for communicating with friends, including Messenger, Viber, WhatsApp, and social media. I am fluent in emojis and stickers. I long to go on a holiday inspired by a picture I have seen online. I have bought more apps than books in the past month. I never leave my house without my phone.

"Like" if you can commiserate with any of these.

These are all the intangible, pesky symptoms of being an iAddict. Authorities on the matter have until now recommended various methods of self-regulation, such as checking email only twice a day, closing or removing troublesome apps, and turning the phone off the rest of the time. But we all know that does not work. I myself have tried that for forty days at a time only to go full throttle the day I set myself free, and I have seen the same in countless students and colleagues. But there is another way . . . one more scientific and realistic than self-regulation.

First, let's dissect the science of addiction and being an iAddict. To be addicted is to be physically and mentally dependent on a substance. Addictions affect the brain through a craving for an object. They lead to a loss of control over its use and continual involvement despite knowing the adverse consequences.

This almost always has to do with some level of pleasure being generated in the brain.

All substances that create pleasure release the neurotransmitter dopamine into the nucleus accumbens, a cluster of nerve cells underneath the cerebral cortex. This is often called the brain's reward system. The original function of dopamine release is actually to keep us doing good things we must do for survival, such as eating, sleeping, and moving. All addictive substances, be they drugs, food, sugar, sex, or gadgets, create a shortcut to the brain's reward system by flooding it with dopamine.

So, when you pick up your handheld device and see or read something you like in any way, the nerve cells of your brain release dopamine, delivering a good, positive, pleasure-filled message to your brain. Your brain records this, altering its future response, making you feel happy in the moment and crave more dopamine. You crave the dopamine both emotionally and biochemically. We cannot change our innate biochemical functions, but we can address the mental ties to iAddiction.

Being an iAddict boils down to one thing: wanting more pleasure. This can be in the form of attention, love, gratification, good news, approval, information, or affection, to name a few. The gadget itself represents a freestanding, always open oasis of digital delight. Every time we check our phones, be it our inbox or our social media feed, we search for pleasure and scroll for gratification. The phone creates an escape from our surroundings—crowded train, annoying line, screaming kids—without even moving. This diversion is often pleasure in and of itself. But then, with only a few taps, we can flee into a world with no hassles, no talking back, no demands; it is a yellow click road to Oz.

Email is its own Pandora's box, sucking our time as we both read and write. Each time we check our email we hold our breath in hope of good news. Despite how much banal email pings back and forth, we clutch onto the eternal dream embedded in it all. We get off on email, hoping, just once, it delivers the jackpot.

Social media complicates the matter further, manipulating our desires by providing a breeding ground for endless potential positive reinforcement (was your Tweet favorited?) and uncomplicated, pure love (how many "likes" did your last post get?). By the time we have taken an average stroll through our phone, our brain's reward center is overflowing with dopamine, and biochemically, physically, and emotionally needing more, turning you into an iAddict one swipe and tap at a time.

The Retox phrase to combat iAddiction is *aparigraha*. *Aparigraha* means "non-possessiveness or non-grasping." It is the antithesis of wanting or grasping for more—more dopamine, more pleasure, more gratification—the cycle that plagues us iAddicts in today's modern world. Aparigraha is actually the fifth of ten main steps the ancient yoga philosophers insisted upon mastering in order to find true happiness and before ever stepping on a yoga mat. Superficially it may appear we are constantly on the phone with good reason, but if we understand aparigraha, we know that it is simply a grasp for more pleasure, which will never actually fulfill us. You see, the more we ignorantly grasp, the less we really have; the

more we look outward, the less we can gaze inward, where our real nature and gratification lie. The more we search for intangible satisfaction, the less we will have tangible happiness.

The biggest risk of being an iAddict is losing bona fide happiness while endlessly hunting down digital distractions. Which can and will happen.

To help you beat iAddiction and find real happiness, right here, right now, I have created a two-part mindset program for you. The first is a daily practice to get your head and heart out of the screen and into reality. The second is a six-step plan for starting a digital detox, whether it is a two-week or two-minute one. I have used both with everyone from high-level execs to teenagers and my husband. Retox mindset for iAddiction has been a huge success for everyone who has implemented it, retraining the brain to not grasp for pleasure where pleasure is not actually found.

RETOX

DAILY PLAN

1. **Step Away.** Put it down. Blow it a kiss. Good-bye.
2. **Walk.** Go for one. This can be a thirty-second walk across your living room, a stroll to the water cooler, a hike in the hills, or a lap around the block. Whatever or wherever you can and want, but do it without your phone.
3. **Interact.** On the walk, interact with someone you see along the way. See a person, and either talk to them or simply wave. Shoot them a smile, comment on something you read, ask them a question, share

a story, compliment their outfit, or just simply lift your chin in an old-school head nod.

4. **Connect.** When you are with a person, make a point of connecting with their eyes as you interact. Look at their face, look at their expressions, and listen or notice their response. Absorb their physical reactions, emotions, and pleasure resulting from you paying physical attention to them, even if it is just a head nod of acknowledgment back.

5. **Appreciate.** Close your eyes, even if only for a second, and let your brain absorb what just happened, a physical engenderment of pleasure, a physically induced rush of dopamine to the reward center, and a desire to do it all again. Without the phone.

TIPS FOR STARTING A DIGITAL DETOX

The above Retox plan for being an iAddict should be a daily practice. Here are six additional steps to help you lead a less addicted life, and maybe even take a short (or long) digital detox:

1. Shower and get dressed before you check your phone.

2. Airplane mode is your friend! Turn the phone off or on airplane mode before bed, in between meetings, during meals, and when you really, truly are not awaiting urgent news.

3. Buy a real newspaper or magazine and let your fingers get dirty from the ink.

4. Delete all non-essential apps from your phone. You know the ones I am referring to . . . Admit it, face your scrolling facts, and delete them!

5. Leave your phone at home or on your desk for one errand a day, in addition to the above practices.

6. Stare into space and let your mind wander for one to three minutes a day.

Retox Soundtrack:
"Hypnotize" —THE NOTORIOUS B.I.G.

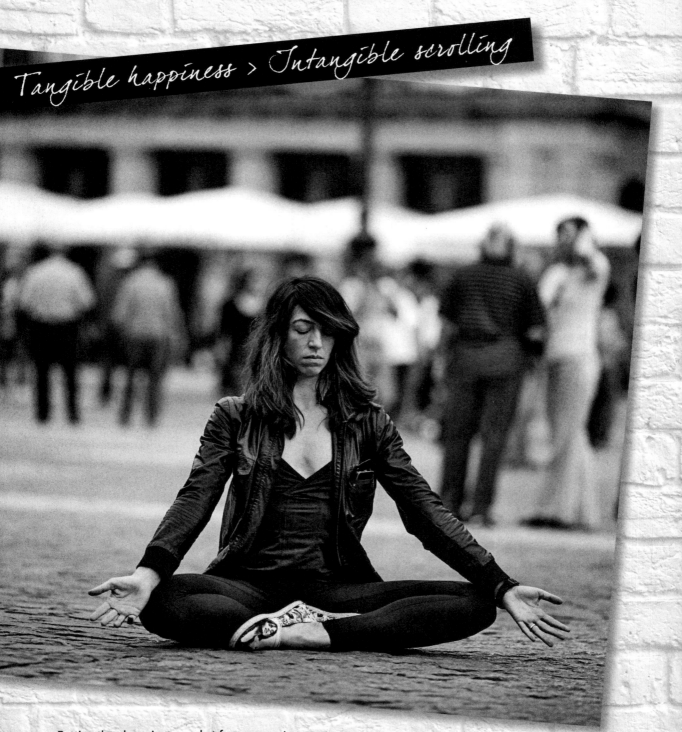

Tangible happiness > Intangible scrolling

Putting the phone in my pocket for a moment.
Texas.

ENERGIZER BUNNY

THE LOW ENERGY SOLUTION

No Pain, No Gain

IN MY EARLY TWENTIES, I worked from 5 a.m. to 6 p.m., sweat from 7 p.m. to 9 p.m., dined and partied till 2 a.m., then got up in one pretty good-looking piece to do it all over again, seven days a week. Without coffee. Those were the days.

How did I do it? How did *you* do it, you may wonder now as you get by only with the help of your afternoon caffeine fix and eagerly curl up on the couch with a Netflix marathon rather than throw back a midnight martini on a workday. Were you superhuman, young, or just crazy? And what's wrong with us now?

Low energy is an overly common phenomenon: the 6 a.m. "Are you kidding me's?!" as the alarm goes off; the 3 p.m. blahs; the 7 p.m. lazy dinner cancellations—they happen almost every day to almost all of us. Feeling sluggish is the norm, high energy a mere mirage in our lethargic, listless minds.

Fear not, you are not old. You are not boring. Your energy is not gone. It is merely hidden under layers of life. It is now up to me, you, and Retox to unearth it.

Let me tell you about Karen, a one-time lover of weekend naps and afternoon sugar rushes who avoided going out at night. In truth, Karen was simply so low on energy all the time that these were not passions, but rather survival necessities. She was always tired, constantly craving a bed, a hit of caffeine or sugar, or a way to escape into one or the other. Which, at thirty-four, made absolutely no sense, and was a tragic waste of a beautiful, vivacious personality the world needs.

When Karen contacted me, she was despondent, dejected, and worn-out. She was sick of being tired all the time, bored with constantly needing energy, and utterly confused about what was the right diet, sleep pattern, or workout to make her feel perky and alive. Relationship after relationship took a hit, as she would be too drained (or lazy) to go out for a drink, dinner, or even a movie. She could not keep a boyfriend, as she would be too tired to maintain healthy intimacy. Her clothes were tight and her skin a mess, as her caffeine and sugar intake had been steadily increasing across daily snacks. And she was just . . . how do I say it? . . . boring and annoying, as she endlessly whined about being tired, and used her low energy as a crutch, thus sucking vital energy out of everyone around her. Honestly, Karen was no fun to be around; I do not even think she liked to be around herself.

202

Luckily, my experience with giving people energy boosts goes back to my time on the trading floor, where our daily 7 a.m. morning meeting was already two hours into the work-day and one hour before any normal person would be clocking in. Everyone around me lived on ginormous Starbucks lattes (with extra shots of espresso), subsisted on greasy order-in lunches and 4 p.m. vending machine runs, and slumped into their chairs a millimeter a minute, simply begging for the day to end. My colleagues constantly chided me about my atypical afternoon snacks—a tomato soup, salad, or half an avocado instead of chips or a donut—my frequent decaf coffees, and my perky chatter. They routinely asked if they could "plug themselves in" to my "natural force." I told them it was partly natural, yes, but really my energy was largely due to how I sweat, ate, and thought. I started sharing my secrets with my colleagues at Morgan Stanley, then my clients of I.AM.YOU., then Karen, and now you. I promise you, these Retox energy-boosting tips work and are better than what-ever number 4D is from the vending machine. They will create permanent changes in your energy, inside and out.

YOGA

It's kind of funny that most people associate yoga with relaxation. I mean, totally go to yoga and relax, be my guest, whatever is going to chill you out. But yoga was never, ever in-tended as a tool for relaxation; rather, it's an instrument for energy cultivation.

Yoga, as we discussed earlier, is meant to harvest and increase your natural energy. The poses, when aligned and done correctly, paired with a proper yoga breath, are de-signed to concentrate and amplify your innate energy reserves. Akin to acupuncture's nee-dles, they are said to uncover energy reserves trapped and hidden across the inner channels of your body, and then bring that energy into the central line, where it can grow and you can thrive. Yoga is actually about shifting and fos-tering your energy, and not at all about chilling it out.

Retox yoga for low energy does not include a twenty-minute Child's pose. Sorry! It instead moves your insides to rejuvenate and feed your outsides. Retox is about uncovering and fostering all the energy you already have, but cannot always find. Let's get started.

RETOX

DESK FIXES

STAND

Stand up wherever you are. Bring your belly button to your spine. Lift your chest. Roll your shoulders up toward your ears then down your back. Inhale, lift your arms up. Do whatever work you need to do while standing, or just stand for a few moments to let your body reenergize.

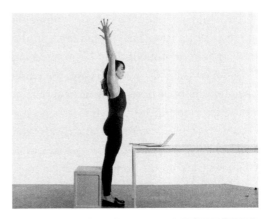

ENERGY BREATH*

Lift your arms straight up and open them into a V. Inhale to a comfortable level. Begin short, sharp breaths out of the nose, where the inhale is simply a reaction to the exhale, as the diaphragm pumps on the abdominal wall. It should feel somewhere between sneezing and blowing your nose. (If you are pregnant, skip khapalabhati.) Keep these up for one minute, energizing your body with each pump.

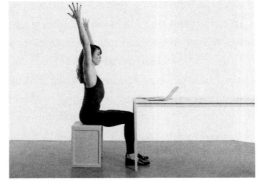

TWISTS*

Inhale, sit up tall. Exhale, twist to the right, bringing your left elbow outside your right knee and your thumbs to your sternum. Hold for ten to thirty seconds. Inhale, back to the center. Exhale, twist to the left, bringing your right elbow outside your left knee and your thumbs to your sternum. Hold for ten to thirty seconds. Repeat left and right.

FLOATING STAFF

Start sitting with your hands by your hips or on the armrests. Extend your legs in front of you and flex your feet. Inhale, press down and lift your hips off the chair. Float here as long as feels good or work toward floating for three to five breaths. Repeat as you like.

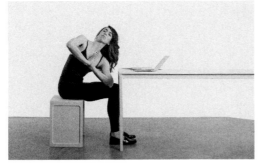

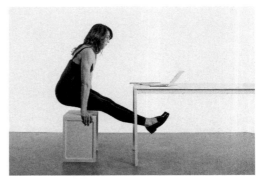

QUICK FIXES

ENERGY POWER FLOW

Start in Plank pose. Inhale here. Exhale, bend your elbows straight back into Chaturanga. Inhale, Up Dog. Exhale, bend your elbows, flip your feet, and come back to Chaturanga. Inhale to Plank. Exhale, Down Dog. Repeat cycle three to five times.

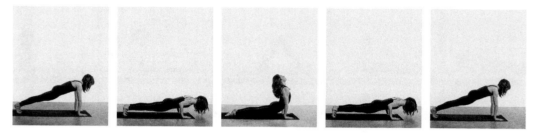

ENERGY LUNGE*

Start standing. Bring your right leg forward into a lunge, and inhale to a comfortable level. Begin short, sharp breaths out of the nose, where the inhale is simply a reaction to the exhale, as the diaphragm pumps on the abdominal wall. It should feel somewhere between sneezing and blowing your nose. (If you are pregnant, skip khapalabhati.) Count fifty-four pumps, then repeat fifty-four pumps with your left leg forward.

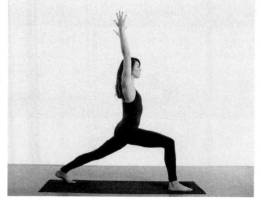

HEADSTAND PREP OR FULL

Start on your hands and knees or in Child's pose. Interlace your fingers and place your forearms on the floor. Bring the top of your head to the floor. Straighten your legs like in Down Dog, bringing your butt in the air. Slowly walk your feet toward your hands, maybe even coming onto your tiptoes. If it feels good and you want to move farther, bring one knee into the body then the other, making a small ball. Do not flick off your toes or jump/hop in any way. If you want to come to a full headstand, straighten your legs up. Do whichever variation feels right; the point is that your lungs and heart are above your head for a bit.

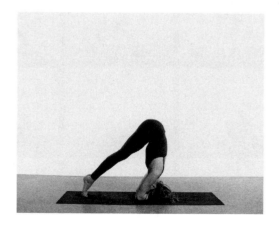

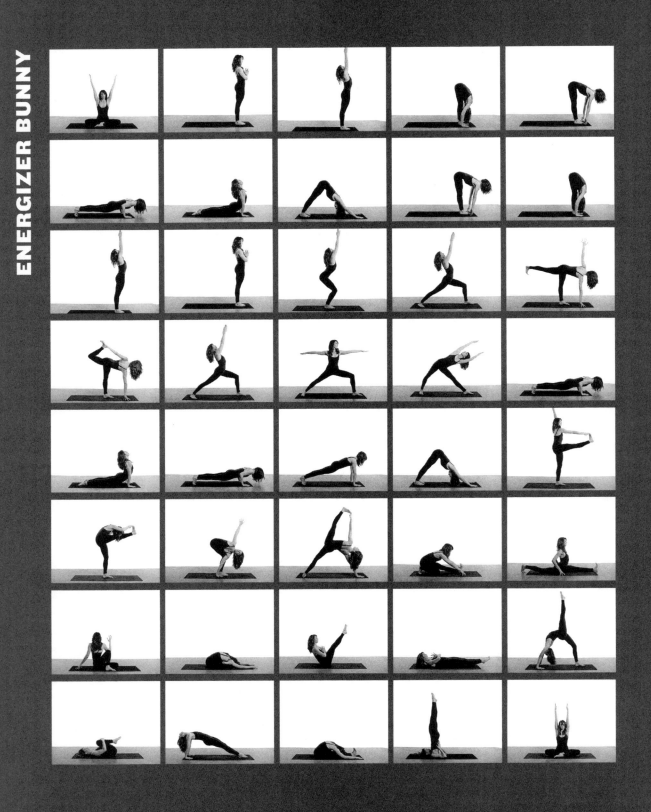

NOURISHMENT

It takes more energy to figure out what you should eat and drink to have energy than whatever you decide on finally ingesting will give you. I am tired just thinking about the process.

Scientifically, energy is actually a very simple concept. It measures the capability of an object or system to do work. When it comes to food, we talk about calories. Basically, a calorie is a unit of heat used to indicate the amount of energy foods will produce in the human body. Aside from what I mentioned earlier in the LSP (page 26), I rarely talk about calories, mainly because obsessing over them usually leads to unhealthy, neurotic eating habits—some of which I, myself, have already wasted too much life suffering from. That said, let's just consider a calorie a unit of energy, and not all calories are equal. To boost your energy, you need to enhance the quality and quantity of calories. Plain and simple.

Retox nourishment for low energy is an optimized plan for efficient, energetic eating. Using these guidelines, you will conserve your vigor for what really matters and soar through the day with a natural oomph no artificial stimulant has ever made possible.

DETOX

The first step of boosting your energy is to dispel and rid yourself of certain nutrition myths that actually diminish your energy reserve and prevent you from being your true energetic self. Adhering to these myths not only saps your energy but can lead to weight gain, bad skin, unpredictable moods, digestive discomfort, headaches, and a litany of other issues you really do not have the time or energy to deal with.

MYTH: ENERGY DRINKS CAN PROVIDE A QUICK, SAFE ENERGY BOOST. I know they are marketed as hours of low-calorie, pure energy in a simple shot, but these bad boys are destroying you from the inside out. Your body is created to process whole, organic ingredients as natural fuel, not to chug chemically created liquids as fake insta-fuel. Energy drinks and shots mess with your body's natural energy production and slowly create a dependence on external, fake energy, rather than a stimulation of your innate internal mechanism. These shots may give you the perception of feeling great, but inside they are sucking you dry. Put them down and let your body start energizing itself like it knows how.

MYTH: LOW-CALORIE FOODS ARE THE BEST CHOICES WHEN YOU NEED ENERGY; THEY WON'T WEIGH YOU DOWN. When staring at the vending machine or snack selection, the low-calorie packages may appear to make the most sense. Yet most low-calorie foods are injected with additives to make them actually taste like something and increase shelf life. Although low in calories, these are the bad, chemical-laden calories that will likely pack on pounds, encourage lackluster thought, foster brain fog, and slow your entire system down. Skip the low-calorie options and go for energy-packed nuts. They may be higher in calories, but remember: calories equal energy, and these high-quality calories provide the fuel that your body needs to function.

MYTH: SUGAR IS THE ENEMY. The truth is, your brain needs glucose to function. If you

207

do not give it sugar, it cannot perform. If your brain cannot perform, you will feel sluggish, tired, and blech. Now, I'm not advocating you grab a handful of gummy bears or a giant frosted and rainbow-sprinkled donut. But sugar in its natural form is an essential component our body needs. Just put down the jelly beans and pick up an orange.

MYTH: PROTEIN POWDER SHAKES CAN PUMP YOU UP. Protein is crucial to maintaining high energy levels, but fake proteins can stagnate your internal systems and thus external output. Protein powders are fake; your body does not know how to naturally process them. As a result, they require more energy to metabolize—energy you could be putting elsewhere. Stick to real proteins such as quinoa, high-quality beef, and eggs and your body will run like a lean, efficient machine.

MYTH: DIET SODA IS AN EFFECTIVE PICK-ME-UP. Diet soda has no calories—that is, energy. It is simply a brew of chemicals and caffeine. And the artificial sweeteners that are "saving" you calories are far from harmless. Aspartame, NutraSweet, and their partners in crime have been linked to cancer. They have also been shown to trigger insulin just like sugar, which sends your body into fat storage mode (especially around the abdomen), engenders water retention in the face, and leads to weight gain.

MYTH: YOU CAN EAT FRUIT THROUGH-OUT THE DAY TO KEEP YOU GOING. Yes, you want some sugar in your diet. But fruit bombing yourself at snacktime is only going to make you more tired than before. The older and more stagnant we get, the harder it becomes to break down all the fructose in fruit, which, unmetabolized, stays in your system and slows it down, making you feel lethargic. Pick one piece or serving of high-water-content fruit such as a slice of watermelon or a cup of blueberries and be on your energetic way.

MYTH: YOGURT OR HUMMUS IS THE PERFECT PROTEIN-PACKED SNACK. Yes, these conveniently packaged options do contain protein and may seem like an easy, clean-energy boost. Yet Traditional Chinese Medicine considers them damp, cold foods loaded with carbs and fat that may make you lethargic. Your "healthy option" may just be draining your energy more.

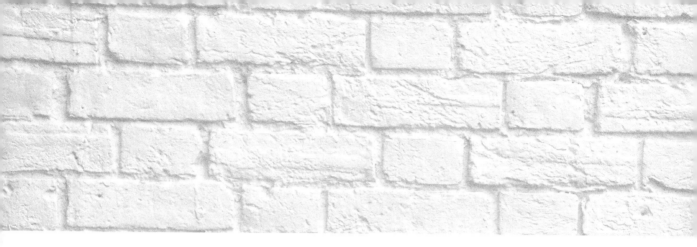

DETOX

Detox the snacks on the left and Retox with the replacement on the right:

INSTEAD OF:	HAVE:
Yogurt	½ avocado
Hummus	½ cup chickpeas
Grapes	Blueberries
Honeydew melon	Cantaloupe
Dried fruit	Fresh fruit
Peanuts	Walnuts or hazelnuts
Coffee with skim milk	Decaf with almond milk
Smoothie	1 apple or ½ banana
Chicken	Fish
Soda	Seltzer with lime, orange, or berries
Black tea	Herbal tea
Latte	Americano with some steamed almond milk
Protein bar	Quinoa Power Punch (see recipe on page 214)
Potato Chips	Quinoa chips
Candy	Raisins or Goji berries, plain or chocolate covered
Chocolate candy bar	Handful of chocolate chips

209

RETOX

These energy-boosting tips will help you maximize your energy levels and potential:

COOK YOUR FOODS. Let's go back to the word *calorie*: It's a unit of heat. Cooked, heated foods are the accessible calories you need; they provide a prolonged, natural energy source. Try having half to all of every meal cooked so that your body can easily tap into the calories and allow you to feel vivacious all the time. Swap raw veggies for steamed or sautéed, and trade juices for soups.

EAT MEAT. I constantly hear of people taking vitamin B shots and iron pills to boost their energy. You know what would be easier, healthier, and more efficient? Just eating a steak. Think about our origins: Our primitive

THE MEAT TEST

I want you to try something: Eat purely vegetarian one day, including a vegetarian dinner. Sleep a normal amount, then track when you get hungry the next morning, what you crave, and how energetic you are. Another day, eat mostly vegetables, per the 2/3 directive in the Keeping in Together chapter (page 37), but include a steak for dinner. Sleep the same amount as the time before, then track when you get hungry the next morning, what you crave, and how energetic you are. You may experience what countless studies have shown: red, protein-packed meat leads to prolonged energy highs and feelings of satiation.

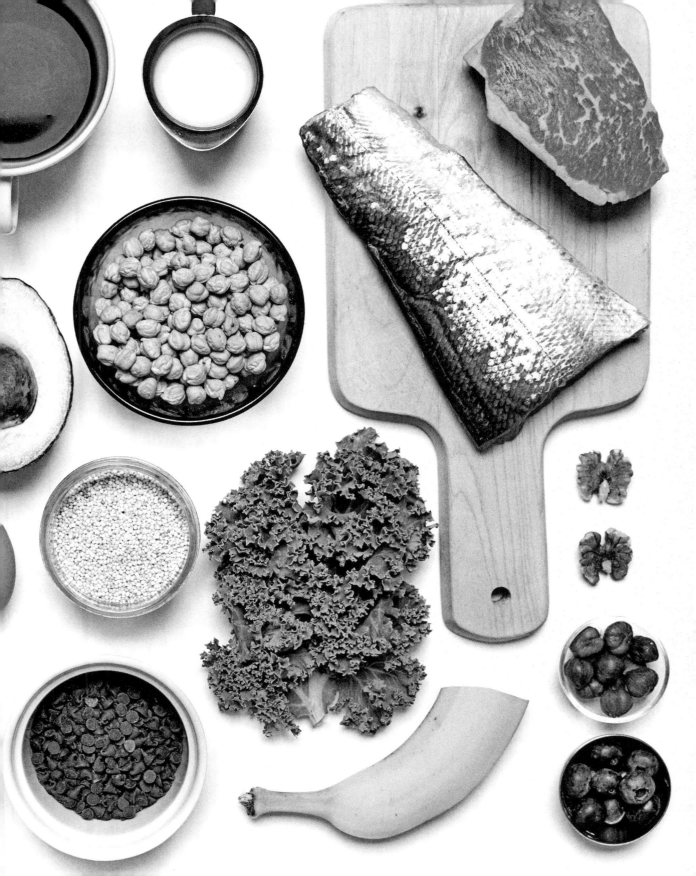

ancestors ate meat with some fruits and grains. Meat was our first fuel. Yes, we have evolved, but not so fast that we no longer need our long-trusted, primary source of energy. The vitamins and minerals in beef are essential to our system. In addition, low energy is often a sign of low iron, a deficiency that red meat can treat. Make sure you eat lean, organic, ideally grass-fed beef two to three times a week, and you will almost instantly notice a surge in your energy.

EAT EGGS. In Eastern medical traditions, eggs are considered the life force. Real, freshly cracked eggs are vital tools to increasing your internal energy reserves so that you have a sustained high throughout the day. Make sure you eat the yoke half of the time and simple egg whites the rest. Also, insist on real eggs, not ones liquefied in a carton, and from free-range chickens naturally fed without soy.

DRINK COFFEE (IN MODERATION). Don't waste energy making coffee the enemy. We all know sometimes there is nothing more effective than a cup of joe. Let yourself have the coffee, I swear it will be okay. But consider making your second cup decaf or half decaf/half regular instead. And instead of filling your cup with milk and sugar, keep it pure and light with almond milk, or drink it black so you get the most out of every sip.

EAT YOUR COLORS. The more colors in your diet, the more sources of energy your body has to pull from. Make sure you have red, yellow, orange, and green in your diet every day, with tomatoes, citrus fruit, lettuces, and more. The brighter your plate, the more vivid and sharp your mood.

MAKE SURE YOU EAT YOUR GREENS! Green veggies are packed with nutrients and hydration, as we well know by now, but also the carbs and sugar your brain needs to think clearly. The carbohydrates in veggies are the type that break down over time, giving you sustained energy boosts as well. When you are feeling low in energy, triple the amount of greens you eat. It is that simple.

DRINK WATER. Often, being tired and lethargic is merely a sign of dehydration. Chug a glass when you are feeling low on energy, and especially before you grab that sugary snack. You may note that the "midafternoon low-energy sugar craving" was nothing more than your body asking for hydration.

SNACKS

Half an avocado

Orange or citrus fruit

Quinoa

Vegetable soup

Almonds and raisins

Three-Bean Salad

I like to make a batch every week and keep it in the fridge.

1 pound green beans, trimmed and cut in half

1 (15-ounce) can garbanzo beans, drained and rinsed

1 (15-ounce) can kidney beans, drained and rinsed

½ red onion, diced

⅓ cup red wine vinegar

¼ cup extra virgin olive oil

Black pepper, to taste

1 tablespoon minced fresh parsley or cilantro

Bring a large pot of water to boil. Add green beans and cooked until tender but still green, 4 to 5 minutes. Drain and run under cold water to stop the cooking. Mix green beans with canned beans and onion. Dress with vinegar and oil and sprinkle with black pepper. Mix well, then top with parsley or cilantro.

Green Energy

1 cup cooked broccoli florets

2–3 cups baby spinach

1–2 tablespoons extra virgin olive oil

1 teaspoon balsamic vinegar

½ avocado, sliced

Mix broccoli and spinach. Dress with olive oil and vinegar. Toss and top with avocado. Enjoy as an energy-boosting snack!

Quinoa Power Punch

You can have this daily as a snack or even as breakfast. It's great as a side dish for lunch or dinner, but to make it a main course, serve over salad or top with an egg or half an avocado.

1 cup cooked quinoa

1 bell pepper, chopped

1 cup fresh, canned, or frozen peas

¼ cup slivered almonds

1 tablespoon olive oil

Salt & pepper to taste

Mix all ingredients in a large bowl.

S² (Steak and Spinach)

You can buy your favorite cut of lean, organic, grass-fed beef, but I always prefer a thin fillet. If you chose a different cut, adjust your cooking time accordingly.

1 (4-ounce) beef fillet

Nonstick cooking spray

1 teaspoon extra virgin olive oil

3 cloves of garlic, thinly sliced

1 (9-ounce) bag baby spinach

Preheat oven to 450 degrees.

Heat a heavy oven-safe skillet over high heat, then spray with nonstick cooking spray or olive oil. Dry beef with a paper towel, then add to pan and cook 30 seconds on each side. Place skillet in oven and cook until the meat is to your liking. Depending on the thickness of your steak, rare is 7 to 12 minutes, well done is 15 to 20. While the beef is cooking, heat oil in a skillet. Add garlic and cook until it just begins to brown. Drop in the spinach and stir. Then cover with a lid and let cook 2 to 3 minutes until wilted. Serve the meat with the spinach, and you will feel your energy boost throughout the next day.

MINDSET

No pain, no gain. This is the premise of most quintessentially American endeavors, and it was the motto on the back of my favorite T-shirt in high school. The original Tibetan yoga philosophers captured the same essence in one word: *tapas*. No, not Spanish food! *Tapas* comes from the Sanskrit root *tap*, which means "to blaze or burn." *Tapas* itself means "discipline, effort, fire, devotion, and suffering through pain." It is a repeated effort, almost like stoking a fire, to achieve a higher goal and become healthy, happy, successful, and free. No pain, no gain.

There are three types of tapas, or effort: that of the body, working hard physically; that of speech, working hard in communicating; and that of the mind, working hard in thoughts and emotions. All will temporarily drain you and make you feel lethargic, tired, lazy, and in need of a boost, but ultimately they will propel you to the next level of you, be that a more vivacious, resilient nature, self-confidence, or an external, more tangible success marker, such as an accomplishment in your work or family life.

The yoga philosophers speak of tapas as the only path to success. It is about working hard, getting tired, and doing it all over again because you know that it is the only way to be a better version of you. It is a burning effort to achieve a goal, a willingness to undertake hardships, put in more energy than you thought you had, and not take the easy way out. In that, you build integrity, strength of character, courage, and wisdom. Through this work you discover your true nature, your true capabilities, the real you. Basically, you must suffer through energy lows to reach any sort of personal highs.

Low energy, say the yoga philosophers, is merely sign of a weak fire. In order to boost your energy, you must stoke the fire. You must endure the low energy waves and simply focus more, applying a constant effort until both the fire and you blaze long and strong without you even thinking twice about it.

Tapas is your fire and your fuel, the cure and the cause. It is all the energy inside you. With this understanding, it is easy to see that the key to boosting your energy is not necessarily to sleep more, do more yoga, and make sure you eat your greens. The Retox secret to energy is as much mental as it is physical, if not more so. It is a practice in effort, with a purpose.

RETOX

This is simple, straightforward, and guaranteed to turn your energy around before you even realize it.

First and foremost, stop saying you're tired. If you keep saying it, it will be. Now, think of someone you love, someone important in your life, or just someone you think could use an energy boost. Bring them to mind.

Now pick one thing you are going to do for them every day. It can be sending them a text to check in, bringing them a flower, picking them up, setting out their breakfast, giving them a prayer. It can be simple and discreet or elaborate and effervescent, whatever comes to mind first.

Pick one thing for one person. Now decide and commit to doing this one thing for them every single day for ten days.

Do not tell them what you are doing. Just stoke your fire for them, and for the energetic you that will result.

Retox Soundtrack:
"Days Go By" —DIRTY VEGAS

Sharing the energy with ten thousand on Central Park's Great Lawn for the Lolë White Tour. **>**

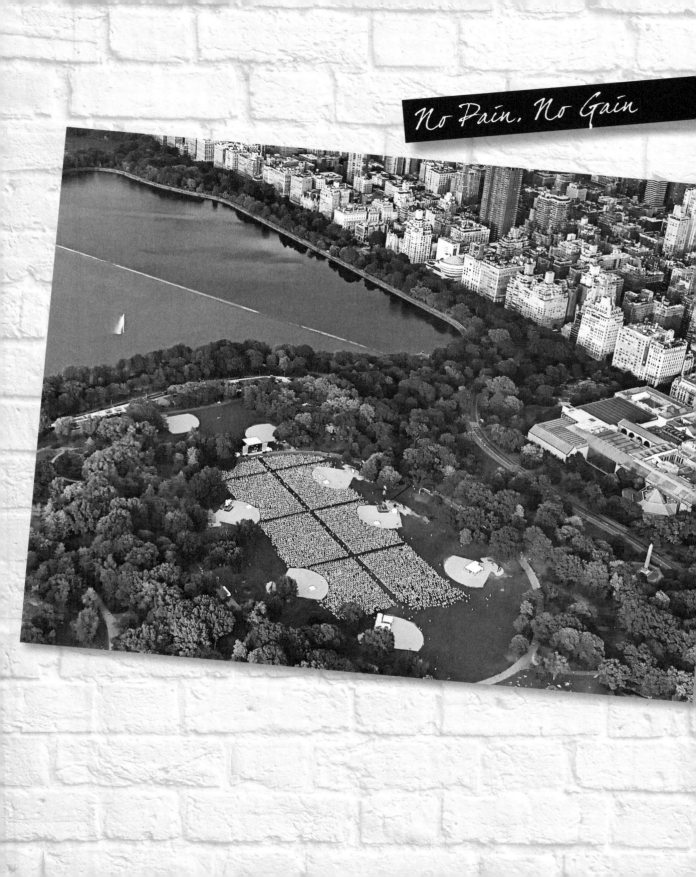

No Pain. No Gain

HUSTLIN' AND BUSTLIN'

HYPERDRIVE

It will all come

I CAME OUT OF THE womb on hyperdrive. As a baby, I never stopped moving, making sounds, or looking for entertainment, even when my pacifier was sufficiently dunked in whiskey by my Texas-bred Polish grandfather. I did not sleep through the night until I was almost two years old and never once napped, no matter what the conglomeration of neighbors and relatives tried in attempts to lull me to sleep. (God, if you are listening and ever bless me with a child, please let him or her sleep.) It must have been quite intense for my parents, especially my mother who was a full-time, high-level exec at IBM.

Perhaps unsurprisingly, at four years old, for the first time, I was told to shut up, stay still, and do nothing. I was running around the front yard inspecting the juniper bushes that lined the left side of the house, when Vicky the babysitter emerged from inside with my little sister. Excited to have someone to talk to, I asked her why the juniper leaves were different from rosemary, and began to explain my recent botanical observations. She instructed me to sit on the front stoop, which, always obedient, I did, and very deliberately told me to not think as much, to ask fewer questions, and to sit still more. I was not pleased.

That evening as my mother attempted to soothe my sister's umpteenth ear infection with a warm clove of garlic (yes, we are a family who followed old wives' tales—and they actually worked!), I asked her why Vicky said what she did. She lifted me onto the kitchen counter, her gold bracelets brushing the white and black tiles, and told me that Vicky was wrong, that questions, thought, and curiosity are extremely im-

portant, that energy and activity are great, and above all, that I should never listen to anyone who told me otherwise. Words cannot explain how clear this day is in my mind—it was probably the first time I was told to go for it, mentally and physically. My next memory around those years is of my mother home full-time, likely so that she could support and guide my natural hyperdrive.

Hyperdrive is a state of fast-paced, perpetual thought and motion. It commences in the mind with a circuitous internal conversation. The voice in the head cycles in loops most often comprised of a series of to-dos, do-quickers, should-have-dones, what-ifs, gotta-dos, and, if lucky, a novel idea. We look to the next thing while doing the current thing, worried about the thing after that. This relentless thought pattern usually causes a physical reaction of constantly doing, constantly going, or as my mother calls it, "Go, go, go."

Modern life not only stimulates hyperdrive—it *is* hyperdrive. Today there is a relent-

220

less pressure to *do*, and to do quickly and effectively, whether that means taking another call, posting something else on social media, checking another round of email, running more errands, or dare I say, pretending to be busy. We are fanatical about accomplishing "things," somehow gauging our self-worth by precisely how many "things" we do. We are a culture obsessed with accomplishments and efficiency, in love with multitasking and racing through to-do lists. It is almost as if you are not on hyperdrive, then you are failing.

The catch is, we collectively exist on hyperdrive, but hyperdrive is taxing our individual existence. It creates an internal physiological engine that pushes us to the extreme, challenging our natural essence. Despite its scientifically proven benefits, we rarely allow our minds to wander, let alone permit ourselves to do nothing and just be. We relentlessly focus on the next goal or task, the next "do" or "must-do" that will somehow complete our self-worth. Worst of all, most often our first breath of the day is the last one we take before trying to fall asleep. Modern society may be fueling the tank, but we are driving the hyperdrive cars.

When I was younger, I never thought there was a problem with hyperdrive. The more we can get done, the better, right? But then, one day when I was thirty, it hit me. Sitting on a park bench in Prague, I had a total breakdown, bawling hysterically into my boyfriend's Budvar, successfully diluting his first Czech beer of our vacation. I had not slept more than five hours a night in ten years, I was working fifteen to seventeen hours a day, five to six days a week, and I was painfully glued to my email. No one was forcing this upon me—I worked entirely for myself at this point. Yet I could not

let go, I could not stop, I could not just say no. I was hyperdriving myself to death.

I am pretty sure my loved ones saw it coming—my parents had been giving me the "slow down" speech for months, and my boyfriend had been turning off my alarm clock a few mornings a week in an attempt to have me sleep in longer (it didn't really work, but was an ingenious idea). Personally, I noticed a shift in my mood from chipper to bitchy, coupled with a fervent desire to cross things off my to-do list, while simultaneously adding to it more and more. I was constantly squeezing in additional appointments in the name of efficiency, consequently sprinting around the city, arriving sweaty and drained in both mind and body wherever I went. My personal yoga practice became a hot mess, with shallow breaths and at an über-accelerated pace—the same class that I taught in ninety minutes would take me forty to do on my own. Above all, nothing I did was particularly fun anymore. Even on vacation in Prague, I couldn't relax and enjoy. I finally realized it was time for a drastic change.

If I kept up this pace, I was going to combust. So I decided to make myself my own patient, using the very same Retox hyperdrive techniques I had just spent months sharing with my client Vanessa, a thirty-nine-year-old financial analyst and television commentator in Manhattan. She slept no more than four hours a night, managed a team of sixty people globally, and literally did not know how to stop. Her biweekly entrance into I.AM.YOU. studio encapsulates it all: She would simultaneously unbutton her blouse while typing on her iPhone, finish a work call on her BlackBerry, gesturing to me, changing into yoga pants, and attempting not to fall while still teetering in her heels.

HUSTLIN' AND BUSTLIN'

Vanessa would abruptly bark at anyone, including me, that she felt she was wasting her time or being inefficient. She lived for speed, multitasking, and "getting shit done," something I can totally relate to.

Yet Vanessa, the epitome of hyperdrive mania, dragged herself to me simply looking to "feel better." Although she initially refused to do or listen to anything I said, she kept coming back for more, even putting her phones away during our sessions and reporting back to me via a rapid-fire email on how she felt every evening. Day by day, I chipped away at her hyperdrive, and before long, Vanessa realized that she was calmer, more effective at work, sleeping better, and happier. To top it off, she had lost a few inches around her waist and thighs, got a promotion, and—it sounds like a cheesy rom-com, but it's true—found true love.

Retox for hyperdrive is not about slowing down, letting go, or doing less. But it is about taking a step back so that you can harness your inner energy and guide it directly to where you want to succeed, in body, mind, career, and life. Here are the tools that I applied to Vanessa, myself, and countless other hyperdrivees across the most chaotic, stressful, demanding cities in the world.

YOGA

Yoga is the quickest way to tell if you are on hyperdrive. If you refuse to close your eyes for longer than twenty seconds, your breath is short and shallow, and you leave or contemplate leaving before Savasana, or you avoid yoga completely, then you are on mental and physical overload. Listen, I get it. Meditation,

annoying non-calorie-burning "stretches," and lying still when you have tons to do is ostensibly a waste of time. As a hyperdrivee, I completely commiserate, but I am begging you to give Retox yoga for hypedrive a chance. It is sort of an I.AM.YOU. house specialty.

You see, most yoga and wellness approaches for this state of being are not designed by someone who is actually on hyperdrive, or who even understands it, let alone deals with dozens of hyperdriven students in the most hypercrazy city in the world, Manhattan, on a weekly basis. Other experts often suggest a regular, long morning meditation and some soft, static stretch-focused yoga . . . which would naturally encourage any person who has anywhere near the baseline activity level we are talking about to either completely banish yoga altogether or simply swoop into class for the "necessary" parts and then rush out. Been there, done that.

Retox yoga, on the other hand, is designed in a way that leverages your hyperdrive cycles, then guides you to a still, calmer state from there. First, I let you go through your circles of mental and physical energy—why fight it? I distract you a bit with funky moves and music, throw in some cardio and strength challenges that force you to focus solely on what is going on, and push you just hard enough so that you have to pay attention to the moment, thus releasing some of the gasoline. With Retox yoga, you eventually arrive at a point where you are patiently begging for stillness, in body and mind, and I oblige. Think of it as a sweaty, moving meditation that manually shifts your internal gears (and will simultaneously help you burn fat, but that's just a multitasker's perk).

222

RETOX

DESK FIXES

LION'S BREATH
Take a deep inhale. Exhale strongly out of your mouth, sticking your tongue out, optionally dropping your head down as well. Repeat one to five times.

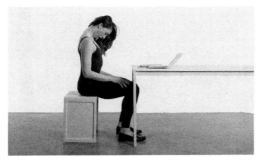

BALLS OF HANDS TO FOREHEAD
Place the heels of your hands on your forehead, either right at the eyebrows or just above them, whichever feels best. Let your fingers relax and press the heels into your forehead with as much pressure as feels good. Breathe through your nose for five to ten breaths.

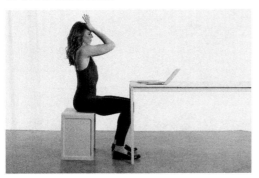

HOVERING CHAIR
Press your feet into the ground and lift your butt off the seat. Hover in Chair pose with your palms on your thighs. Hold three to ten breaths or as long as feels good.

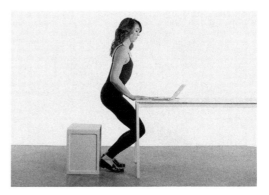

ANGLED STANCE
Stand up and place your hands on the desk or table. Bend forward to a 45-degree angle. Press down on the desk and engage your triceps. Inhale, press hard enough that your feet float off the floor an inch or so. Try to catch some air for one to three breaths, then repeat as feels good.

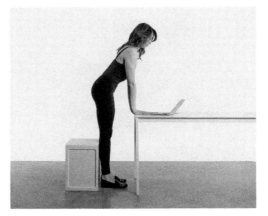

Bonus!

RANDOM STARE
This is as easy as it gets. Put down whatever you are doing and just take a look around. Gaze wherever your eyes land. Stay as long as you like, breathing naturally.

QUICK FIXES

HYPERDRIVE FLOW

Start in Plank pose, with your shoulders over your wrists, your elbows straight, and your body parallel to the floor. Inhale here. Exhale, bend your elbows straight back to a 90-degree angle, making sure your shoulders are no lower than your elbows. Inhale into Plank pose, straightening your elbows. Repeat one to three times.

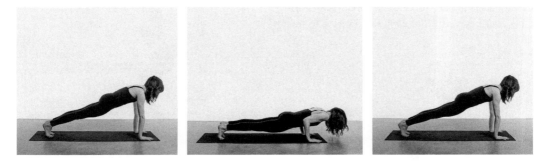

THREE-LEGGED PLANK

From Plank pose, lift your right foot up as high as possible. Hold one to five breaths, then put it down and repeat with the left foot. Make sure your wrists are under your shoulders and your elbows are straight, abdomen lifting the whole time.

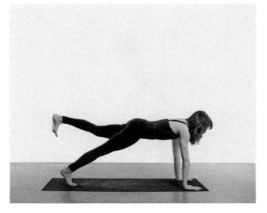

WIDE STRADDLE

Start sitting with your legs spread as wide as possible into a V. Flex your feet. Inhale, sit up tall. Exhale, fold forward in between your legs. Either reach your arms forward, palms on the floor, or grab your big toes. Try to reach your chin to the ground. Hold here five to ten breaths, actively using your arms and flexing your feet.

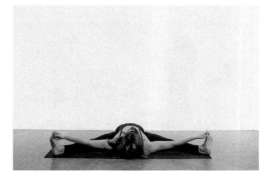

224

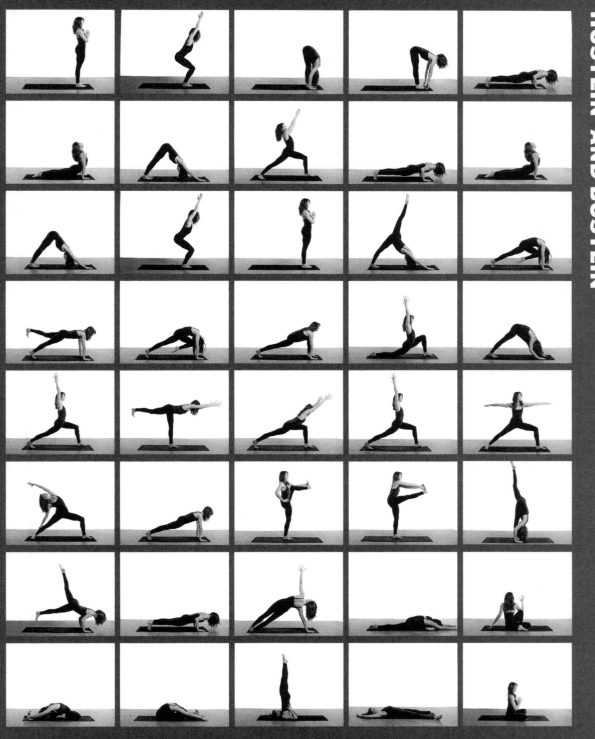

NOURISHMENT

Soon after my not so minor Eastern Bloc meltdown, I got it together and created a new paradigm for an intense, but not hyperdriven, existence, which lasted until the infamous WP took over—wedding planning. I had sworn to myself that I would never become *that* woman, and my fiancé and I made a pact to not fight during the WP process, so in theory all was dandy. Yet one day, after I had a rather, let's say, "animated" phone call with a wedding vendor while standing on the corner of Fifth Avenue and Nineteenth Street (so sorry to any of you who may have walked by), I caught myself racing out of a juice store, $13 bottle of green juice in hand, eager to gulp down my 4 p.m. "lunch" for the third day in a row. I chugged the first bit, but then stopped dead in my tracks and realized that, indeed, I was on hyperdrive again. I dropped the bottle in the trash and decided to sit for a proper meal of a couple slices of pizza and a salad at the joint on the corner. I had to nip the hyperdrive in the bud before I turned into a crazed, emaciated bridezilla.

Like with everything while on hyperdrive, general nourishment tends to be extreme. Either we eat too fast, or we don't eat at all. Often we do not even register what we have or have not ingested, inhaling anything as we actively do something else. All of this wreaks havoc on our digestion, by slowing it down when we do not eat then demanding too much from it when we finally do, and can often lead to intense Alien Baby bloat, headaches, and more.

Retox methodology provides you with clues that you may be on hyperdrive and tips to combat them, followed by recipes that will not only feed you on your crazed days, but also soothe you as you prepare them.

DETOX

Avoid these habits, or use them as clues to your hyperdrive:

1. You "forget" to sit. Almost everyone on hyperdrive "forgets" once in a while, even the biggest of eaters like me.
2. At least one meal a day is eaten while walking, commuting, or in the car. If you are eating in a public setting while in transit, you are guilty of hyperdrive as charged.
3. You finish your plate before anyone around you. You are eating so fast that you stare bewildered at those around you, wondering how they could take so long.
4. You barely chew. Forkfuls scarfed down go from the plate to your stomach almost in one fell swoop.
5. You can't remember what you ate the day before. Food has moved so low down your priority list that you simply cannot remember, or do not care to remember, how you fueled yourself hours before.

RETOX

Here are some tips to help tame your hyperdrive tendencies:

1. Eat three meals a day plus snacks. Recipes for quick grab-and-go ideas follow.
2. Stop and sit at a table. Sit and partake in normal humanity.
3. Take a breath between each bite, thus slowing down the entire pace of your meal. Have this be the new pattern: inhale, insert forkful, chew, three deep full breaths, repeat.
4. Reduce coffee, green and black tea, as well as all caffeinated sodas (sodas should be cut out generally anyway!). Caffeine almost makes you feel high when you are on hyperdrive; try to cut it out or at least keep it to just one cup before noon so that your body can attempt to obtain a normal rhythm for the rest of the day.
5. Cook or bake once a week. Use cooking and baking aromatic, delicious foods as a moving meditation to manually shift you into a more balanced gear, nourishing your body and mind at once. Pasta sauces and baked goods are the best.

SNACKS

Almonds

Popcorn

Carrots

Clementines (easy to peel)

Soup (if you don't slow down, you will burn yourself)

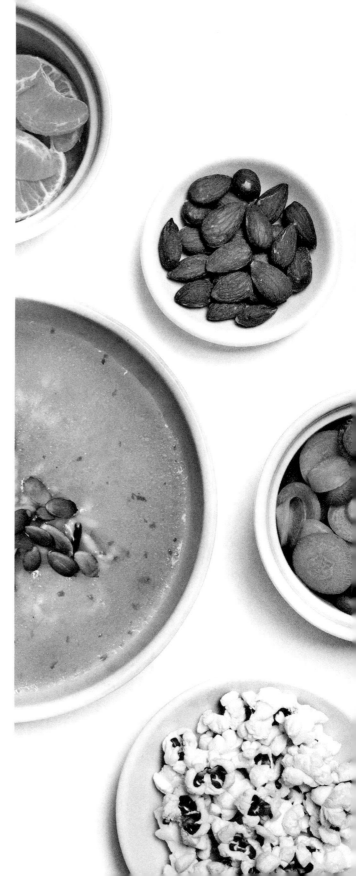

RECIPES

Dice-and-Dash Mushroom and Spinach Frittata

Grab a slice each morning on your way out the door so you are fueled for whatever the day brings.

1 teaspoon extra virgin olive oil

1 (10-ounce) container sliced mushrooms

2 cups baby spinach, thoroughly rinsed and dried

6 eggs

Salt and pepper, to taste

Hot chili flakes (optional)

Heat oil in a large pan over medium heat. Add mushrooms and spinach. Let cook while you crack the eggs into a bowl and whisk. If you would like to use egg whites, use 12 egg whites, or use half and half (3 full eggs, 6 egg whites).

Before the vegetables are fully cooked, add the egg mixture to the pan. Season with salt, pepper, and hot chili flakes, if you like. Cover with a lid for 10 minutes or until eggs are fully cooked. Flip over onto a plate when it is done, and cut it into slices.

Cali Chopped Salad

You can make this for yourself or create it at a salad bar.

1 head romaine, finely sliced

1 pint cherry tomatoes, sliced in half

½ cucumber, chopped

1 stalk celery, chopped

½ carrot, chopped

½ cup canned garbanzo beans, drained and rinsed

½ avocado, diced

DRESSING

1 tablespoon Dijon mustard

¼ cup extra virgin olive oil

2 tablespoons balsamic or red wine vinegar

Throw all salad ingredients into a large bowl. In a small bowl, whisk together all the dressing ingredients until the dressing starts to thicken. Toss the salad with the dressing and enjoy every bite.

Pasta al Pomodoro

Pasta al dente has been scientifically proven to be leaps and bounds better for you than overcooked pasta. Don't keep the pasta in the water for more than 12 minutes as it may become mushy.

1 tablespoon extra virgin olive oil

2 cloves garlic, thinly sliced

½ white onion, diced

3 cups chopped tomato

3 pinches salt

1 (16-ounce) package pasta of your choice

Parmesan cheese (optional)

Heat oil in a large pan over medium heat. Add garlic and cook for about 2 minutes, then add onion and cook until the onions are completely soft and translucent. Add the tomatoes to the pan, along with salt, stir and cover. Whatever you do, do not hyperdrive and lift the lid, just let it all simmer there over medium heat. After about 10 minutes, give it a stir, cover, and let it continue to simmer.

While the tomatoes are cooking, fill a large pot with water and bring to a boil. Salt the water and add pasta, cooking according to package directions.

Once the tomatoes are fully cooked and their juice has created a sauce, pour freshly boiled and drained pasta into the pan with the sauce. Stir, sprinkle with Parmesan if you like, and enjoy!

Chocolate Chip Cookies

Baking has a soothing element, and the smell of these cookies is heaven! Lick the bowl while you wait for the cookies to bake and let the smell infuse your body.

2 eggs

1 teaspoon + extra splash pure vanilla extract

¾ cup brown sugar

¾ cup white sugar

2 sticks unsalted butter, softened

2 cups flour (your choice: all-purpose, whole wheat, or almond)

1 teaspoon salt

1 teaspoon baking soda

½ cup flaxseeds (optional)

½ cup chopped walnuts (optional)

1 (12-ounce) bag chocolate chips (semisweet, milk, or dark)

229

(recipe continues)

Preheat oven to 350 degrees.

In a big bowl, mix together eggs, vanilla, brown sugar, white sugar, and butter. Mix until smooth. Slowly add in flour, salt, and baking soda. When the dough is smooth, you can decide to go omega and add the flaxseeds and/or walnuts. Stir together well. Add in chocolate chips, and mix.

Use a tablespoon to scoop out the dough, form into balls, and place on a cookie sheet lined with parchment paper or another nonstick element. Bake 12 to 15 minutes.

MINDSET

As an innately hyperdriven teenager addicted to sweat, endorphins, speed, and forward motion, tennis was the closest thing to a stagnant inferno I could have imagined. Trapped and netted in, unable to communicate or interact with anything other than a metal waffle on a stick and a fuzzy, inanimate ball. Yet my parents insisted I play, claiming it would be "good" for me, and as usual, they were right.

After suffering through weeks of tennis camp (aka hyperdrive agony), where they hollered at me to "slow down" every other shot, I oddly became fond enough of the sport to join the high school team, ultimately captaining it and heading to the Northern California state championships. I am no Steffi Graf, but I started to discover the rhythmic nature to tennis, one that forces you to slow down, stop, and, above all, be patient.

My natural tennis instinct is to swing into the ball as fast as possible, sprint back to center court before the stroke is complete, bounce around, prep for the next shot, then quickly swing again, look up at where it's going before I have finished the stroke, get annoyed at myself, sprint back to center, kick myself for not playing well, and repeat. Talk about hyperdrive!

This hyperdriven tennis process ultimately led to balls popping straight up or smack into the net, with endless anguish and words not suitable for print here spewing out of my mouth. There is nothing enjoyable about the game in these times, for me or anyone around me, just as there is truly nothing pleasurable about hyperdrive. Focusing on where the ball is going rather than the stroke sets you up for a bad shot and a bad match. Yet my father, the very man who dragged me onto my first tennis court, solved the problem for me, reminding me that the only way to play well is simply to slow down, follow through, and be patient. Funny that's what the ancient Tibetan Buddhists said about life, too.

Kshanti, or "patience" in Sanskrit, is considered one of the six qualities necessary to achieve happiness, health, and success, or as the Tibetan Buddhists call it, enlightenment. It comes along with kindness, generosity, joyful effort, stillness, and wisdom, yet for me and most of my clients plagued with hyperdrive, patience is the most challenging. Patience, says Tibetan Buddhist theory, is not about becoming apathetic, indifferent, or detached—hitting the ball perfectly over the net and winning are definitely the goal—but rather about systematically breathing through the process and not getting angry when it does not go right.

For someone on hyperdrive, patience likely seems not only insane, but unnecessary, an absolute impediment to efficiency, efficacy, and optimization. Yet as I have learned over the years, patience is the single most important ingredient to wellness and success, whether you care about enlightenment or not.

Without patience, you miss everything going on around you, and every future opportunity coming your way. You can stay on hyperdrive all you want, but without a dash of patience and a dose of Retox, you will likely drive by everything you are gunning for without even realizing it. Thankfully, I have a solution.

RETOX

The easiest thing to do for hyperdrive is to lie on the ground and just stare, ideally at the sky, but the ceiling works as well. Seriously, just plop yourself down, let go of what you are holding—both your thoughts and your emotions, and as if in some Woodstock-style high, just look up blankly. This will force your mind to just be, activating your default mode and spurring on all sorts of internal nourishment and creativity. Doing this just a minute a day will nurture your mind and body into their ideal gears.

For something a bit more potent, I want you to try one of the simplest of ancient Tibetan Buddhist meditations aimed at engendering kshanti and abating hyperdrive:

Take a comfortable seat, wherever you are and however feels best. You can sit at your desk, on the floor, at the table, on the train . . . Just make sure that your spine is reasonably long and you are not totally slouching. Let your arms relax and hands rest gently on your thighs or knees, wherever feels most comfortable, and let your eyes softly shut.

Bring your attention to the tip of your nose, and start to notice your breath. Breathe through your nose naturally, maybe even starting to feel the air flutter across your upper lip on its way in and out. Just sit, relax, and breathe.

Once you are comfortable and noticeably breathing, start to follow your breath with your mind, inhale and exhale. Once you get used to your breath, I want you to add in a mental saying:

Inhale, *patience*.
Exhale, *it will all come*.

With each breath, you are permitting your brain to disengage from the never-ending loop, allowing in clarity while energizing your entire being, paving the way for a truly optimized and efficient path for your body, mind, and life.

Retox Soundtrack:
"9 to 5" —DOLLY PARTON

Ready to smack the ball. California.

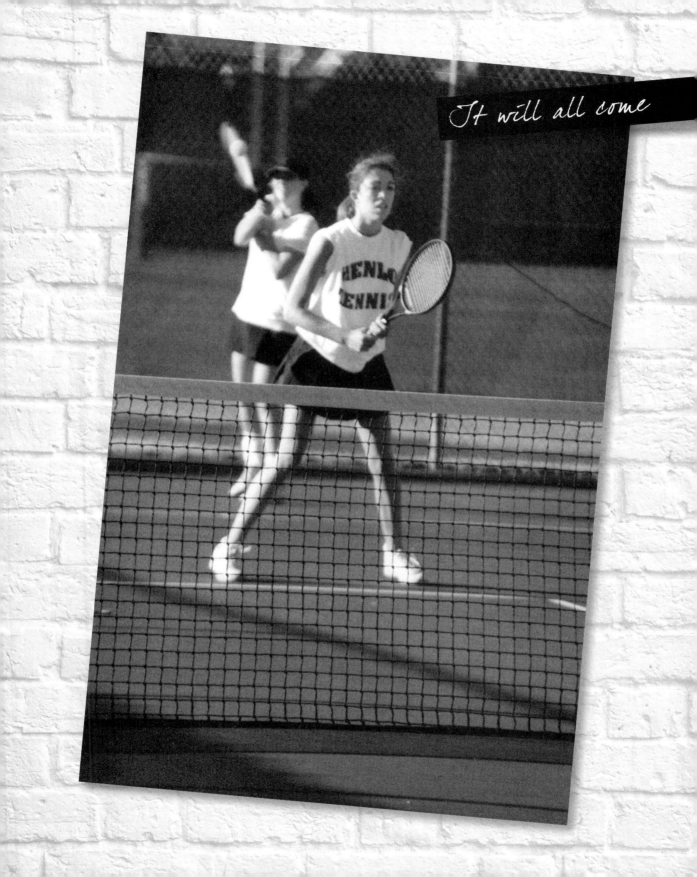

It will all come

MENTAL STDs

MANAGING STRESS

AND ANXIETY

Focus on breathing, not spazzing

I DO NOT THINK THERE is one person I know who is not plagued by an STD. I bet you have one, too, as do I. It is nothing to feel shy or awkward about; STDs are the norm these days, almost a badge of honor.

Stop stressing! The STDs I am talking about are Mental STDs—or stressfully transmitted diseases. The hallmarks of Mental STDs are extreme stress and anxiety. Most often stress is concern over controlling the present moment; anxiety is concern over controlling the future. Stress affects 75 percent of Americans and 60 percent of individuals worldwide. Anxiety is the most prevalent mental disorder in America, affecting over 40 million adults. In China, 86 percent of the workforce is said to suffer with acute stress, and 91 percent of Australians say they suffer from high stress in at least one area of their life. Mental STDs are, unfortunately, all the rage.

What's fascinating about Mental STDs is that they affect the entirety of you. They start in the mind, then permeate your entire system, leading to a litany of undesirable physical and mental conditions, from weight gain to acne, back pain, insomnia, poor memory, headaches, diarrhea, a weakened immune system, infertility, cancer, and straight-up bitchiness, just to name a few.

At the epicenter of these STDs is the brain. When you encounter a stressor, be it an intangible perception—like a thought or worry— or a tangible stimulus—such as coming face-to-face with a man-eating tiger or, in today's world, a pissed-off boss or screaming child—the brain activates the sympathetic nervous system, setting off a fight-or-flight response. This is a natural reaction embedded in us since the beginning of time so that we can eat, grow, live, and survive. This state is characterized by an increased heart and respiratory rate, tense muscles, slowed digestion, and sharpened senses. Basically it preps us to attack or make a run for it. When the fight-or-flight response is triggered, the hypothalamus, located just above the brain stem, secretes corticotropin. This stimulates the pituitary gland, also known as the master gland and located just under the hypothalamus, causing it to secrete adrenocorticotropic hormone, thus activating the adrenal glands. This is where Mental STDs start to get interesting. The adrenal glands sit directly on top of your kidneys, meaning the stress has already moved out of the brain and into the middle of your body. When the brain sends the message of stress, the adrenals go at full throttle, producing and releasing adrenaline and cortisol, the main hormone related to stress. Cortisol gives us energy by converting protein and releasing stored sugar, and adrenaline amps us up by making us more alert and focused. The combination, managed entirely by the adrenals, truly makes us ready for fight or flight, and sets off a chain reaction of events that affects every area of your brain, and thus system.

The fight-or-flight response is beneficial when we're actually in danger. It enables us to outrun that tiger or handle an adversity that befalls us. The problem is that these days the response is triggered constantly, both for real dangers and not. The constant stress we're under keeps the adrenals firing and leads to adrenal fatigue, a condition that causes extreme tiredness, sweet and salty cravings, hair loss, and general aches and pains, among other things.

The thing is, the world out there isn't gonna change; we're constantly under stress and Mental STDs are here to stay. Yet there is not one part of your body, mind, or life that is not affected by the biochemical and physiological reactions caused by stress and anxiety, making a 360-degree Retox cocktail the ideal pour.

Alex, a recent divorcée in Ohio, has two kids under the age of eight, a full-time corporate job, and a new, serious love interest. As if the angst and fighting leading up to her divorce were not enough, Alex now has to juggle a new significant other; alimony to her ex; a chaotic and stressful work environment; balancing time for herself, her kids, and her new relationship; and, well, raising energetic, inquisitive children. Mental STD much?

When I first met Alex, she complained of frequent headaches, neck and shoulder pain, and hair loss. She said she had trouble falling asleep and wondered if lack of sleep was causing memory issues—she was constantly forgetting things and even once forgot to pick the kids up from daycare! She experienced heartburn and stomach bloat often and was carrying at least twenty extra pounds around her middle. After hearing about all she was dealing with, I knew I needed to attack the stress and anxiety head-on, from all angles at once, in true Retox form. At the beginning, Alex was too anxious to even hear what I was saying, but also too stressed to have the energy to really question it, which, thankfully, worked in my favor.

We used yoga to boost her adrenal function and remedy her insomnia, weight gain, memory loss, and digestive issues; we started with at-home yoga routines twice a week and "homework" poses to do for thirty seconds at work, in the shower, or after the kids had gone to bed. I wrote out a menu plan that worked for both family and work life, aimed at cleansing and strengthening the organs most affected by stress, namely the liver, kidneys, and adrenals. And I used Retox mindset action plans to create a habitual method to address life stressors before they set off an acute fight-or-flight reaction.

Alex felt relief after our first session, and to this day, Retoxes on a regular basis, claiming that she now feels better than ever. The surrounding stress inducers have not changed; the method of dealing with them has, which is precisely the Retox cocktail I am about to share with you.

YOGA

I don't know about you, but when I am stressed and someone tells me to relax, I freak out. Even worse is when I walk into a fitness class hoping to sweat out the Mental STDs and the teacher is from la-la-land, prattling on about relaxing and "letting go" instead of putting us through a regimen that will get our blood pumping. Both merely increase my stress levels, make me more anxious, and assure me of a Mental STD for the rest of the day. Perhaps you can relate.

Stress and anxiety create a hyperactive brain/body state. The common anti-stress "re-laxation" yoga that goes straight into a chill, stretchy, attempted meditation is too much of a shock for most systems, and can create additional stressors for your body to process— which is why some people (me, and maybe you) cannot de-stress automatically in a Pigeon pose. Retox has a process, akin to a recipe, to combat Mental STDs with yoga.

The first step is selecting poses and breath structures that will balance hormones and relieve main muscle and organ groups. The second step is to move, shake, and sweat out the adrenaline coursing through your system, thus deactivating the fight-or-flight response. The third is to finally chill.

With this Retox yoga recipe, your body and mind can beat the STD from the inside out. Your adrenals rest, muscles release tension, mind quiets, and entire body rediscovers its intended natural state of homeostasis.

RETOX

DESK FIXES

ADRENAL RELEASE
Place your hands on your mid back, fingers facing down. Try to align your hands with your kidneys. Inhale, imagining the breath going toward your hands. Exhale, gently press the heels of the hands into the back. Breathe. To take it a bit further, inhale counting to five. Exhale, counting to five. Repeat for thirty to sixty seconds.

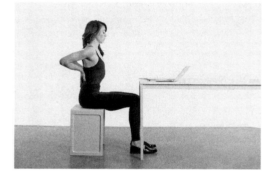

STRESS-BUSTING LION'S BREATH
Take a deep inhale. Exhale strongly out of your mouth, sticking your tongue out. Drop your head, optionally shaking it out as you exhale. Repeat one to five times.

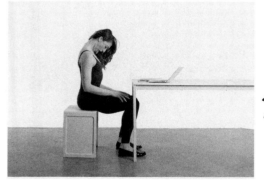

GENTLE TWIST*
Inhale, sit up tall. Exhale, twist to the right. Look over your right shoulder. Hold here five breaths, then repeat on the other side.

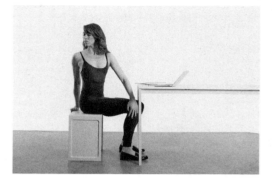

BRAIN STIMULATION
Place your hands on top of your head. Inhale, directing your breath with your mind's eye up into your hands. Exhale, here. Repeat three times, then simply hold and breathe into your entire skull, from the brainstem up toward your hands.

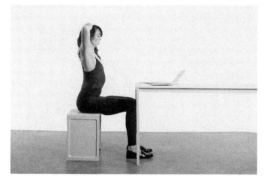

Bonus!

TONGUE RESET
Simply relax your tongue and let it release toward the back of your mouth. Stay like this as you work, drive, wait in line, or listen to a call, and just be.

239

QUICK FIXES

ANTI-STD FLOW

Start in Down Dog, feet hip distance apart, hands on the floor shoulder-distance apart, bottom in the air, and legs straight. Inhale into Plank pose, bringing your body parallel to the floor. Exhale into Down Dog. Inhale into Plank. Exhale into Down Dog. Repeat five to ten times.

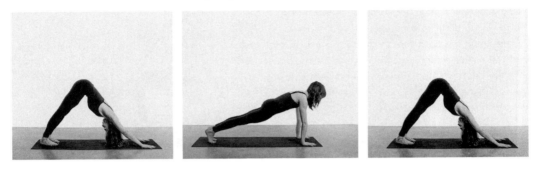

TWISTED FORWARD FOLD*

Start sitting on the floor, legs open into a V. Inhale, lift your right arm up. Exhale, reach and grab your right leg or foot, letting the elbow fall to the floor or on a block, or even to your thigh. Inhale, lift your left arm up. Exhale, reach and grab your right leg or foot as well. Twist and drop your head, twisting and breathing where it feels good for five to ten breaths, then repeat on the other side.

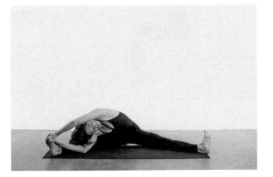

ADRENAL ROLL

Take a thick towel or blanket and make it into a long, tight roll. Place it on the floor and lie down on it, with the roll under your kidney band/adrenals, or middle back. If it feels good, take your arms alongside your ears. Relax and breathe here as long as you can.

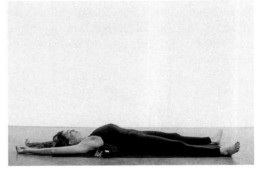

240

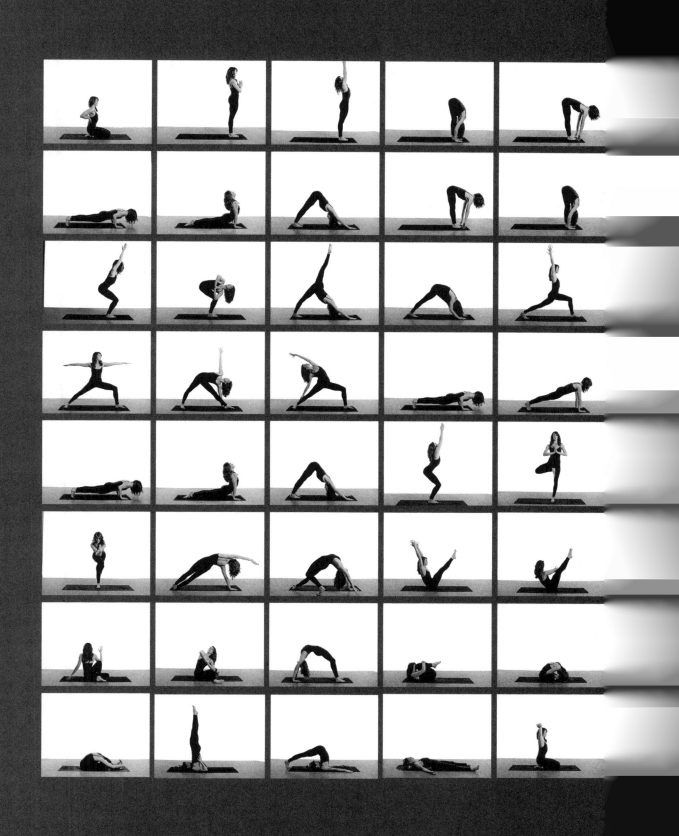

NOURISHMENT

If you have a Mental STD, food is your penicillin. When and how you eat is as important to managing stress and anxiety as what you actually ingest. These Retox tips will help quell your STD, replenish your overworking adrenal glands and liver, and inspire you to eat your way calm.

DETOX

DITCH THE DOGMA. Whether you realize it or not, adhering to some self-imposed nutritional dogma is probably stressing you out. Unless you are clinically, severely allergic, forget the latest trends and just eat the real, whole foods your body is asking for, even if they have the "dreaded" gluten, meat, dairy, or sugar. We have been eating these foods for centuries—they are not inherently bad. So give your mind one less thing to worry about.

EAT UP! When your body goes for long periods of time without food, the adrenal glands release cortisol and adrenaline, the stress hormones we have been discussing. Meaning, if you do not eat, you biochemically stress out your system even more. Make sure you regulate your blood sugar by eating every two to three hours; this is important even if you are not hungry. Always have a solid breakfast, and try to get into a normal eating pattern with ample snacks.

WATCH THE CLOCK. Your adrenal glands follow a natural circadian rhythm you need to heed. Eat breakfast between 6 and 8 a.m., or at least before 10; lunch around noon; and

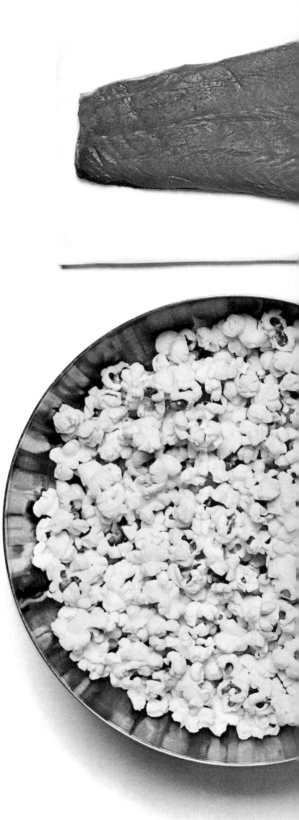

242

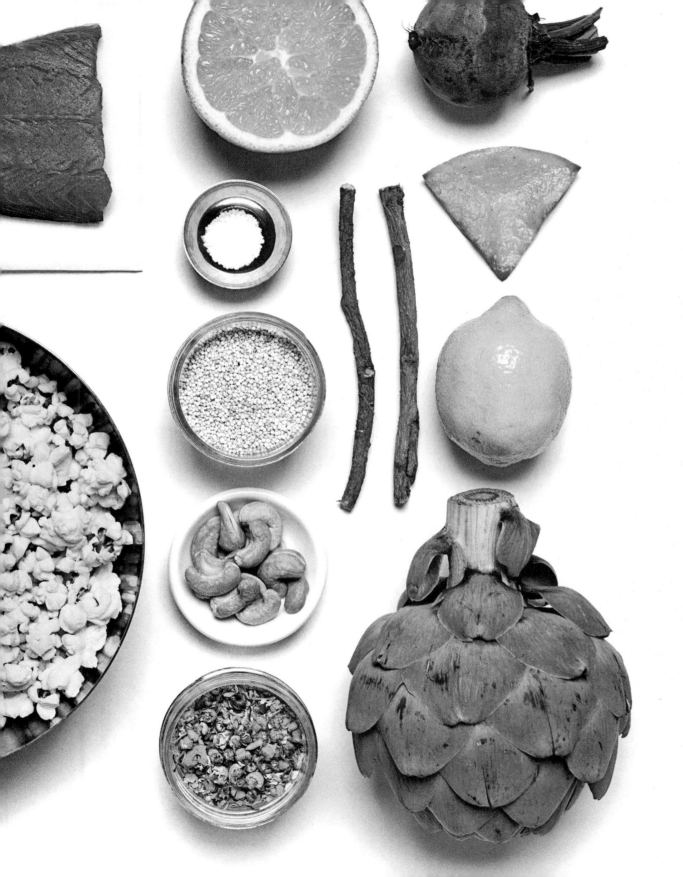

dinner around 6 to 7 p.m. if you can. If work gets out late or you have a social engagement, have a light "pre-dinner" of real, solid foods before your later full meal. This will soothe your system while simultaneously helping your adrenals recover.

COMFORT FOOD ISN'T ALL THAT COMFORTING. I know when you are stressed nothing is more appealing than a brownie, ice cream, chips, and fries, but typical comfort foods are usually quite heavy in saturated fats and calories. These will bog down your system and may even make you feel gross and guilty about eating them, which could, in turn, create more stress as you anxiously try to squeeze in an extra workout to burn them off. When you are suffering from a Mental STD, try to eat clean without junk food.

CHUCK THE CAFFEINE. The scent of a perfect cup of coffee or tea can initially soothe your mind, but the caffeine in them will just add to the adrenaline, and thus anxiety, you are already experiencing. Switch to decaf during extreme Mental STD outbreaks and give your body a break.

JUST SAY NO TO JUICE. I see more stressed-out people juicing than you can even imagine. And you know what? It does not work. Replacing a solid meal with a juice leads your body to think you are starving it, sending it into fight-or-flight, and thus starvation, mode. In addition, running around like a lunatic with a juice bottle without taking a moment to sit, breathe, and, heaven forbid, chew adds additional stress and anxiety. Eat real foods when you have a Mental STD; your body is already in agony as it is.

HAVE THE MUNCHIES. Munching and snacking is a common nervous behavior, and can actually be therapeutic to balance blood sugar, as noted above, as well as distract your cortisol- and adrenaline-full energy. Feel free to snack away, but with good foods that will help your adrenals, liver, and hormones calm down. Berries, oranges, and edamame are good choices. This type of munching will keep you busy and distracted without packing on pounds or adding more stress.

RETOX

Now that we know the "how," let's focus on the "what." Rather than give you a long list of foods to eat that you can probably find on a blog somewhere—and may or may not actually be beneficial—I am going to categorize foods based on how they affect the two parts of your body most affected by stress: the adrenals and the liver.

ADRENALS

As discussed at the beginning of the chapter, when you have a Mental STD, your adrenal glands go into overdrive. You thus need to nourish them. The best way to do so is to cut the caffeine and eat regularly and include the following foods in your diet:

QUINOA. Quinoa is a complex carb that will help regulate your blood sugar levels. Eat half a cup as a snack or side dish, make my Quinoa Pea Buster (page 246), or add to salads or stir-fries.

CHAMOMILE. Sip on chamomile tea throughout the day. It has a naturally soothing effect on the body.

SALT. Yes, this is one of those times you need salt. When your adrenals are working extra because you are stressed-out, they create cortisol. When cortisol levels rise, a steroid hormone called aldosterone decreases. Aldosterone helps your body maintain salt and water in order to regulate your blood pressure and electrolytes. In fact, if you are getting dizzy or lightheaded during these times of Mental STDs, you may have low levels of aldosterone. So salt it up! Add an extra pinch of salt into what you cook (always preferable to raw salting), or sprinkle some high-quality sea salt on your foods. Have salted cashews, crackers, and popcorn around as well to snack on.

ORANGES. Adrenals need vitamin C to do their job, including the production and regulation of hormones. In addition, stress wears down your immune system, so extra vitamin C will give it a boost and help prevent you from getting sick. An orange with breakfast or as a snack throughout the day packs a healthy dose of vitamin C.

LICORICE ROOT. Licorice root contains plant hormones that mimic the effects of cortisol, meaning you can trick your body into thinking you have enough without your adrenals going crazy. Either try a tablespoon of licorice root extract daily, or find some organic, pure licorice root candies or black licorice with high levels of the root and munch away.

SLEEP. Z's are not food, I know, but sleep will be your number one nourishment factor for replenishing your adrenals. If your adrenals are fatigued, you may have a tough time falling asleep, but you have to try to get to sleep. Get into bed thirty minutes earlier or set your alarm thirty minutes later, even if it means commuting to work with wet hair for a while. Your body will thank you.

LIVER

Stress and anxiety are as draining on the liver as alcohol. In Traditional Chinese Medicine, the liver is the main organ to process stress, or *ya li*. It regulates the flow of all qi, or energy, throughout your body. When you have a Mental STD, you need to make sure you nourish your liver, feeding it what it needs to be strong and at ease.

ARTICHOKES. Artichokes are one of the most powerful cleansing and strengthening agents for the liver. Eat them as snacks or as a starter, or sip on their juice with the recipe on page 93.

BEETS. Like artichokes, beets are great for your liver. Add some slices to your salad or plate whenever you can.

GIVE UP THE GOODIES. Temporarily, at least. Avocado, sugar, chocolate, coffee (even decaf), and alcohol—all things I, for one, crave when I am stressed-out—are immensely tough on your liver. Yes, even the avocado. Give them a rest for a bit and you will notice within a couple of days how much lighter and brighter your body feels.

PROTEIN. Your liver needs additional nutrients to be extra strong during Mental STD outbreaks. Make sure you are having a small portion of organic and wild fish or beef at least once a day.

LEMON. Your liver produces bicarbonate, a base that reduces acid. When you are stressed and your liver is on overdrive, its ability to regulate your body's acid levels are hindered, especially if you are downing the alcohol, coffee, and sugar. Keep slices of lemon around to garnish your meals and drinks to balance it out.

SNACKS

- Quinoa chips
- Corn tortilla chips
- Water with lemon and cucumber slices
- Oranges
- Licorice

RECIPES

Quinoa Pea Buster

Quinoa for your adrenals, peas for your liver.

- 1 cup quinoa, cooked
- 1 cup peas, fresh or frozen
- Juice of 1 lemon
- ¼ cup extra virgin olive oil
- Salt, to taste

Put quinoa in a large bowl. Stir in peas, lemon juice, olive oil, and a pinch of salt. Serve as a snack, side, or topped with salmon or an egg if you need a bit more oomph.

Grilled Cheese

Melted cheese has been shown to relax the system, especially when combined with carbs. The veggies are to tone your liver.

- 2 slices bread of your choice
- 1 slice cheese of your choice (Gruyère, Monterey Jack, and Cheddar work best)
- 2 slices tomato (optional)
- 1 artichoke heart (optional)

While warming a pan or panini grill, assemble the sandwich of bread and cheese, adding tomato and/or artichoke, if desired. Place in the pan or grill, and cook until cheese is melted. Eat as is, or with a side of sliced cucumber like my mom used to make for us, and enjoy.

Superfood Pisto

This is a Retox version of one of my favorite Spanish dishes.

1 tablespoon extra virgin olive oil

1 medium onion, chopped

3 cloves garlic, minced

6 large tomatoes, chopped

Salt, to taste

1 large green pepper, chopped

2 zucchini, chopped

½ cup peas, fresh or frozen

1 cup cooked quinoa

Freshly grated Parmesan (optional)

Heat oil in a sauté pan over medium heat. Add onion and garlic and cook until the onion is translucent. Be careful not to burn the garlic. Add tomatoes and a pinch of salt, cover, and let simmer for 15 minutes. Add peppers and zucchini, cover again, and let cook until vegetables are soft, about 7 minutes. Add peas and quinoa, stir, and cook until warmed. You can top with freshly grated Parmesan if you'd like and a side of crusty bread. Enjoy!

Pasta Senza Stress (Stress-Free Pasta)

2 tablespoons plus 1 teaspoon extra virgin olive oil, divided

Salt, to taste

4 ounces dry pasta (I like penne best)

1 (6-ounce) salmon fillet (wild salmon is always your best choice)

1 (14-ounce) can artichoke hearts, chopped

Freshly ground black pepper, to taste

Fresh mint or basil, for garnish (optional)

Bring a pot of water to boil. Add 1 tablespoon olive oil and a pinch of salt to the water and cook pasta according to package directions, 10 to 12 minutes. While the pasta is cooking, heat 1 teaspoon olive oil in a small skillet over medium heat. Sauté salmon fillet, cooking 4 minutes on one side and 3 minutes on the other. When pasta is cooked, drain and pour into a shallow bowl. Add artichoke hearts, remaining tablespoon of olive oil, black pepper, and mix. Place salmon on top of pasta and top with more black pepper and fresh mint or basil, if desired.

MINDSET

Not to stress you out or anything, but Mental STDs are the bubonic plague of our time. They circulate in pretty much every societal setting and industry, and run rampant across all socio-economic and global realms. Given their prevalence and how easily transmittable and transferable stress and anxiety are between us, these Mental STDs are like today's version of the Black Death, a slow, anxious, stressful one.

But you know what the scary part is? Stress is the new happy. We as a society have an almost sick obsession with stress, wearing Mental STDs like a badge of honor on our chests, a proof of our self-worth and consistent contribution to humanity. Just think about how often "stressed" is incorporated into the answer of the very simple question, "How are you?" It seems like if you're not stressed you must not be doing enough or are not important enough. As I mentioned earlier, most stress and anxiety are about control—the former over the present moment, the latter over the future. Yet Tibetan yoga theories teach us that there is actually nothing you can control in the present moment aside from your mind. You cannot control your surroundings, the outcomes of any action, or any moment in the future. All you can control are your thoughts and perceptions; you can only control your mind.

Panic, stress, and anxiety never pay. But staying focused and calm when everyone else is flipping out does. Which is why Retox is so important.

The world out there will not change. It is real, it is intense, and it is unapologetically busy. But it is also serene, organized, and open to endless possibilities. It is up to us to create the peace that is already inside us to find the tranquility in the world surrounding us. It is up to you to eradicate your stress and anxiety, and up to you to prevent it from plaguing your being and everyone around you, for that matter. No one can take your stress away except for you; no one can quell your anxiety except for you.

This is an easy and effective Retox technique that I have used on myself and hundreds of I.AM.YOU.ers plagued by Mental STDs. This technique helps reduce stress and anxiety and quiets the mind so we don't create more. Think of it as a massive dose of Retox Xanax.

RETOX

Take out a yellow legal pad, large notebook, or blank sheet of paper. Yes, old-school, real paper, and a pen (OMG!). Now I want you to start listing everything you have to do. Call the doctor. Mail the checks. Buy toilet paper. Email the report. Schedule a meeting with your boss. Research summer holiday flights. Anything and everything. Think of it as a giant to-do list.

Keep writing everything, line by line, item by item. Spill it out on the page.

When you are done, take a step back, and tear the page out. Place it to the side and begin to rewrite the list, but this time, categorize in some way that makes sense to you. Usually, I put calls in one area, skip a couple lines (because inevitably something else will come up), emails in another, tangible deliverables for work in another, errands in another, and so forth.

Essentially rewrite the list in segments. When you are done, take a step back, but leave your notebook open, pen next to it.

Everything on that page is what you are stressed and anxious about. And it is all there, in one place. And it all fits on a page and is actually not that stressful if you just look at the individual line items. What you are stressed about is the amalgamation of them all, and the potential future items that may be added to that list, and their outcomes.

So, instead of freaking out in your mind in endless anxious unproductive circles, focus on the list, and go through it calmly in whatever order calls you. Go through item by item, and as you complete something, take your pen and strike a line through it. Cross it off the list; take it out of your Mental STD basket.

You will soon notice the list getting shorter, calmly and peacefully, and that you are miraculously STD free.

Retox Soundtrack:
"Knee Deep" —ZAC BROWN BAND & JIMMY BUFFET

MENTAL STDS

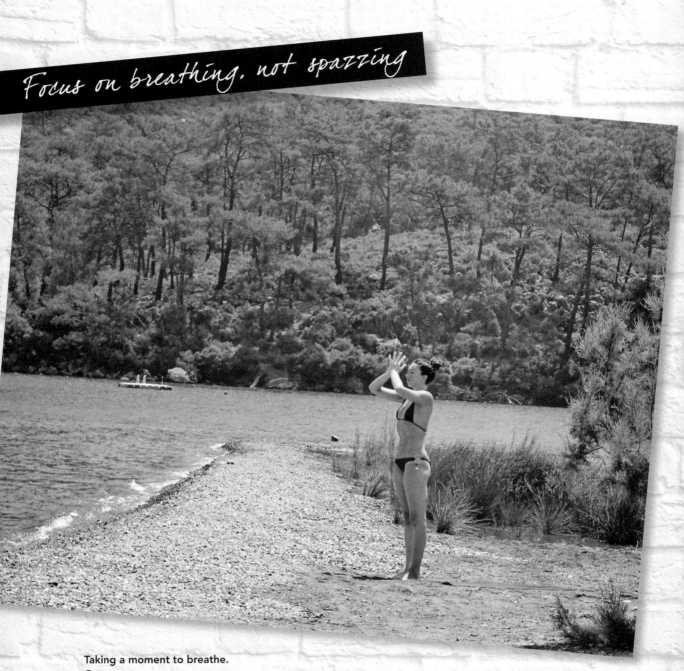

Focus on breathing, not spazzing

Taking a moment to breathe.
Greece.

DANGLING WO(MAN)

I trust change

ON SEPTEMBER 14, 2008, LIFE was good. I was brunching with friends to pre-celebrate my birthday, sipping prosecco and ready to dive into plates of pasta under a pristine NYC skyline. I distinctly recall reflecting on how happy I was. I was kickin' ass at work, goo-goo gaga over my boyfriend, and squeezing out everything NYC had to offer. I loved my job, my man, my city, my life. It had all come together. Twenty-eight was going to be an awesome year.

On September 15, 2008, my actual birthday, life was a hot, horrible mess. Lehman Brothers crashed and filed for bankruptcy, sending the financial industry into total disarray. Morgan Stanley's stock price plummeted to single digits, cutting the value of my hard-earned savings by more than three-quarters in less than a day. The firm quickly lost many vital clients and softly announced a series of upcoming layoffs. My hardworking parents lost a chunk of their savings. And I found out my boyfriend's mother had stage four cancer. Life was officially a disaster.

I went from a state of security and happiness to a black hole of upside-down uncertainty in less than twenty-four hours. I did not know if I would have my job at the end of the week—or if the industry would even exist, for that matter. My boyfriend had returned home indefinitely to take care of his mother, dozens of people I knew had lost their jobs, and my grandmother lost half her retirement. Life on the trading floor epitomized an inferno, with relentless screaming, panic attacks, and desperate shouts for help. I was confused, scared, exhausted, and painfully suspended in uncertainty. I felt like a dangling woman, at the mercy of life and its unknown, endlessly changing circumstances, nothing more than a weakling hanging on by a thread.

Dangling Woman is a term I coined for the way we feel in ambiguous and uncertain phases of life. When you are dangling, you feel like you have no ability to dictate your future, largely because you have straight-up no idea where to go. You are confounded about where to add energy and how to steer the ship of life that is you. You feel like you are swaying between endless options in your career, health, and personal life, unable to discern where, when, or how to land. You feel lost, out of control, and anything but strong and firm. You swing between potential outcomes and opportunities, and suffer from an overarching sense of doubt and hesitation, one often laced with fear. You are somewhere between where you currently are and where you want to be, neither of which you may be able to define. Sound familiar?

The demands, stress, and constant flux of today's existence have made Dangling Woman (or man) a ubiquitous and totally modern life phenomenon. Sometimes dangling arises from a career challenge or shift in your personal life, other times from familial changes or health trials, but either way, it is torturous. You feel stuck but floating, swaying between one thing and another, without knowing what that other thing is or where you will land. You feel removed from everything going on, yet acutely sensitive to any random occurrence that could possibly affect you. As a result, you dangle in your present reality, afraid to take action and fearful that you will never land on solid ground where you can experience joy, confidence, success, or certainty again. You question your self-worth and purpose, maybe even your entire life.

This was certainly the case for my client Jeff, who it seemed was dangling from a thread many miles long. Jeff ran his own company based in Colorado, while his wife was a high-level lawyer in New York City. As an entrepreneur and his own boss, he worked from their Manhattan apartment, but regularly traveled out West to ensure the offices and production ran smoothly. He hadn't been to an I.AM.YOU. class for a few months, and when I finally saw him again, he looked haggard, confused, unhappy, and unhealthy. I could tell from his eyes and discombobulated energy that he was dangling, which he confessed to me a few days later.

Jeff was miserable and bewildered in both his job and his personal life. The constant travel tired him out and detached him from the people and places he loved, not to mention the daily details of his business. Although he was an entrepreneur, he wanted to change his business and career, but there was no clear answer presenting itself as to how, let alone to what. On the personal side, Jeff was no longer connecting with his wife of six years, who worked twelve- to twenty-hour days, and afterward often went out until sunrise rather than coming home, even when he was in town. They had been discussing divorce, but were still living together and making facades of being happily together when out in public. Fights were common between them, and a thick tension pervaded it all. Jeff was trying to be positive and patient, attempting to get control of something, or at least glimpse a silver lining of opportunity, but he was firmly confused, questioning all the decisions he had ever made. He was a bona fide dangling disaster.

Jeff had Retoxed with me once before, recovering from some serious weight and kidney issues, ultimately losing thirty pounds and getting a clean bill of health, so he was willing to give Retox techniques a shot at addressing this dangling crisis. My first step was to get him on a regular yoga schedule, even if it was just five minutes a day. Then I injected his diet with new foods, as I will discuss in upcoming pages, and changed his eating habits entirely. Finally, we talked about strategies he could use day in, day out to stay grounded and techniques he could utilize as scaffolding to fall back on when his dangling state started to really get out of control.

A year later, Jeff is happier than ever in a loving, connected relationship with his wife.

He sold his first business for a healthy chunk of change, and now runs a new one out of New York City. He dangled for a while, but he has come out like a gladiator on top of the world.

YOGA

Here's the thing: When you feel your life is not where you want it to be, your external experience is simply mirroring your internal intangible body. If we cure the inside, we heal the outside.

As we discussed earlier, the intangible body and all the energy within it is said to run through thousands of channels in your body. The majority of Eastern philosophies and traditions of medicine teach this—from acupuncture (which uses needles to move the energy) to Daoism (which uses just breath) to yoga (which uses postures with breath). When things are safe, secure, successful, and grounded in our lives, our energy moves easily through the three main channels in the middle line of the body, as we have discussed. When things are going rock-star-gladiator-I-rule-the-world, the energy is said to be all in the *uma*, the most central of these three channels, known in other yoga traditions as the *sushumna*. But most of the time, especially when we are dangling, the energy is scattered across thousands of channels all over your body, nowhere near your central channel, creating a disarray in your physical body and mind.

The goal of yoga for the Dangling Wo(man) is to bring the energy to the central channel, thus giving you strength, focus, and a more grounded state. Here are some things you can do to help you cut the dangling thread and land on your feet, smiling.

RETOX

DESK FIXES

V POWER BREATH*
Raise your arms up into a V. Open your thumbs and index fingers out. Inhale to a comfortable level. Begin short, sharp breaths out of the nose, where the inhale is simply a reaction to the exhale, as the diaphragm pumps on the abdominal wall. It should feel somewhere between sneezing and blowing your nose. Keep your arms and hands up while pumping for thirty seconds to a minute. Repeat daily. If pregnant, keep your arms in a V and breathe normally.

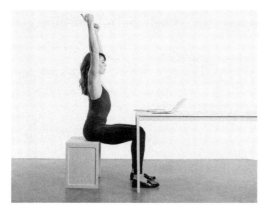

SEATED ANGLED LUNGE
Lean forward to 45 degrees in your seat. Inhale, reach your arms alongside your ears. Look at the tip of your nose. Breathe here.

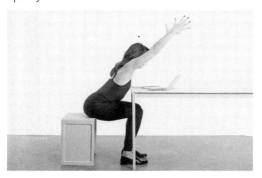

FIST BACKBEND
You can do this sitting or standing. Interlace your hands behind your back. Straighten your elbows and stretch across the front of your chest. Inhale, reach your sternum up; exhale, arch back. Find whatever size backbend feels comfortable Stay here and breathe for as long as is comfortable.

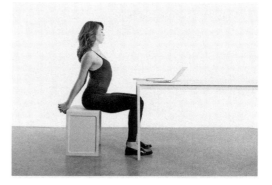

POWER ARMS
Either sitting or standing, inhale and bring your arms up alongside your ears. Exhale, interlace your fingers but point your index fingers up. Pull your hands up, creating more space from your hips to your index fingers. Drop your chin slightly and breathe.

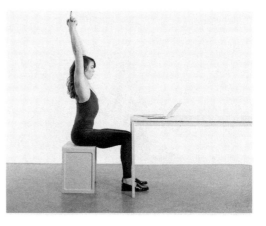

QUICK FIXES

ANGLED LUNGE

Start standing with your left foot forward, knee bent to 90 degrees and right leg straight behind you. Reach your arms alongside your ears. Angle your body forward to 45 degrees. Pull your left hip back and hover your abdomen over your thigh, keeping your back leg totally straight. Hold five to twenty breaths, then repeat on the other side.

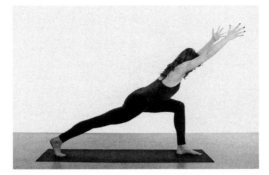

TREE

Start standing. Inhale, bring your right knee into the chest. Exhale, place your right foot on the inseam of the left leg, above or below the knee but not on it. Press your inner thigh into the foot. Bring your hands to your heart. Hold here five to ten breaths, then repeat on the other side.

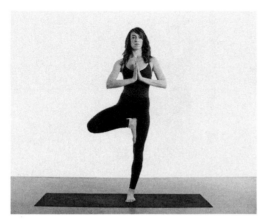

INCLINED PLANE

Start sitting with your legs extended in front of you. Place your hands on the floor by your thighs. Inhale, lift your butt and legs off the floor, pressing your hands and feet into your floor. Exhale, drop your head back and breathe here five to ten breaths.

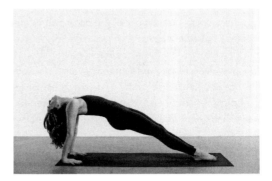

FETAL POSITION

Lie on your back and bring your knees into your chest. Roll onto your right side. Rest your head on your right arm. Breathe here.

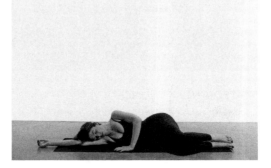

256

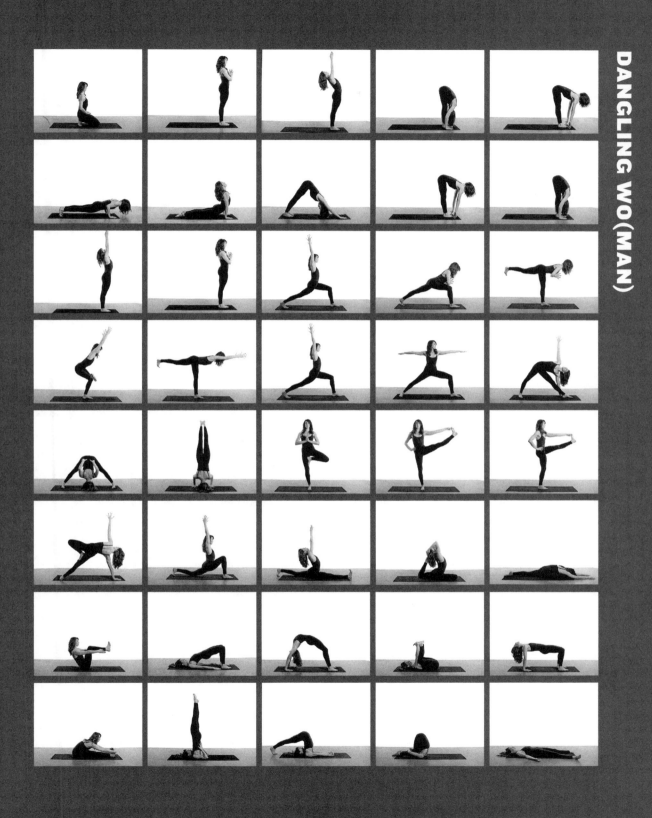

NOURISHMENT

When you are dangling by the threads of your mind, you need to invest more in the roots of your body. One of these roots is nourishment: what you eat and how you eat it.

DETOX

MEALTIME. I know it may feel like if you eat on the go you will be saving time and thus be able to work more on creating solutions that will settle you down, but it will actually only intensify your feelings of dangling and uncertainty. Sit down and have a meal. Enjoy at least one leisurely meal a day: Find a quiet booth in the corner of the coffee shop or read something fun during lunch, plan to have dinner with a friend, or enjoy a picnic in the park. Whatever you do, do not eat in the car or while you are walking or actively working. This will only unsettle your entire digestive system, taking you further from stability.

NO JUICING. Avoid juices when you are dangling. Aside from being raw and usually had on the run, their nature keeps your body light and floating, which is exactly what we are trying to remedy. If you are into the liquid veggies, have them as a cooked soup instead.

RETOX

COOKED FOODS. As a Cali girl, I love my salads, believe you me. But when you are feeling uncertain and lost, you need stable and cooked foods to keep your body grounded. Make sure you have two meals a day made up of cooked foods. Whether it's a veggie omelet or a grilled

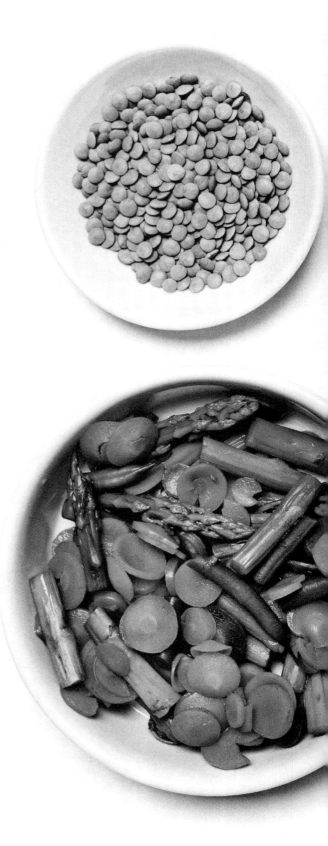

258

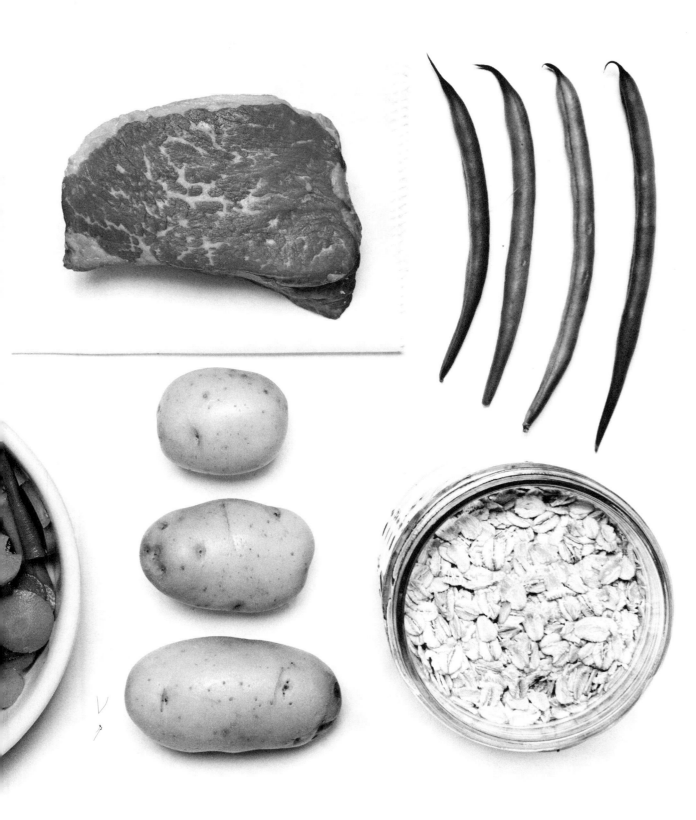

steak with a side of greens, have something warm and soothing.

BREAKFAST. Personally, I do not love breakfast, but it is imperative for overall body health and most imperative if you are dangling. Try a bowl of oatmeal, which will help lower your blood pressure and ground your system for the day to come. Or pick something that will support the foundation of your body, like a Spanish omelet. And make sure that you do not eat it in the car, on the train, or while walking. If it is at your desk, at a meeting, or with your kids, fine, but sit and eat it somewhere, somehow.

DON'T WANT TO COOK? No problem at all. Make smart choices when ordering in and going out. When you are looking at the take-out menu or the choices at the restaurant, look first at the sides. Pick out two cooked vegetable sides first, then go back and pick your main. That way you will ensure that you will have some cooked nutrients to help you stand on your feet.

RECIPES

Chata's Veggie Lentil Soup

1 tablespoon extra virgin olive oil

1 clove garlic, minced

1 onion, chopped

2 stalks celery, chopped

2 carrots, chopped

1 tablespoon salt

1 cup lentils

3 cups water or vegetable stock

Heat oil in a heavy pot over medium heat. Add garlic, onion, celery, and carrot. Add salt, stir, and cover. When the onion starts to get golden around the edges, about 10 minutes, add the lentils and water or vegetable stock. Stir and cover. Let simmer, covered, until the lentils are cooked, about 15 minutes. For the I.AM.YOU. secret, smash the lentils with a masher or fork in the last couple of minutes, take a taste, and add more salt if you like.

Lemon Chicken

1 boneless, skinless chicken breast

2 tablespoons butter

Juice of 1 lemon

Salt and pepper, to taste

Heat a small skillet over medium heat. Add butter and let it melt. In the meantime, squeeze lemon over the chicken breast. Place chicken in the pan and cook 4 minutes per side, or until chicken is cooked through. Season with salt and pepper and serve with a side of veggies.

Beef Patties

It does not get easier than this.

1 pound ground organic beef

Salt and pepper, to taste

Make the beef into 4 patties or buy them premade. Cook on the grill or in a pan to your liking, which even if it is well done will be no more than 5 minutes. Serve with a side of veggies.

Mom's Mashed Potatoes

This takes a bit of effort but is so worth it. One bite of these and you will feel safe at home again.

6 potatoes, peeled and diced

1 stick salted butter

2 tablespoons milk

2 tablespoons salt

Bring a large pot of water to a boil. Add the potatoes and boil until they are soft and cooked. Drain and place back in pot. Add butter and milk and mash with a hand masher or, if you want your potatoes to be light and fluffy, whip them with an electric hand mixer.

262

MINDSET

The post-Lehman days in the fall of 2008 were some of the most stressful I have ever lived. There was not one moment in which I felt calm, secure, or capable; I legitimately think I aged five years for every day I spent on the trading floor after the crash. Not knowing what to do about it all besides panic (or drink), I threw myself into my yoga studies more intensely than ever, which is when I first realized that the Tibetan yoga philosophers are the gladiators of the mind, masters of sense and rationality.

They have a saying, *Dak Chik Rang-Wan-Chen Ki Dak Mepa*, or as I like to simply translate it: "There is no such thing as an unchanging thing."

The best way to grasp this idea is to think of clouds. Clouds are made up of thousands of particles that are constantly shifting and changing. The particles are clear and malleable, impossible to physically grasp. These are constantly changing, empty particles, yet our mind pulls them together and forms something we see from afar as a solid, congealed mass. We see one cloud, but in reality it is millions of translucent particles floating, moving, and changing in space. By the time we even start to realize this, the cloud has shifted and morphed, taking on a whole new form.

Like clouds in the sky, the nature of our world and our being is constantly changing. Nothing actually exists in a way that does not change, and everything you see, touch, and do is innately transforming. Just like a cloud will not take a permanent, solid shape, neither will your reality. It is impossible, because as the ancient Tibetan philosophers taught us, there is simply no such thing as an unchanging thing.

Once you truly understand this, you will never feel like you are dangling again, because you will know that dangling, or being in constant flux and transformation, is life's true nature. This is your strongest weapon, one that will convert you into a gladiator for life.

RETOX

Take a comfortable seat, wherever works for you.

> As you inhale, say to yourself, *I trust me.*
> As you exhale, say to yourself, *I trust change.*

Repeat this with your eyes closed as you sit, breathing in and out through your nose for as long as feels good. Do this every day. If you want to take it to the streets, say the sequence to yourself as you walk, drive, or commute. You are you. And it will all come. I promise.

Retox Soundtrack:
"Sultanas de Merkaillo" —OJOS DE BRUJO

DANGLING WO(MAN)

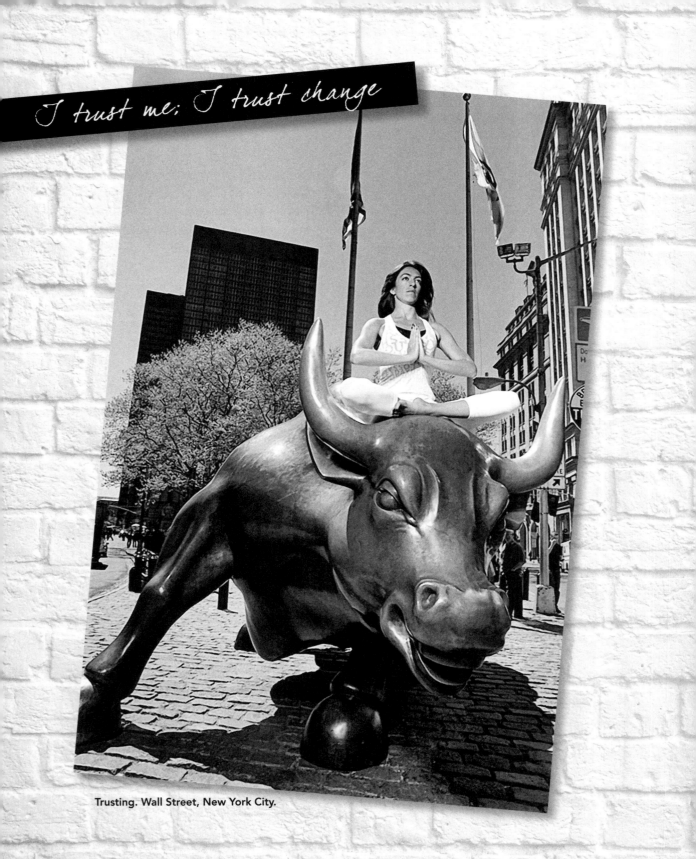

I trust me; I trust change

Trusting. Wall Street, New York City.

THE BLUES

SADNESS, LONELINESS,
AND LOW MOODS

Plant the seeds you want to grow

WE ALL EXPERIENCE THE BLUES from time to time. I routinely have days when I am down, feeling like a failure, and wondering when, and if, something good will actually happen. If you don't believe me, I'll post a picture of my puffy eyes on Instagram next time, or just ask my mom who always knows something's going on from the second I begin to utter the phrase, "Hi, Mom," on the phone. I would call these moments of lack of self-worth and sadness nuts, but they are actually pretty normal; we are human after all.

Despite our best efforts to live a balanced, happy life, sometimes we are the main characters in our own country-music ballad, overcome with sadness and loneliness, bad relationships, feelings of inadequacy, and a lack of self-confidence. Sometimes the songs are especially tough—family trauma or a breakup, a layoff at work or major shift in life or health—and send us into a spiral of sadness, unwilling and unable to smile, jump out of bed, and laugh into the bright side. We feel hopeless and consistently fatigued, uninterested in what used to make us excited. We walk around on the verge of tears, and long to hide in a deep, dark cave alone forever.

If this sounds familiar to you, you are not alone. But if you have these feelings every day for two weeks or longer, and they are impacting your ability to manage at home and at work or school, then you may need treatment, and you should be assessed by a skilled professional. If you are having suicidal thoughts, please contact a medical professional or at the very least tell a trusted friend or family member.

You don't have to stay stuck in a pit of sadness or depression. There are tools that can help you; I can help you. There is hope, and you will smile again. Just read Suzanne's inspiring story and know that there is a way out.

Suzanne is one of the most beautiful, radiant people I have ever met. She is as athletic as she is creative (*extremely* is the adjective for both), Tina Fey–style hysterical, generous, and caring. She is the full package. But life was not treating her like that when I met her. In fact, she was getting bitch-slapped through a multiyear rough patch across all of life's fronts that would just not let up.

A few weeks after taking her ring shopping, her live-in boyfriend of seven years broke up with her out of the blue as she was getting dolled up for a date night. Just like that, from the couch in the other room. A month later, he realized he made a mistake, proceeded to beg for her back, called up all of her friends and family for support, and endlessly professed his undying love for her. She took him back, only to have him dump her again the next morning via text message.

If that wasn't enough, things were less than rosy on the job front. Two years earlier, she was in a dead-end job with an abusive boss. Her friends and family saw how miserable she was and convinced her to quit. Fortunately, she soon got a job with a start-up doing work she enjoyed. Eight months into the new job, she was laid off as part of a general downsizing, and despite hitting the pavement daily she had not been able to find a new job. When we met, her best friend had committed suicide, her dog had cancer, she had gained twenty pounds, and she had almost no savings left. I can't make this up. She was jobless, man-less, money-less, overweight, and completely down in the dumps. This gorgeous girl was finding it tough to find a reason to live, yet she desperately wanted to be happy again.

Like many in her position, Suzanne had dabbled in cocktails of Prozac and Zoloft, and bought and read every self-help book out there. She said in retrospect she noticed the various methods made her feel better for a bit as she flipped though their pages, but that inevitably the positive gain wore off. She got super into yoga, tried meditating for an hour every day, became a vegan, and worked her butt off every day . . . but nothing was working. She could not find the "true happiness" or that miracle that every book was promising, and she did not have the patience for any more tactics that would waste her time.

Through a long web of social media friends of hers, she began following @iamyoustudio

on social media, and one of my posts struck a chord. She emailed me asking for a coaching consultation, which we set up. Soon after, we began Retoxing, starting with mindset and nourishment practices, and some Quick Fixes as daily yoga homework. I gave her solutions that would actually help her, and she truly put them to work.

It was hard, but Suzanne did it. She healed herself, in mind, body, and life, by applying Retox techniques day in, day out, and through them created her own true happiness. She now has a totally kick-ass job at a much better company, a man who not only loves her but inspires her every day, has picked up a bunch of new hobbies and friends, and is more beautiful than ever.

The blues do not last forever, but they are a bitch. You can heal yourself, you will heal yourself, you have to heal yourself; the world needs you. These Retox tools will work, and I will hold your hand the whole way. If Suzanne can do it, so can you. I promise.

YOGA

There is nothing more disheartening than someone wasting your time, or something you invest time in not working. Which is why, starting now, we are cutting the yoga crap and getting straight to it.

General yoga will not cure your loneliness or bad moods forever. In all honesty, if the class is not vigorous or guided, it could actually make you feel worse, allowing you too much time to calmly think in a "relaxing" silence, thus pushing your mind into the oblivion of the dark side. Like your sweaty candlelit spin class, it may make you feel somewhat better, which is awesome, but when Retoxing, I demand lasting results.

Low mood is a combination of biochemical and mental shifts inside you that need to be addressed with a precise combination of breath linked with anatomically focused movements so that you can heal and become radiant again from the inside out. Each tool I give you in the yoga section is selected because it stimulates your lungs, raises serotonin (your natural Prozac) and adrenaline (your natural energy) levels, and lowers levels of monoamine oxidase, or the enzyme that breaks down serotonin. The full sequence helps create endorphins, which are the ultimate happy drug. There is a focus on backbends, as they are believed to help with depression in Traditional Chinese Medicine, and specific breaths linked with all so that your mind cannot wander into whatever it is that is dragging you down.

Should we get better together?

RETOX

DESK FIXES

LION'S BREATH BACKBEND

Cross your forearms over your head, holding elbow to elbow. Inhale, sit up tall. Exhale strongly out of your mouth, sticking your tongue out as you arch your back slightly into a backbend. Repeat one to five times.

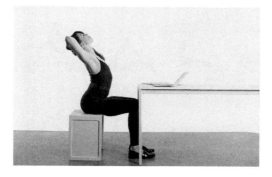

DEEP TWIST*

From Bright Breath with your wrists crossed overhead, drop your left arm outside your right leg and take your right arm behind you. Look up and hold five to ten breaths. Recross your wrists above your head, then repeat on the other side.

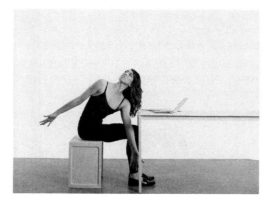

BRIGHT BREATH*

Lift your arms and cross your wrists above your head, fingers up. Bring the back of your head toward your arms and even find a slight backbend in the upper back. Inhale to a comfortable level. Begin short, sharp breaths out of the nose, where the inhale is simply a reaction to the exhale, as the diaphragm pumps on the abdominal wall. It should feel somewhere between sneezing and blowing your nose. (If you are pregnant, skip khapalabhati and breathe normally.)

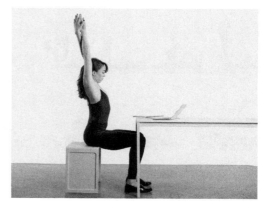

BIG BACKBEND

Place your hands on the back of your chair or interlace your hands behind your back. Straighten your elbows and stretch across the front of your chest. Inhale, start to arch your back. Exhale, use the weight of your arms to create a deeper backbend. Do this sitting or standing and hold five to ten breaths.

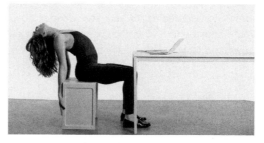

QUICK FIXES

SUN SALUTE B

Start standing with your feet together and your hands touching at your chest. Inhale, bend your knees, lift your arms up, and look up in Chair pose. Exhale, fold forward and straighten both legs, bringing your forehead to your shins. Inhale, extend your spine and look forward. Exhale, Chaturanga or Plank pose. Inhale, Up Dog. Exhale, Down Dog. Inhale, place your left foot forward, right heel down, arms up and touching in Warrior 1. Exhale, place your hands down, step back and lower into Chaturanga or Plank. Inhale, Up Dog. Exhale, Down Dog. Repeat on the other side. Then inhale and step or jump your feet between your hands. Exhale, fold forward. Inhale, bend at the knees, arms up for Chair pose. Exhale, come to standing, legs straight, hands to your heart. Repeat entire cycle two to five times.

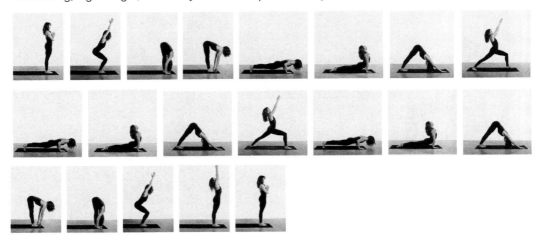

BABY COBRA*

Lie facedown with your legs straight, palms by your chest, and elbows bent. Inhale, lift your chest and engage the muscles of your chest and arms, almost feeling as if you are pulling your chest forward while dragging your hands back. Exhale, press the tops of your feet into the floor. Stay here for five to ten breaths. To go a little deeper, clasp your hands behind your back, straighten your elbows, and lift your chest up farther.

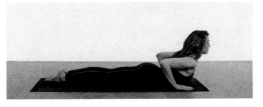

WHEEL

Start lying on your back with your knees bent and your feet hip distance apart. Place your hands alongside your ears. Inhale, press into the floor and lift everything up. Exhale, let your head dangle. Hold here five to eight breaths, then repeat one to three times. If this is too much for you, keep your arms by your torso and just lift your bottom and lower back up into Bridge pose.

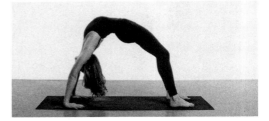

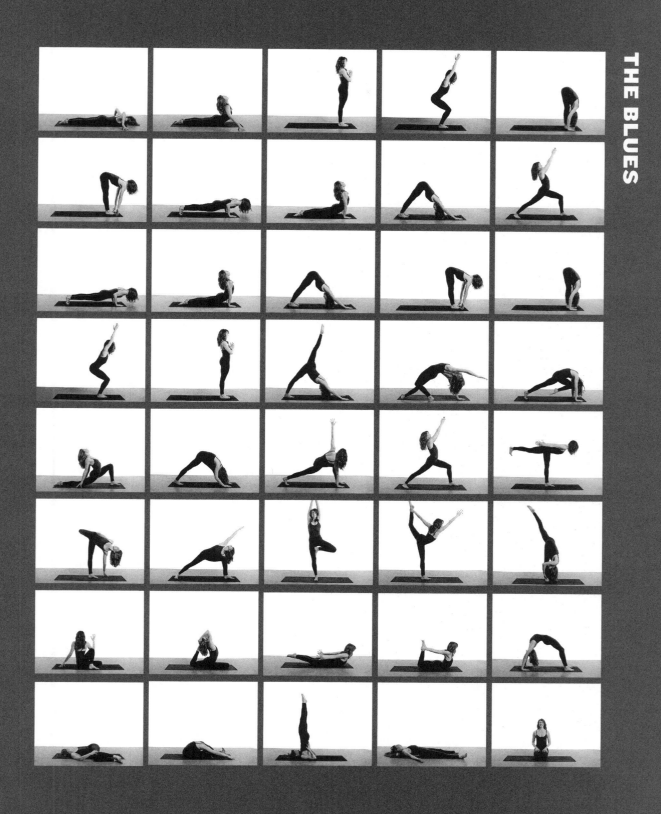

NOURISHMENT

I know you want to wallow in chocolate and ice cream. I also know other times you have no interest in eating at all. That may make you feel sort of better in the moment, but I can help you eat your way to happiness. Seriously.

Many nutritional imbalances have been shown to make people prone to sadness and unable to recover for longer periods of time. In fact, studies are now showing that when you balance your diet with certain nutritional foods, feelings of sadness, depression, guilt, loneliness, desperation, and loss of energy can be alleviated. This, combined with choosing foods and recipes that are enjoyable, make up the Retox nourishment plan that will increase your happiness serving many times over.

DETOX

First, we have to get rid of blues-inducing food habits.

PUT DOWN THE CRAP. Eating the ice cream, candy, chips, chocolate, and other junk food may soothe you in the moment, but it is not the solution. The chemicals in processed foods have been shown to make you 58 percent more susceptible to depression. In addition, the fat and empty calories will probably make you gain weight, which will likely make you feel even worse. Basically, you are shooting yourself in the foot by diving into a hot fudge sundae.

TREAT YOURSELF TO TREATS. Given that, do not cut out every food that makes you happy. Instead, look at these as treats—little nuggets and morsels of happiness that you get

272

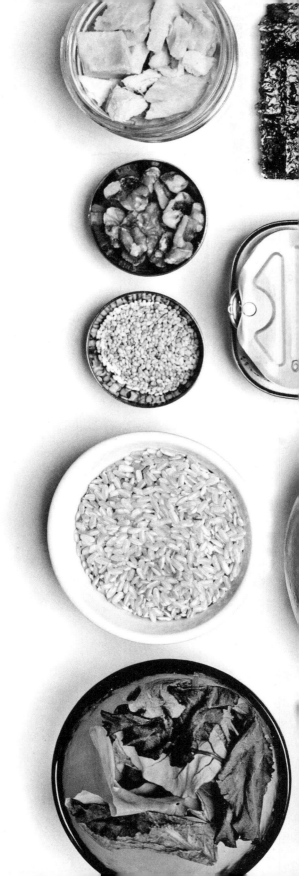

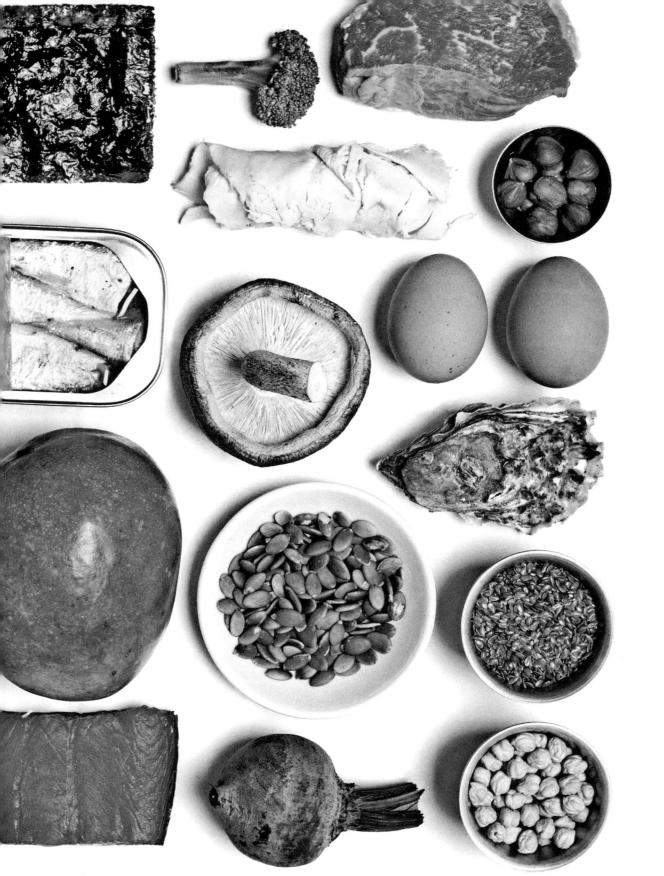

to look forward to within the context of all the other good stuff you are eating already.

SKIP THE SKIPPING. Not eating is not the solution, either. Your body needs nutrients to create the hormones to make you happy, healthy, and strong. If you do not eat, you will not be happy. So even if you do not want to, you have to. Schedule meals in like a meeting or appointment and force yourself to show up.

EAT WITH OTHERS. Eating is not just about the food itself; it is an experience. Plan out meals with others that you like or uplift your spirit, maybe even someone funny. Walk with a coworker to pick up your lunch, schedule dinners and brunches with your friends, and make eating a social engagement you participate in.

RETOX

Now you are going to bombard your system with biochemical happiness generators. Deal?

AMINO ACIDS. Serotonin, your natural happiness drug, is made from amino acids. If you increase your intake of certain amino acids, you can increase your happiness. Some high amino acid foods to lift you are mango, beets, kelp and spirulina, sesame seeds, hazelnuts, chickpeas, turkey, and brown rice.

OMEGA-3. A recent study showed that populations that ate more fish had lower levels of depression than those that do not. The reason behind the happiness? Omega-3s. Omega-3 fats are essential fats, meaning they cannot be manufactured by the body and must be ingested. Try adding omega-3-rich foods to every meal, such as salmon, fresh tuna, sardines, oysters, walnuts, flaxseeds, and brown rice.

VITAMIN B AND FOLIC ACID. People who have low levels of vitamin B and folic acid tend to react in a less positive way than those who do not. Studies have even shown that they are more likely to be sad and down. Add these nutrients to your diet by including the following foods, which are rich in both: beef, lentils, eggs, broccoli, dark leafy greens, and pumpkin seeds.

VITAMIN D. Ever notice that people in sunny places always seem to be smiling? Biochemically it is because they get more vitamin D from its best source: the sun. The rest of us who are not lucky enough to live in a sun-drenched paradise need to make sure we eat more vitamin D, which is actually hard to find in significant levels in common foods and is not easily absorbed via vitamins. These foods contain natural vitamin D and should be paired with a few minutes in the sun: shiitake mushrooms, sockeye salmon, catfish, tuna, and free-range eggs.

SNACKS
Mango
Hazelnuts and walnuts
Pumpkin seeds
Hardboiled egg

274

RECIPES

Breakfast of Cheerful Champs

Eat a wedge of this frittata for breakfast every morning.

8 organic eggs

1 tablespoon extra virgin olive oil

1 cup baby spinach

1 cup shiitake mushrooms, diced

1 cup chopped broccoli

Salt and pepper, to taste

Crack eggs into a large bowl and whisk. Set aside. Heat oil in a large oven-proof pan over medium heat. Add spinach, mushrooms, broccoli, and salt and pepper, and cook until the vegetables are soft. Pour eggs into pan and cook, undisturbed, until the sides set, about 2 minutes. Cover and cook 10 to 13 minutes until set. Slide onto a plate and cut into wedges.

Happiness Salad

2 cups baby spinach (or mixture of leafy greens)

½ avocado, diced

1 cup beets, diced

¼ cup hazelnuts

2 tablespoons extra virgin olive oil

1 tablespoon balsamic vinegar

Put spinach, avocado, beets, and hazelnuts in a bowl. Dress with oil and vinegar. Toss and enjoy.

Peppery-Crusted Tuna

1 (5-ounce) piece of wild tuna

Juice of 1 lemon

¼ cup coarsely ground black pepper

¼ cup sesame seeds

1 tablespoon extra virgin olive oil

1 clove garlic, thinly sliced

Put tuna in a bowl and cover in fresh lemon juice. Place pepper and sesame seeds on a flat plate. Dredge tuna in pepper/sesame seeds and coat completely.

Heat oil and garlic in a small pan over high heat. Add tuna to pan and cook 1 minute per side. Serve with a side of sautéed spinach or a side salad dressed with extra virgin olive oil and lemon juice.

275

Brown Rice Risotto

1 tablespoon extra virgin olive oil

2 cloves garlic, minced

1 large tomato, chopped

3 handfuls baby spinach

1 cup mushrooms, chopped

2 cups broccoli florets

Salt and pepper, to taste

2 cups cooked brown rice

Pinch saffron

Grated Parmesan (optional)

Red chili flakes (optional)

Heat oil in a large skillet over medium heat. Sauté garlic until it just starts to turn golden. Add tomato, spinach, mushrooms, and broccoli. Season with salt and pepper and cook until vegetables are soft. Add rice and saffron and stir, allowing the juice of the vegetables to soak into the rice. Serve warm or cold, sprinkling with Parmesan and/or red pepper flakes, if you like.

Retox Nachos

I know I said no comfort food, but Retox comfort food is totally fair game.

1 tablespoon extra virgin olive oil

2 cloves garlic, minced

2 cups baby spinach

½ pound organic ground beef

½ white onion, chopped

1 tomato, chopped

½ avocado, diced

Sour cream, sliced jalapeños, fresh cilantro, for garnish (optional)

Sesame blue tortilla chips

Heat oil in a pan over medium heat. Add garlic and cook until just turning golden. Add spinach and sauté until wilted, about 5 minutes. Remove from pan and let cool on a plate. In the same pan, add ground beef, breaking it up with a wooden spoon as it cooks. When the meat is cooked through, remove and place on top of the spinach. Top with onion, tomato, and avocado. Garnish with a dollop of sour cream, jalapeños, and cilantro, if desired. Serve with tortilla chips and dive in!

MINDSET

Life is precious and you deserve to be happy immediately, so I am going to come right out and say it:

> Your reality is a reflection of your thoughts. Your world is a reflection of your mind.

You can quickly and easily transform your reality into one that is bright and beautiful by shifting your thoughts. If you shift your thoughts, you will transform your reality. If you overhaul your mind, you will change your world. The key to exiting the blues and making it onto the big happy stage of life is changing the circle of thoughts that your mind is stuck in. It's these thoughts that define your world and your existence in it.

RETOX

Take out a paper and pen. Close your eyes for a bit and breathe through your nose, sitting up straight. Then slowly open your eyes and go through these five steps:

1. **Scan.** On one side of the page, write down all the sentiments bothering you and keeping you down. Write down their origins, details, and the adjectives your mind is using to describe it all. Your emotions, from anger to frustration, loneliness to simply sadness. Write it all down. On the other side of the page, write down all the things you want to feel, everything you want to achieve or have in life, and everything you do not have now that is making you feel down. Write every-thing that comes to mind on the corresponding side of the page, as banal or ridiculous as it may seem. Write down anything that goes through your mind.

2. **Pinpoint.** Go through the sentiments you do not like and actively cross them out with a big X or a scribble. Be aggressive about it! Then flip over the paper and look at the places you want to be—happiness, employment, pregnancy, a raise, self-confidence, love, whatever—and circle those. They could be just general emotions such as "smiley" or "happy," or perhaps they are precise in terms of a position, job, or person. Regardless, circle the ones that you want. Flip the page, and cross out more of what you don't want. Then go back to what you want and circle more.

3. **Declare.** Now repeat out loud or in your mind what you circled; say it over and over to yourself, maybe while you are doing yoga or running, or while you are on hold or walking through the house. Perhaps you tell a friend or parent, perhaps you keep it to yourself, but I want you to repeat what you circled in your mind and out loud. These declarations are what start making the change to what you want official.

4. **Give.** This is the secret sauce. Now give someone the very thing you have declared you want. In doing so, you are planting the seeds for it to come to you. So for instance, if you want someone to shower you with presents, surprise someone with a little gift, even just a cookie from the bakery or a single flower. If you want money, donate some money away. If you want friendship, be a good friend. If you want attention

from your spouse, drizzle them in extra affection and love.

5. **Breathe**. At least once a day do this exercise:

Inhale, saying: *I will be happy.*
Exhale, saying: *I am already.*

Every day go back to that list. Mentally and physically cross out what you do not want, and re-circle and declare what you do want. Do this actively with pen and paper and then stealthily in your mind no matter where you are, incorporating the repeated breath visualization as well. The repetition will train the muscle of your mind and guide your thoughts into the reality you hoped for in the world you have dreamed of. It is possible, it will happen, and it will happen through the conduit of you.

Retox Soundtrack:
"Boom Boom" —JOHN LEE HOOKER

Feeling safe and happy. New York City. Photograph by Mick Rock.

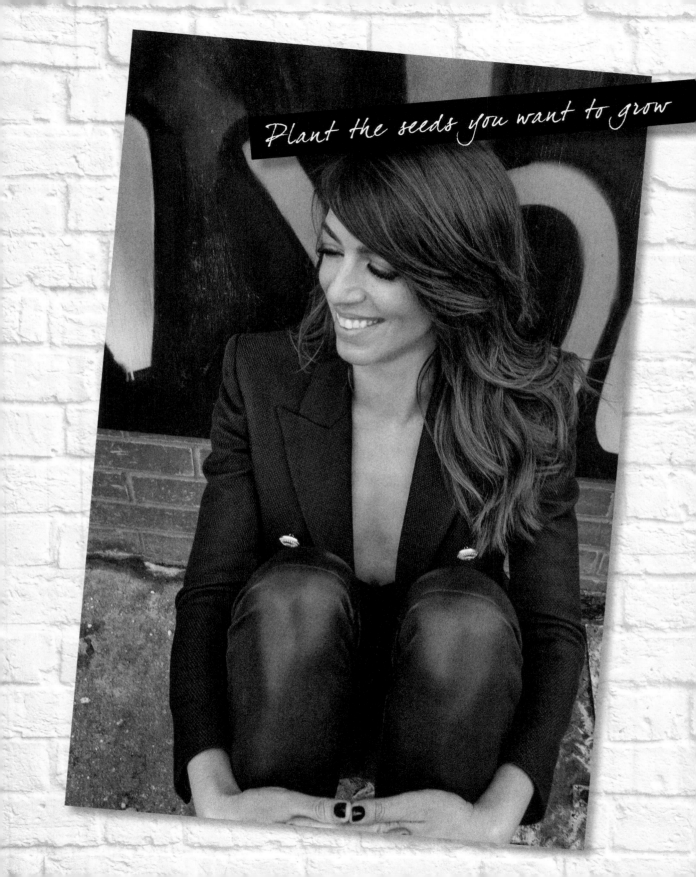

Plant the seeds you want to grow

I'M FAT

CREATING YOUR IDEAL

BODY AND MIND

I am what I choose to see

ON MONDAYS, I WEAR MY fat clothes. Am I fat on Mondays? No, but I definitely think I am, which is precisely why I have a Monday I'm Fat wardrobe—baggy shirts, loose pants, big sweaters, and long, wide, loose yoga clothes. It is all there in my closet, set aside and ready for my fat days. The whole thing is fairly ridiculous, because there is no way I could technically go from feeling all-American girl sexy on Sunday to obese and gross on Monday, but as far as I am concerned, on Mondays, I'm Fat, and that's that.

Now, don't take this the wrong way, and don't hate me, but what makes my Mondays truly absurd is that I have never actually been fat. I have been overweight, yes, many a time, and sometimes fuller than my liking, but not fat in the way I have felt or seen myself in the mirror. This is partly due to genetics, but mostly due to the fact that exercise has been integral to my daily life, my whole life, just as has eating vegetables at every meal and avoiding processed food. My parents raised me that way out in Cali, and it stuck. This fitness and food combo has kept me healthy and strong despite all my fairly intense epicurean indulgences. So I know thinking I'm fat is a bit nuts, but it is honest. Granted this book would probably sell better if I were to tell you some story about how I was massively overweight then decided to start yoga; gave up meat, gluten, and sugar; and ultimately lost forty pounds.

But that wouldn't be true and, as I hope you know by now, I am all about straight-up, honest facts. Which is why you can't hate me for sharing the truth. Okay?

Interestingly enough, the fattest I have ever felt was when I was the skinniest. Back in 1999, as a sophomore in college, I convinced myself that I was really, really fat. And man, did I believe me. I dropped myself down to eight hundred calories a day, deliciously made up of coffee, Sour Patch Kids, frozen yogurt, mustard, and some canned tuna with pickles—totally Michelin-star caliber. I ran seventy to eighty miles a week, walked everywhere, and glared at my "fat" stomach in the mirror every chance I got. I did not have a scale, so I cannot say how much I weighed, but I do know that as a five-foot-eleven athletic nineteen-year-old, my size 2 and 4 clothing was supremely baggy, something that made me enormously content.

My parents and close friends kept telling me I was too skinny, attempting creative ways to beef me up, but I did not pay any attention to them, let alone understand why they were not seeing what I was seeing. I was fat and needed to be skinnier. Maybe then I would be as successful and hot as my Princeton peers.

I kept up this unhealthy shenanigan for almost a year. Then one day, on my daily run under a spectacular blue sky, I collapsed to the ground in agony. I half hobbled, half crawled back to the car and took myself for X-rays and an MRI. I had broken my femur. The doctor told me no running for three months. At most, I could swim without kicking, but her recommendation was for complete rest. I freaked out. I was going to get *so* fat now. The world was over.

A few days later, the doctor called me back to her office. Initially I was quite excited; maybe she was going to tell me that there was a misdiagnosis and the pain was just a bruise of some sort, that I could continue running. No such luck.

She sat me down on a pleather green chair in the university medical center with a grave look on her face. She said, "Lauren, I want to tell you something. You broke your femur not because you are running too much, but because you are not eating enough to support your body." She continued to explain that the way my bone broke was 100 percent due to malnourishment, and if I did not make a change, my entire body would fall apart and I would never be able to run or play sports again.

I heard her loud and clear. Never running again was not an option, so I knew I had to eat better. Life had given me a warning—it was now time for me to get it together. I was not fat. It was all in my mind.

Sometimes we think we are fat, but we are not. Other times we are overweight, but we let ourselves think we are bigger than we actually are. Both states send us into a tailspin of self-harassment, guilt, unhealthy habits, and, worst of all, self-criticism and negative self-talk. We get trapped in the weight of our minds, unable to see who we really are, driving ourselves mentally haggard as we beat ourselves up, forgetting to take care of the very self we are hating. We need to break the mental funhouse mirrors. Only then can we become our ideal self in our ideal body.

I'm Fat is not about a number on a scale. It is about our self-perception and how we interact with it. It is about a physical feeling we have of being more overweight than we are, and the corresponding mental afflictions and ensuing physical bulwarks that that creates. Often I'm Fat is totally irrational and fluctuates from one day to the next, a mere sensation engendered by something we ate, stress, water retention, hormones, a random comment, or how we slept. Other times we really do need to shed some pounds, but we cling to the mental and physical burden of our inflated image, so despondent that we can't do anything. We metaphorically become weighted down, unable to just start right now and lose those extra pounds. Whether we have some weight to lose or not, our mind tips our emotional scale in a direction that holds us back from being who we are meant to be—radiant, glowing, and light inside and out.

In the following pages, I am going to share with you yoga tips and a full sequence to burn off both literal and figurative fat; nourishment tips to manage not only those days you feel fat, but the days before in which you may be engendering that feeling without knowing it; and a mindset plan to keep you out of the I'm Fat abyss. I have applied these methods to myself and hundreds of clients across the nation, and I have seen how they have transformed our relationship with our mind, body, and life from the inside out.

YOGA

Okay, people. I know the image of yoga is easy and soft, an activity more to complement an intense workout than a workout in and of itself. Well, that yoga isn't Retox yoga. Retox yoga, when done properly, will make you sweat; it will make you firm and chiseled; it will make you strong inside and out. Retox yoga is for you, so that when you look in the mirror you see your true beauty.

284

RETOX

DESK FIXES

STRONG BREATH*

Lift your arms straight up. Open them into a large V. Inhale to a comfortable level. Exhale and begin short, sharp breaths out of the nose, where the inhale is simply a reaction to the exhale, as the diaphragm pumps on the abdominal wall. It should feel somewhere between sneezing and blowing your nose. (If you are pregnant, skip khapalabhati; just hold your arms and breathe normally.) Keep these up for one minute, energizing your body with each pump.

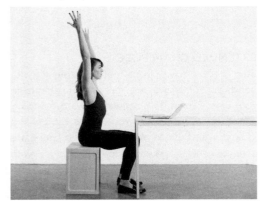

CHAIR LIFT

Start sitting, breathing normally. On an inhale, lift your butt up. Hover over your seat in the air in a quasi Chair pose. Hold five to ten breaths, or hold one breath and repeat ten times.

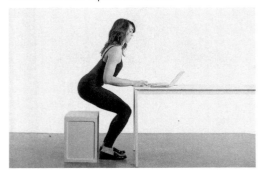

CHAIR ABS

Sit up tall and lift your arms alongside your ears. Inhale fully. Exhale, lean back, keeping your back straight and engaging your core. If this is too much for your lower back, reach your arms forward or keep them on your thighs. Hold here one to five breaths, then repeat as it feels good.

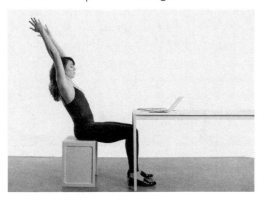

WARRIOR ARMS

While seated, extend your arms out to the sides. Spread your hands wide and engage through your fingers. Contract your triceps and hold here, five to twenty breaths. You can also do the Strong Breath in this pose.

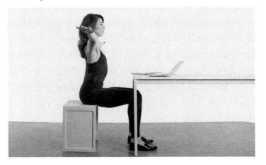

285

I'M FAT

QUICK FIXES

ABS WITH BLOCK*
Lie on the floor and lengthen your arms along your ears. Hold a block or books between your hands on the floor. Take your legs to 90 degrees. Inhale, flex your feet. Exhale, drop your heels toward the floor. Maybe that is only a few inches, or maybe to 45 degrees as shown in the photo, or perhaps all the way to hover just an inch off the floor. This will depend on the health of your back, strength of your core, and more than anything, what feels natural and possible. Inhale, lift your legs back up to 90 degrees, lifting your butt up this time. Exhale, bring your toes to touch the block or floor behind your head. Inhale, come back to 90 degrees where you started. The slower you do this the better. Repeat five to ten times.

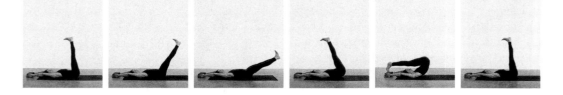

FAT-BUSTING PLANK*
Start in a forearm Plank or normal Plank pose. Exhale all the air out. Inhale to a comfortable level. Begin short, sharp breaths out of the nose, where the inhale is simply a reaction to the exhale, as the diaphragm pumps on the abdominal wall. It should feel somewhere between sneezing and blowing your nose. (If you are pregnant, skip khapalabhati; just hold a plank and breathe normally.) Engage and lift your thighs. Press down through your hands. Let yourself shake, but place your knees on the floor if it is too much. Keep up the pumps for thirty seconds, then come to Child's pose with your knees on floor and your chest resting on your thighs.

EXTENDED CHAIR POSE
Start standing with your feet together. Inhale, bend your knees and take your arms up alongside your ears. Exhale, fold halfway forward, bringing your torso to hover over your thighs. Sit low and look at your thumbs. Make sure your knees are over your ankles and your arms are engaged, with the abdomen actively lifting off the thighs. Hold here five to twenty breaths.

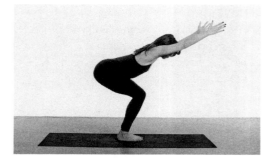

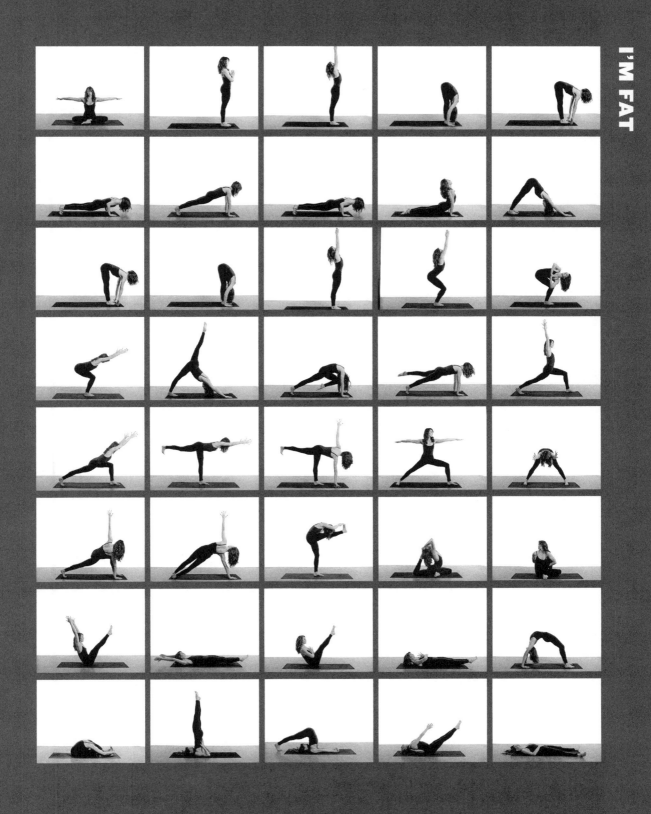

NOURISHMENT

Feeling fat is the worst. It can lead to anxiety, depression, self-torture, and guilt, all with a backdrop of low self-esteem and just wanting to hide. Although I'm Fat is rooted in the mind, many times we actually are a bit fat in our bodies, our clothes are tight, and we just feel gross. In both instances, we tend to struggle to make the right food choices, instead succumbing to the crap we know we are not supposed to eat or chasing the latest diet craze, cutting out random items in a desperate attempt to gain some control. In more severe I'm Fat episodes, we decide to either binge or purge, both subconscious modes of self-flagellation. Guess what? These will all just make you feel, and be, fatter.

Back in college, my mind thought I was fat, so I rationalized an extreme way of eating that made me skinny on the outside, but this unhealthy eating didn't address how I felt on the inside. In fact, it made me feel gross, perpetuating I'm Fat even more. I was lucky to have been scared straight when I was, and I swore to myself to never eat typical I'm Fat foods again. These days when I am having an I'm Fat moment, I know I first must figure out why, and then I address it, all of which I am going to share with you just like I did with Kelly.

Kelly was a vivacious young SoCal gal living in Manhattan. She was a perfectionist who worked in sales ten hours a day followed by working out for two. She came into the studio for a simple I.AM.YOU. yoga class one night, having heard it was the best workout in town, and immediately afterward, she bought a class package and signed up for one-on-one coaching. As I always do, I asked her to list three goals for the coaching program, to which she answered, "Lose the extra weight on me, get skinny, and be healthy." Valid desires, except that as a five-foot-nine rail-thin size 6, I really could not see the pounds she was talking about, so I decided to focus on her third request, being healthy.

Within one week of working together, I realized that Kelly suffered from I'm Fat like so many driven women I know. On some days, her diet was littered with all sorts of I'm Fat tell-tale foods like the ones I used to eat—frozen yogurt, green drinks, canned tuna. On other days, it was crowded with combinations of foods that physically made her feel fat in the waist and face, even though she thought they were helping her shed pounds and stay skinny. It quickly became apparent that she needed a diet makeover.

When Kelly first heard my plan, she was very reluctant, but I promised I would take her from I'm Fat to "I'm smokin'" in a matter of weeks. Fortunately, she decided to put her trust in me. First, I had her almost triple her daily caloric intake. Kelly had been food phobic for so long that this was a struggle for her, but when she started adding food that satiated her and saw that she wasn't gaining weight, she was on board. Then I had her stop being a vegetarian. She hadn't eliminated meat for ethical reasons; she just thought it was a convenient way to go low fat. I also had her give up her precious green juices and encouraged her to let go of every nutritional dogma she had read about (and she seemed to have read every diet book out there!). By the end of the month, Kelly was chiseled in her arms, back, abs, and thighs, supremely energetic, and feeling better than ever. In the end, she actually gained five pounds, yet dropped an entire clothing size, and she no longer thinks she is fat. The best part? Kelly does not torture herself anymore and allows herself to eat all the foods she loves. She's even lightened up her workouts in the name of rest and recovery a few times a week. If she and I made the shift, so can you.

Okay, maybe you can't relate because the number on the scale is actually higher than it should be. But that doesn't make your I'm Fat days any less unrealistic. Take Gail. A stay-at-home mom of three, she had put on extra weight after each pregnancy, and now she was forty pounds overweight. Her doctor had told her she needed to drop some weight, but Gail didn't need a professional to tell her that. She knew it just by looking in the mirror. She tried several diets, and some of them even worked for a time, but inevitably the number on the scale wouldn't budge, her pants would feel tight, and Gail would lock herself in the bathroom crying because nothing fit her.

She started coming to class because she thought yoga would be a way to ease into working out. She felt too big to do anything more strenuous. Well, after her first class, she realized just how much of a workout a Retox yoga class can be, but I wouldn't let her give up. I asked her to let me help her. We talked about her eating habits and it quickly became apparent that Gail was a serial dieter. She jumped from one diet to the next, always looking for the magic formula that would shed the weight, and always disappointed when she still felt as fat as ever. She also admitted to bingeing from time to time, but always on "foods"

she thought would keep her from gaining weight—things like frozen yogurt, dry cereal, pickles, and ice cream sprinkles . . . yep, that's right, not the ice cream, just the sprinkles. You may know what I am talking about. . . .

The first thing I did was ban these "binge" foods. They might be low fat or nonfat, but they are loaded with sugar and chemicals and are just plain gross. Then, just like Kelly, I made Gail forget all the diet dogma. Bread, dairy, red meat . . . nothing was off limits. There was no more "bad" or "good" food. Instead, I asked Gail to keep track of how certain foods made her feel.

Slowly but surely, Gail learned to trust her body to tell her when she was hungry and what her body needed. She no longer binged and the weight was coming off. She continued to do yoga and now is longer and leaner, more toned and more flexible. She still has more weight to lose, but when she looks in the mirror, she sees someone who is making great progress, and more than that, she sees her true self and likes what she sees.

Working with Kelly, Gail, and countless other clients, along with my own experience, has revealed to me some common dietary habits that people who suffer from I'm Fat tend to display. Look at the list below and see how many of these things sound familiar to you:

- You put hot spices and mustard on everything. You use hot sauce, chili powder, pepper flakes, or mustard at every meal.
- You "love" pickles. You routinely snack on them, and it's not uncommon to eat an entire jar in one sitting.

I'M FAT

- Celery is another of your go-to snacks. You love its crunch and the fact that it has negative calories—you literally use more calories to eat it than it actually contains.
- You depend on your coffee. You have at least one a day but usually more, and often one as a substitute for a meal.
- You regularly juice. You believe you are totally full and satisfied after a week of juicing and that juice is an actual meal.
- You're never without a piece of gum. You go through at least a pack of gum a day.
- Diet soda is a mainstay in your diet. You consider it its own food group.
- You fear bread and pasta. The thought of taking a huge bite of either one freaks you out, literally. So sometimes you pretend you are allergic.

DETOX

There are foods that alone or combined make us feel fat, which almost always lead to my I'm Fat Monday wardrobe. These foods and food combinations tip the scale and can cause you to feel fat when you really, truly are not, so try limiting or omitting them for a while until your mind resets itself and you recognize the beautiful person you really are.

CHICKEN. Unless you know where it is coming from, try to lighten up your weekly dose. The hormones in mass-produced chicken, even free range, affect not only the quality and taste of the meat, but are stored in your fat tissues and have been shown to affect your entire system, from your immunity to fertility, weight gain, and water retention. Scrap chicken for one or two weeks, substituting it with fish (wild, non-Chinese farmed) or more veggies.

NUT BUTTERS. Have you ever thought about how many nuts you need to grind to get one tablespoon of nut butter? Yes, almonds, cashews, and peanuts all have their nutritional benefits and protein, but a glob of them is not always necessary. They will figuratively, and perhaps, literally, stick to you, especially if you are not burning it off soon after. Go for a handful of nuts rather than nut butters.

KALE. It's green, and I love the stuff, but it is also very, very hard to digest. You may be downing the kale aiming for slim beauty, but it could be slowing down your digestion and making you retain water as your system fights to break it all down. When you are feeling fat, swap kale for more easily digested greens like baby spinach and lettuces, such as butter lettuce, red leaf, Bibb, and romaine.

FRUIT. Fruit is good for you, yes, but not if you are exploding a bomb of sugar and carbs in your system every day. As we get older, we lose the ability to metabolize fructose, the sugar in fruit, so if you are not running around burning it off, it ferments in your body and makes you feel fat. Try to lighten up on the fruit and stick to lower sugar fruit, such as blueberries, raspberries, apricots, and cantaloupe, and give mango, papaya, pineapple, bananas, apples, and pears a break for a while.

SOY. Soy products such as tofu and soy milk can cause you to bloat around the abdomen. They have also been shown to lower the level of testosterone in your body, a steroid hormone shown to reduce belly fat and increase muscle production. A few simple drops of soy sauce can make you suffer from I'm Fat for days to come. All you ate was sushi, so why do you feel fat? Now you know. Cut out the soy and you will feel and look more svelte in a jiffy.

SALADS. I love salad. That said, many of the salads you order in restaurants can pack on the pounds and, even worse, create I'm Fat sensations without you noticing it. And how much does that suck—thinking you are being healthy but actually instigating I'm Fat? When you get a salad, remember these points:

- Pick one source of protein for it or skip the protein entirely to give your digestive system a break. Garbanzo beans, nuts, or tuna are ideal if you go the protein route.
- Go light on the high-sugar vegetables, like beets and corn.
- Do not make cheese a regular ingredient unless you are really craving it or it is your protein source for the day.
- Beware the kale base.
- Skip the fruit. This adds calories and fructose to your salad, disrupting your digestion, causing bloat, and slowing your metabolism.
- Pick your dressing wisely, but absolutely dress the salad. I cringe every time I see someone get a salad without dressing or just use balsamic vinegar. You must soften the raw vegetables with olive oil in order for your system to easily digest them. You are tearing apart your intestines otherwise, maybe even feeling bloated and, even worse, fat as a result. Also you need some fat to enable the absorption of certain vitamins in your salad. That said, most premade dressings are loaded with sugars and additives, even the "healthy" ones. Creamy dressings are an obvious no-no, but a lot of the times vinaigrettes have sugar, honey, and even ketchup as ingredients along with too much salt, another I'm Fat instigator. Go for good olive oil along with balsamic vinegar, red wine vinegar, or lemon juice.

COCKTAILS. I love a good drink, believe you me, but often those perfect glasses of glory are laced with sugar, agave, honey, fruit juice, and even sodas. Drink clean, sticking to vodka and gin, swapping out mixers with soda water, and choosing wine over elaborate cocktails. This will help prevent a hangover, too.

PROTEINS. We absolutely need protein to survive—just remember my fractured femur if you forget. But we do not need an excess of animal protein like many industries want us to think. Try replacing one serving of daily protein with a vegetable. Perhaps even shift your diet to no more than one animal protein a day, having either eggs in the morning or fish or organic beef in the evening. Or have two plant-based proteins a day, such as quinoa or chickpeas.

In addition, avoid mixing proteins during a meal. Meaning, if you are having a steak for a main course, get a salad to start instead of tuna tartare, or if you are adding tuna to your salad, scrap the beans. Each protein is digested by your body in a different way, so having two different ones in a meal makes it tough on your system to do what it needs to do. Above all, avoid fake, processed proteins like bars and powders. Your body does not know how to break them down.

HUMMUS. Hummus is high in protein, yes, but also very densely caloric. Half a cup usually has over two hundred calories, twenty-four grams of fat, and thirty-five grams of carbs. Couple that with the bread or snacks you are eating it with and your likely relatively sedentary lifestyle, and hummus is bound to make you feel fat. Try cutting it out for one or two weeks, then only eating it if you really want it, and as a small garnish with crudités early in the day, so you can burn it off and put its protein to use.

YOGURT. There are many studies claiming yogurt helps increase your metabolism and burn fat, but an average serving of yogurt has 150 calories, 18 grams of carbohydrates, and 80 grams of sodium. If you are not burning that off, it will definitely make you feel like it is sticking to you, and thus make you feel fat. In addition, in Traditional Chinese Medicine, cold dairy products are said to slow your digestion, and with it your metabolic process, which could actually make you a bit thicker than you would like.

RETOX

You want to stop feeling fat? Here's all you have to do: Eat fat and eat regularly. Seems counterintuitive, but it's true. Your body needs fat to burn fat, and needs energy to repair, grow, and function. Omitting fat and meals from your diet does nothing more than tell your body to go into starvation mode, and thus hold on to your fat stores. Eat, eat, eat. You will be so much hotter as a result.

SNACKS

Slices of Avocado
Egg, however you like it
Tuna
Raisins
Box of blueberries
Sliced tomato (salt optional)
Cup of broth or veggie soup

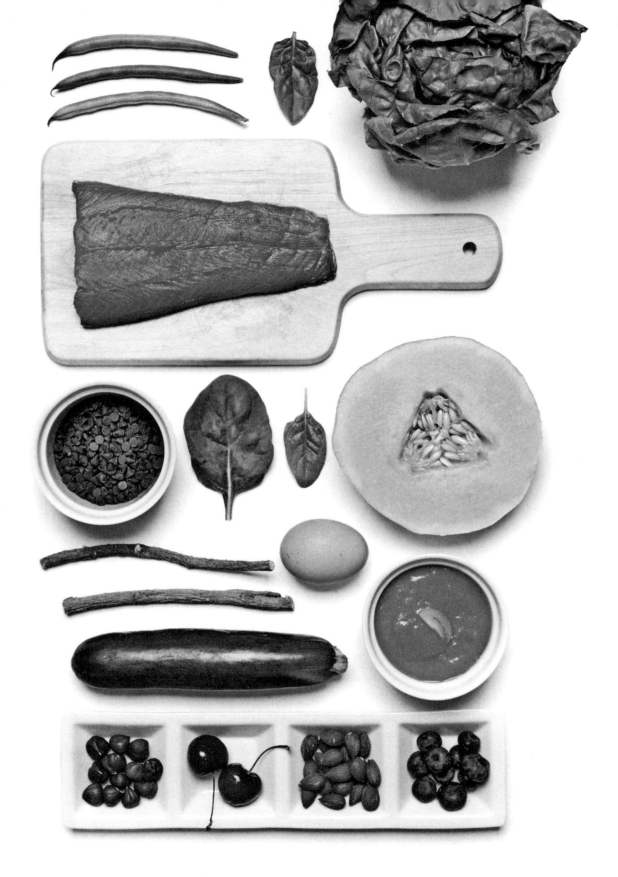

RECIPES

Slimmin' Salad

We use butter lettuce in this recipe because it is the most easily digestible of the lettuces.

3 cups butter lettuce

½ cup grape tomatoes, cut in half

¼ red onion, diced

1 carrot, grated

1 cup green beans, cut in 1-inch pieces

½ cup canned garbanzo beans, drained and rinsed

½ tablespoon Dijon mustard

1 tablespoon extra virgin olive oil

1 tablespoon red wine vinegar

Black pepper, to taste

Place lettuce in a large bowl. Add tomatoes, onion, carrot, green beans, and garbanzo beans. In a small bowl, combine mustard, olive oil, and vinegar. Mix well and pour over salad.

Slimmin' Salmon

You can make this salmon in the oven or on the stove top. The choice is yours.

1 (6-ounce) salmon fillet

1 teaspoon extra virgin olive oil

Juice of ½ lemon

Freshly ground black pepper, to taste

4 garlic cloves, cut in half

Preheat oven to 425 degrees.

Line a baking pan with tin foil. Put salmon, skin side down, in the pan and sprinkle with olive oil, lemon juice, and black pepper. Surround the fish with garlic and place the pan in the oven. Cook until the salmon is cooked through, about 12 minutes.

If you would rather cook on the stove top, prepare salmon the same way. Heat 1 teaspoon olive oil in a skillet over medium heat. Add salmon, skin side up, to the pan. Cook until golden on one side, about 4 minutes. Flip over and cook another 3 minutes, until salmon is cooked through.

Zucchini Sauté

Zucchini has diuretic properties and is straight-up delish.

4 zucchinis

2 tablespoons extra virgin olive oil

½ yellow onion, chopped

2 cloves garlic, minced

Chop zucchinis in rounds or quarters. Heat oil in a skillet over medium heat. Add onion and garlic and cook until both just start browning. Add zucchini to pan, stir, and cover. Let cook until zucchini is soft, about 15 minutes, stirring occasionally. Serve with a slice of avocado on top for a tasty main dish, or simply serve the zucchini as a side to fish or beef.

Chicken Soup

A cup of Retox chicken soup has all the energy and nutrients you need to keep you going throughout the day and make your body strong from the inside, out.

1 large chicken breast with bone, organic preferred

½ white onion, chopped

2 cloves garlic

1 stalk celery, diced

1 large carrot, diced

3 cups water

½ teaspoon salt

Bring water to a boil. Add all ingredients. Let cook for 20 minutes or until chicken is tender. Drink the broth alone or shred the chicken into the broth for a full-on soup.

MINDSET

I am not going to sugarcoat it: Believing that you're a fat cow today, when yesterday you didn't feel so bad, is just you being straight-up stupid. You don't look significantly different than you did yesterday. Feeling fat is all in your mind. And it is exhausting, draining, and ultimately a waste of energy. Even if you do have a few pounds to shed, telling yourself you are fat and beating yourself up about it does nothing to help you reach your goals. In fact, beating yourself up is only going to trip you up.

If you are anything like me, I'm Fat launches a fierce game of ping-pong in your mind, one in which various iterations of "I'm fat/I'm not fat," "Don't eat/I'm hungry," "I look horrible/I look great" take center court, truly bogging you down, making you stressed and borderline crazy.

I'm Fat is a mental matter, one in which we see ourselves as tangibly fat through our intangible mind. It is about self-perception versus true nature, and aligning the two is at the core of my Retox mindset teachings. I know that in those moments when your mind takes control, your perception of reality becomes skewed, making it so, so hard to instigate a positive change, let alone see the truth, one in which your beauty, strength, and sexiness can radiate. But it is possible, just like it was for my friend Caroline.

Caroline is a young mother from Oklahoma. She quit her job after her second daughter, deciding instead to focus on the hardest job of all, motherhood. We met on a community service project in the Navajo Nation and instantly bonded over life, love, and, well, nachos. Caroline had been fit her whole life, but sometime after the birth of her second child, she let herself go. She initially was too tired to lose the baby weight, unable to find the energy to work out or cook healthily while juggling two kids and a household. But that was five years prior. Since then, Caroline had trapped herself in an I'm Fat rut, convincing herself that fat was the new her, and there was just nothing she could do about it. She let herself gain over twenty pounds and routinely tortured herself with crash diets that produced zero sustainable results. After simultaneously starving and gorging herself into bitchiness, she gave up, convincing herself that she was fat for life, and retreated into a needless overweight depression. I had to help her. I had to tip the scale of Caroline's mind and help her rediscover the true, fit her.

This Retox plan based on Tibetan yoga theory helped Caroline shift her perception away from self-deprecating torture to the thin truth. She used it every day, right after sending the kids to school or to bed, and slowly gained the inner strength to shape her body into what she wanted it to be, without the diets, scales, and exhausting regimen. She used her mind to put her body on a plan to beauty, ultimately losing all the stored-up baby weight and more.

RETOX

The Retox mindset plan for I'm Fat is an easy, breezy one, two, three. Sit in a quiet place and read the meditation below, taking a moment to close your eyes and reflect whenever feels right.

THERE IS NO SUCH THING AS AN UNCHANGING THING

I may feel fat or look fat to myself now, but it is not forever. It will change, my body will change, I will change.

My body changes every nanosecond of every day. The me of a minute ago is different from the me of now. If I want my body to change, I must guide it in that direction and it will follow. If I want to stop feeling fat, I must take a moment to understand that everything in the universe is changing, and thus so will I. I am not stuck in this state permanently; nothing and no one is. It will change, my body will change, I will change.

EVERYTHING EXISTS AS I PERCEIVE IT

The more technical phrase for this in Tibetan is *Majamika Sva Tantrila*, or the raw data is there but not until you perceive it; it appears and exists only by appearing to an unimpaired state of mind.

Think of a typical Rorschach inkblot test. When people look at the blob of black ink on a page, the results vary—some see rabbits, others see flowers, others see faces, others see sexual imagery. The blob is the same; our individual perception of it is different.

I see me as fat right now, but someone else may see me as perfect. I, in fact, may see myself as sexy and perfect tomorrow, too, if I let myself. My current perception is the only thing making me fat. The fatness is not coming out of the mirror toward me; it is coming from my mind. I am labeling myself "fat."

It is up to me to change my perception. From there, I can shift how I label my self-image and transform how I exist to myself and the world around me. Everything exists only as I perceive it, so if I perceive skinny and beautiful, that is what I will be.

I AM NOT FAT

I am me, a constantly changing, always developing, completely malleable and radiant me. I am me, so go start to create the me I want to see and feel. I am not fat.

Sit, read, and reread these lines a few times. Then write them down on a small piece of paper or a notecard and put it by your bed or in your bag. Look at them every day, and read them out loud or quietly to yourself. If you want an extra punch, schedule them into your phone as daily reminders, so that you can get out of your head and into the real, radiant, gorgeous you.

Retox Soundtrack:
"Shake It Off" —TAYLOR SWIFT

297

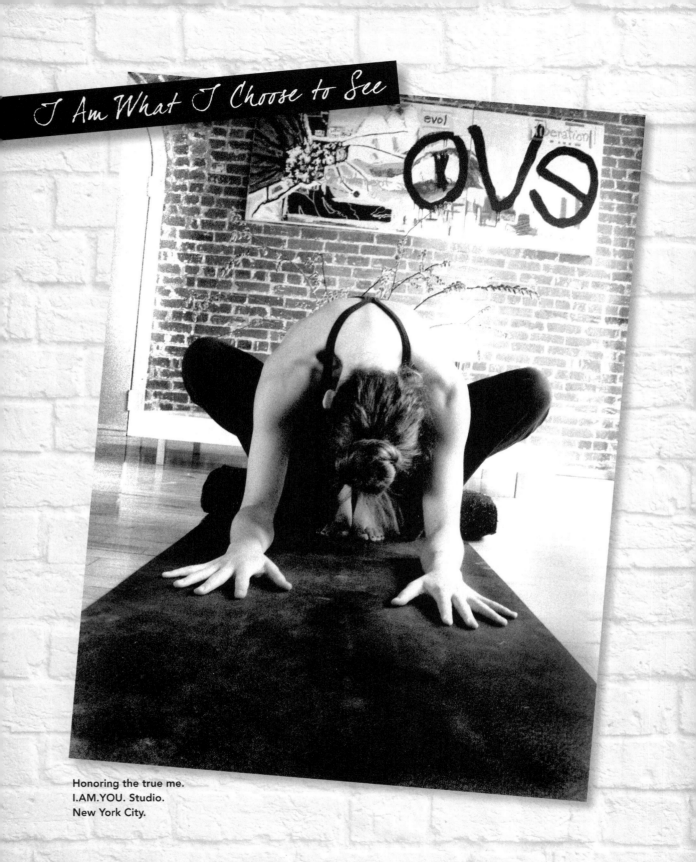

I Am What I Choose to See

Honoring the true me.
I.AM.YOU. Studio.
New York City.

I HAVE TO

CIRCUMVENTING

SOCIETAL PRESSURE

Design the life you want and you will want the life you have

WINE AND I GO WAY back. In fact, our intimacy dates to long before my first sip. Back in the seventh grade, inspired by the infamous *I Love Lucy* episode, I decided to do my annual science project on the fermentation and making of wine. Like my then hero Lucille Ball, I smashed combinations of grapes in buckets with my feet, adding different levels of yeast and sugar to each batch, ultimately studying their fermentation as they aged in glass bottles in the garage. I labeled it Laurennay (like Chardonnay, get it?) and used my grandmother as my official sommelier. Almost ten years later in college, I wrote my thesis on wine, specifically the impending battle between Tradition and Modernity in the Rioja and Tuscany. While my friends sat in dark underground labs running regressions for their projects, I gallivanted around Spain and Italy with a few thousand dollars from the university in my pocket. Needless to say who had more fun . . .

Neither of these in-vino-veritas studies was meant as a rebellion or boondoggle; I took them extremely seriously, winning second prize at the regional science fair and getting an offer to publish my thesis. The university had originally wanted me to write on Chinese immigration law and its impact on the global economy, and although that would have looked impressive on my résumé, I had absolutely no interest in it. I have never been into doing something because I thought I had to, or simply to check projects off a society-imposed to-do list, half bored, half stressed, and totally uninterested.

Mental and physical to-dos are the foundation of what I call I Have To. I Have To encap-sulates the personal and societal pressure to do specific things, and to do them in a particular way. *I have to go to an Ivy League school. I have to get an MBA. I have to get married before I am thirty. I have to cut out sugar and gluten. I have to run a marathon. I have to have kids. I have to breastfeed. I have to make my baby's food from scratch. I have to quit my job to be a good mother. I have to dress conservatively now. I have to move to the suburbs. I have to. I have to. I have to.*

Honestly, who says you do? Why do you feel so obliged to accomplish that or carry out that task?

When we have our heads buried in our "I have tos," we miss what is actually going on around us. Life passes us by while we are checking off things we think we have to do to be successful and happy. We start to attach specific achievements to perceived happiness, relating societal approval to accomplishment. The problem is, I Have To often prevents you from actually *being* you.

If you continually shackle yourself to a list of to-dos, ones that you think will make you happy just because society says they will, you are shoehorning yourself into some manufactured image of you as opposed to existing as your true self. While you chip away at what others have outlined as the path to success and happiness, one of two things will happen: Either life will pass you by, or you will be miserable. Perhaps both. My student Krissie serves as a perfect example of this state, as well as a model of successful Retox recovery.

Krissie suffered from intense I Have To syndrome. A good ol' Midwestern gal, Krissie moved to New York City right after graduating from college for a job in investment banking. Although passionate about interior design, she thought a career in banking was the "right" path for her. After suffering through banal PowerPoint presentations, Excel spreadsheets, and twenty-hour days, six days a week, she went to business school, because that's what everyone in banking does. There, she met a man, endlessly nagged him about proposing, picked out the two-carat diamond solitaire she wanted, threw a ridiculously opulent wedding, and got married by the time she was twenty-five. Soon after the wedding, she quit her job and moved to the suburbs where they bought a house, got a dog, and started family planning. She had checked off almost everything on her life to-do list in a few years, and she was actually feeling pretty good about it. Yet she was not happy.

Everything Krissie did, she did because she thought she had to, not because she actually wanted to. By the time she came to me, she was thirty years old and miserable. Through her tears, she told me that her life was a mess (despite the house, dog, cars, rich husband, and, I have to say, amazing wardrobe). We soon began to apply Retox methods to help her find her true self, her own dreams and passions, her own desires and personal, unadulterated wish list. She used my mindset plan every morning, threw down a mat alone or with me three times a week, and freed herself from her self-imposed restricted diets to give Retox nourishment a try.

Slowly but surely, Krissie began to smile, recovering a bounce in her step and a desire to truly live. While Retoxing, she realized she was miserable in the burbs, missed working, and wasn't quite ready to start a family. The catch is, her husband felt much the same. They had both pressured themselves into following a path that society had laid out for them, rather than following a path that would actually make them happy. Ultimately, Krissie and her husband moved back to the city, where she pursued a degree in interior design. She now runs her own business, has decided to wait to have kids, and is more passionately in love with her husband, and life, than ever.

Just because you think you *have to* does not mean you actually do. Like Sinatra sings, you have to do it your way—and I would add that you have to do it with passion and integrity. Here are some tools to get you on your way—*your way.*

YOGA

I.AM.YOU. Retox yoga is categorized under vinyasa. It flows through a sequence of poses all linked by the breath. The practice as a whole is meant to represent our fluid journey from birth to death, from Child's pose to Sava-sana, Corpse pose.

Most of us struggle to be smack-dab in the present moment, or as so many modern gurus have called it, the Now. Instead, we are usually ensconced in I Have To, continually focusing on the next step, goal, or I Have To achieve-ment. We let details and future to-dos fill our minds, losing sight of the journey as a whole. Sometimes we look up, like Krissie, and think, "How did I get here?"

When practiced correctly, I.AM.YOU. Retox yoga is one of the most powerful tools for remedying "I have to." It compels you to be in the moment and forces you to be exactly where you are, twisted and sweaty on a two-by-five piece of rubber. If your mind drifts toward something else, you, like me, will likely topple over. If you force yourself into a pose because you think you have to do it, you will, like I did

in a headstand almost ten years ago, hurt your-self. (Which, by the way, sucks. I broke three bones in my foot and was in a cast for six months because I thought I had to nail a head-stand then and there.) I Have To does not work for yoga.

I prescribed the following poses and longer sequence for Krissie. She did them daily, and slowly but surely started to feel a drastic change in her self-awareness, which ultimately led her to ditch I Have To and move into "I want to." They will help you do the same, creating a regular space for you to just be you, and tune in to what your body and mind actually need and want.

Try all the Retox poses suggested on different days so you can decipher what it is your body wants and needs. If something does not feel right, simply do not do it and skip to the next thing. Just make sure that you are steadily breathing, in and out through your nose, in one uninterrupted stream. Let the yoga do its job and guide you exactly where you should be, in body, mind, and life. All I want you to do is focus on the moment and breathe.

RETOX

DESK FIXES

SHAKE IT OUT

Take a deep inhale. Exhale strongly out of your mouth, sticking your tongue out. Drop your head and shake it out as you exhale. Repeat one to five times.

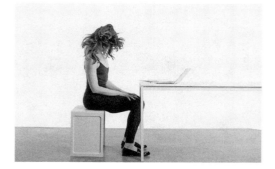

FREEDOM TWIST*

Sit comfortably in your chair, your back tall and straight, your feet flat on the floor. Inhale, reach your left arm up. Exhale, twist to the right. Look over your right shoulder and make sure both sitz bones are on the chair. Bring your right arm behind you if it feels good. Breathe here, then repeat on the other side.

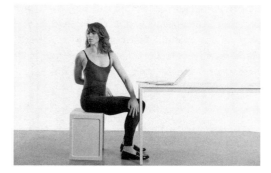

FREEDOM RELEASE

Come to the edge of your chair. Bring your feet together and drop your knees wide. Fold forward, resting your arms and hands where it feels comfortable and dropping your head. Inhale fully through your nose. Exhale out of your mouth, sticking out your tongue if that feels good. Hold here five to ten normal breaths.

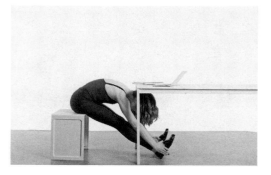

FREEING BACKBEND AND BREATH*

Place your hands behind you wherever feels good. Inhale, lift your chest up. Exhale, start to find a backbend in your upper back. Drop your head back if it does not hurt your neck. Breathe here naturally or begin short, sharp breaths out of the nose, where the inhale is simply a reaction to the exhale, as the diaphragm pumps on the abdominal wall. It should feel somewhere between sneezing and blowing your nose. (If you are pregnant, skip khapalabhati; just hold the pose and breathe normally.) Stay here, breathing or pumping as long as it feels good.

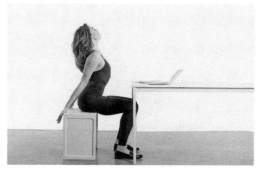

303

QUICK FIXES

SUN SALUTE A
Start standing with your feet together and your hands touching at your chest. Inhale, extending your arms overhead. Exhale, fold forward and bring your forehead to your shins. Inhale, extend your spine, look forward. Exhale, Chaturanga or Plank pose. Inhale, Up Dog. Exhale, Down Dog. Close your eyes and hold here five breaths. Then inhale and step or jump your feet between your hands. Exhale, fold forward. Inhale, reach your arms up, look up. Exhale, hands to your heart. Repeat five to ten times.

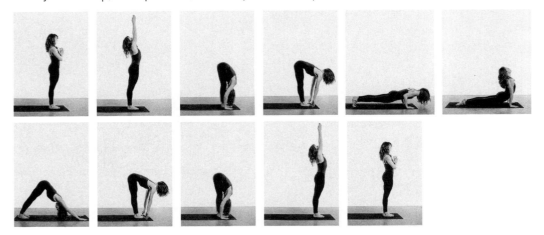

LUNGE TWIST*
Start with your right foot between the hands on the floor, your left leg straight behind you. Your left knee can be lifted off the floor unless it is too much. Inhale, extending your right arm out to the side. Exhale, extending your right arm overhead and spinning your chest open. Hold five to ten breaths, then repeat on the other side.

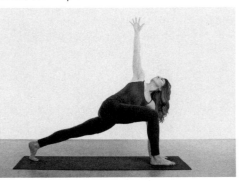

HEADSTAND PREP
Sit on your knees and interlace your hands into a fist. Place your forearms and fists to the floor. Keep your elbows no wider than your shoulders. Place the top of your head to the floor, back of your head touching the wrists. Straighten your legs to Down Dog legs, but in the air. Stay here and breathe. Optionally walk your feet in, and maybe lift your legs up into a little ball or into a full head-stand. Keep your feet on the floor or up in air. Hold here and breathe for ten to twenty breaths.

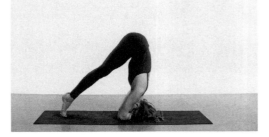

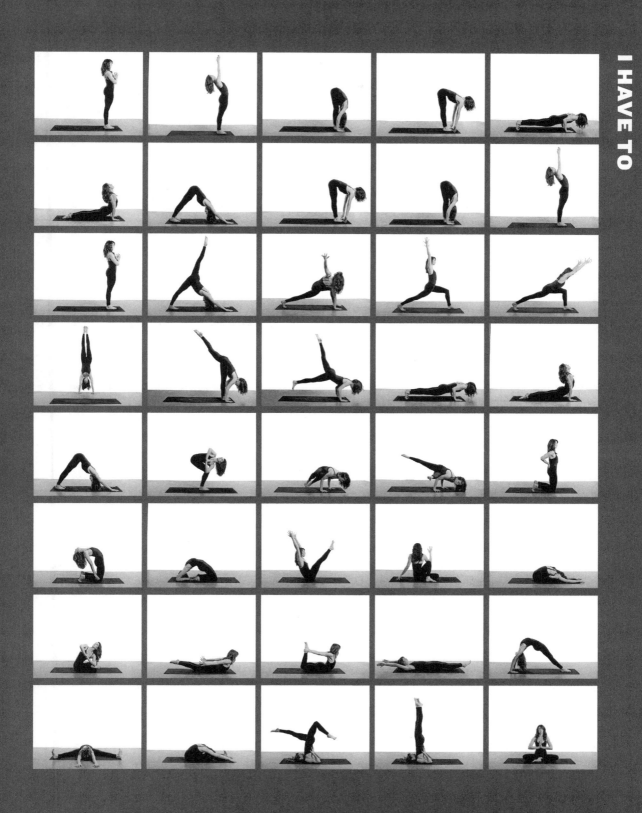

NOURISHMENT

Now it is time to get totally crazy.

I want you to throw out all of your food doctrine for a week. Unless you have a clinically proven medical concern or true allergy, give up all your rules. Forget about no sugar, no gluten, no meat. Essentially, give up giving up what you have given up. I have only three guidelines for you to follow.

DETOX

1. No fast food or processed food
2. No soda
3. No skipping meals

RETOX

Now one simple thing:

Eat what you crave.

Whatever it is, whatever time of day. Yes, you read this correctly.

When I suggested this plan to Krissie, she practically broke into a panicked sweat, but thankfully believed enough in me to give it a whirl. Throughout the process, she realized she was drinking juice because she thought she had to, even though she hated the taste and dent on her wallet. She noticed that kale, although the trendiest food of mankind, gave her massive stomachaches and that she was dying for a burger.

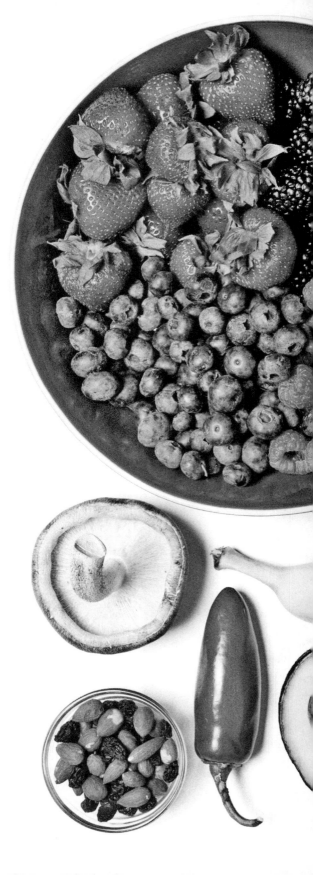

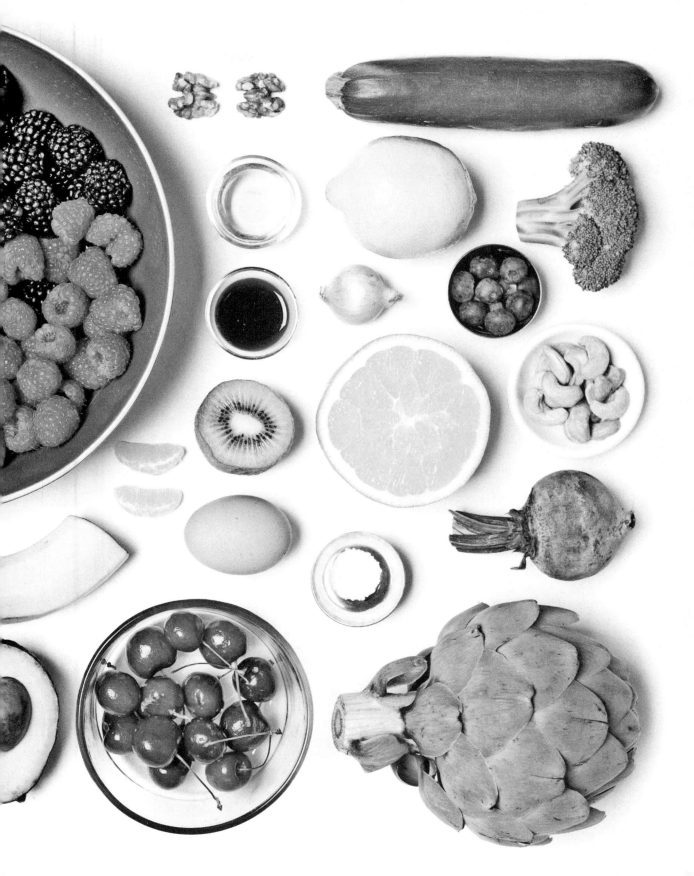

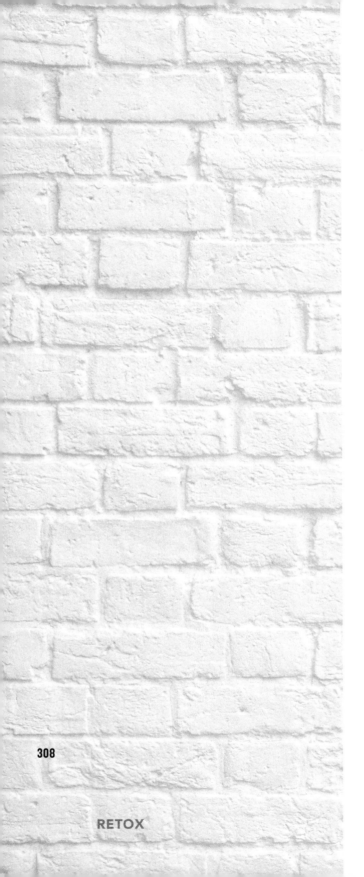

By throwing away her nutritional and dietary "I have tos," Krissie began to notice what her body actually needed and wanted, as opposed to what her mind forced it to have. She ended up losing weight, improving her digestion, and finding straight-up joy in eating. She let go of the pressure to follow certain current dogmas and started to follow the cravings of her natural self, the one that had been hidden under years of "I have to."

So are you ready?

Starting tomorrow, write down every single thing you eat and drink and how you feel before, during, and after you eat it, so you have a record to look back on and see when you felt best and when you could have felt better.

MINDSET

I had just returned to campus after a glorious semester abroad in Florence. I was floating about campus in all my new leather gear, indulging in my new coffee habits without a care in the world aside from learning, reading, writing, living. *La dolce vita.* One day a friend sat down with me for an afternoon macchiato (yes, I was on a mission to convert the masses) and asked how my interviews were going. I responded, "Interviews for what?" He answered, "Lauren!!!! Summer consulting and banking internships! You haven't been prepping or interviewing? What are you thinking?" I put my coffee cup down and had a mini panic attack. Interviews for consulting firms? Am I supposed to be doing this? Shit.

Sure that I totally screwed up my future, I scrambled, setting up interviews with several consulting firms and boutique investment banks in Manhattan, even though I had absolutely no desire to work at any of them. Every time someone would ask me why I wanted to work at their firm, or why investment banking was my dream job, I was at a complete loss. I would head back to the train station, indignant over the pointlessness of these interviews and wondering what I was doing with my life. As I waited for the train in Penn Station, I would stand at the newsstand and flip through magazines, daydreaming of a job in writing or publishing. More often than I should admit, I would rip out the first pages of publications I liked. I was obsessed with journalism and secretly prayed I would be able to dump this consulting/banking charade and pursue my interest in journalism over the summer. The tear-outs provided a pre-Google list of potential contacts.

Perhaps needless to say, after three months of constant interviewing for jobs I actually did not want, I did not get an internship. I was dejected, yet relieved, and decided to start cold-calling the contacts from the ripped-out magazine pages. Fortunately, I got offers for internships at three publications, one of which I took, leading me into a dream Manhattan summer of writing articles, editing, and working on business development for the coolest new magazine in town.

Every morning on my stroll through Soho to work, I realized that during that dreadful interviewing process I had been trying to force myself into a job I did not want, a job that did not fit who I was and who I wanted to be. It can be hard to separate what you really want and what you think you want or should want. I am lucky in that, even when I got momentarily sidetracked, I was eventually able to follow my heart: I interned at a magazine when everyone else was buried in an investment bank; I washed dishes and worked as a waitress while my classmates were interviewing at consulting firms; I studied literature instead of economics to get myself to Wall Street; I skipped business school to head straight to entrepreneurship; and I waited nine years to get engaged, eleven to get married; and I couldn't be happier. I'm proud to say, I have done it my way, following the rules of the game, but never forcing myself to jump through the "normal" societal hoops unless I wanted to.

The thing is, everyone maps out their life journey with different markers. Some people focus on career advancement, others on personal landmarks like marriage and parenthood, others on degrees, and still others on random adventures. The only wrong journey is one that does not make you happy, one you do not enjoy building, or one you are not proud of. The ancient yogis would call this process *vinyasa krama*.

The essence of yoga is vinyasa krama. *Vinyasa* comes from the Sanskrit roots *vi*, which means "sequence," and *nyasa*, which means "selected or placed." Together *vinyasa* means "a joining or linking mechanism." *Krama* means "an uninterrupted process," a sequence of changes or events that occurs from moment to moment. Together, vinyasa krama is your life journey, an uninterrupted sequence of movements or events that create your body, mind, and life experience.

When we have I Have To, we interrupt the natural succession of events in our life, and instead impose what our intellectual, hypersensitive modern mind thinks needs to happen. We focus so much on formulating and constructing the next step that we thwart the organic evolution of life. Our life journey is one that is discovered as we go, one that will fulfill us more than anything we could fabricate. When we try to control our personal vinyasa krama rather than ride its waves, we obstruct our true spirit, our true destiny, and, within that, life's beauty.

The essence of life, like yoga, is in the progression of transitions that unite one experience to the next. If you simply focus on doing what you want, and doing it well with passion and integrity, all the rest will fall into place. You will get there, and you will get there your way.

RETOX

The Tibetan Buddhists say that in order to be enlightened, or as I say, to be successful and happy, you have to have peace and joy in your steps. They also say that the heels of the foot represent the past, the balls represent the future, and the middle of the foot is the life path. They go on to explain that time only exists in the sense of the future and the past; the rest is vinyasa krama, or life itself. Not surprisingly, they created a walking meditation thousands of years ago. I have adapted this to today's times and I Have To, creating the ultimate Retox solution.

Stand up and get ready for a walk. This can be a long leisurely walk, a short jaunt to the water cooler, or even part of your commute through the parking lot or subway platform. Before you go anywhere, notice your breath and make sure it is through the nose.

Now start walking, coordinating your steps with your breath.

> Inhale and step on the middle of your left foot, saying, *What makes me happy?*
> Exhale and step on the middle of your right foot, saying, *Go get it.*

Repeat the breath, the sayings, and the steps. When your mind wanders, bring it back to your stride.

Do this for as long as you are able to in your schedule, and rest assured that your mind will be cleared of any distractions or "I have tos."

Retox Soundtrack:
"My Way" —FRANK SINATRA

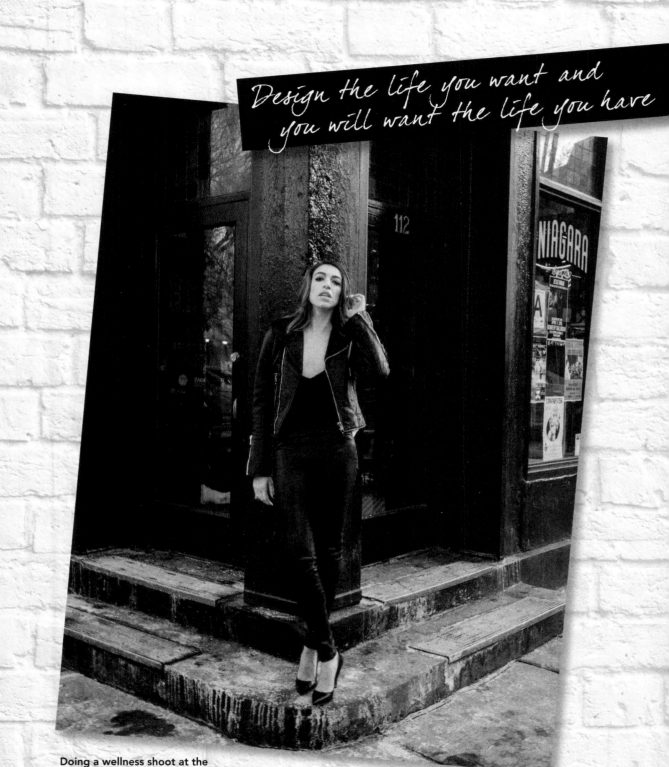

Design the life you want and you will want the life you have

Doing a wellness shoot at the classic New York City rock bar Niagara. Photograph by Mick Rock.

CRUSHIN' IT

CREATING AND

MAINTAINING SUCCESS

Roll with the Punches

MY FIRST YEARS AS AN entrepreneur were fairly brutal. I cried more in the initial twenty-four months of I.AM.YOU. than in my entire seven years on Wall Street, and I am not a crier by nature.

One of my more intense tear festivals came around seven months after launching my business. I had hired a web team to transition me from the first, basic website to the full monty. I knew my target audience and the brand I wanted to showcase. I knew the look I was going for: black-and-white, edgy, and clean. Now all I needed was for them to code it all into an ecosystem for the digital landscape. Simple, right? I wish.

After months of painful back-and-forth, the web team presented the final site, at which point my mascara instantly started tracking down my cheeks. What they had created was nothing like I requested or envisioned; it had bright purple and neon blue, annoying pop-up windows, messy navigation bars, and a litany of other issues. I was distraught, defeated, furious, and, above all, panicked. This disaster had cost me a small fortune. I was doomed for failure.

I spent the day agonizing over what to do. Launch the site I hated and misrepresent the brand I risked everything for and dreamed of creating? Dip further into my savings and remake an entirely new site? Give up and plead for my job back on the trading floor? Or just cry on the couch? I went for the last option; it seemed easiest for a failure like me. When my boyfriend arrived home from work, I showed him the site, and proceeded to go off on what I had actually been shooting for versus that . . . mess. With watery eyes, frenetic Italian American hand gesticulations, and animated rambling, I began to flesh out how I had wanted it, starting at the very beginning. He told me to pause so he could order a pizza and grabbed a stack of white paper from the printer. Over the next few hours and slices, I drew out exactly what I wanted the site to look like and the user experience to be. I then took this stack of drawings to a new web company, Free Association, who built not only what I envisioned, but enhanced that to a user experience far beyond what I had thought possible. All within my budget.

The moral of the story is not about the pizza, or my tears, but rather that achieving success isn't easy. It's tough, it's confusing, it's frustrating. Success means something different for each of us, and from there can take on a unique form each day. It can imply launching your own business or getting the kids to bed on time. Overcoming an illness or learning a new language. Providing for your family or closing a deal. Falling in love or breaking up. Nailing a headstand or sleeping through the night. Getting a promotion or quitting your job. Whatever it is, only you can define your success; it is too individual, too personal, too ephemeral, too amorphous for anyone other than you to do. But no matter what your personal success is, we all ride the same roller coaster to get there. There are highs and lows, days where we end up completely banged up, feeling punches of all shapes and sizes, and others where we are flying high. It's a ride like none other, and irrevocably goes with the territory of getting where you want to be.

In those same initial I.AM.YOU. years of prolific tears, I also ricocheted off walls and sidewalks in elated ecstasy at accomplishments of all magnitudes, from teaching my first sold-out class to getting my first item of press. These precious moments, these successes, are the ones that we all strive for across all our individual careers and paths of life. These are the euphoric victories that inspire us to keep going, the triumphs we try to amass to propel us forward. This is the sweet feeling of success, or as I like to call it, Crushin' It.

In entrepreneurship, as in all walks of life, from motherhood to medicine, love, the corporate realm, and even body acceptance, you have to live with and through the ups and the downs, the highs and the lows. But how do you *actually* get there? How do you succeed, and then maintain that success when you have it?

Dream + Hustle = Success

You need to have a dream to know where you want to go. And then you have to take action to get there.

Success is a journey. Yes, chasing and capturing the highs are part of it, but the only way to get where you want is to accept the inevitable lows and keep going. No matter what comes your way, you keep your eyes on the prize and forge ahead. So Crushin' It is all about rolling with the punches.

There are two types of punches you have to get used to as you head to the top. First, the tangible ones, the ones that you can clearly see the consequences of: getting passed up for a promotion, missing a sales quota, getting dumped, failing to secure the deal, seeing your kid throw their dinner on the floor. Each represents a direct hit, a solid punch you can trace in a material, linear way. Then there are the intangible punches, the ones you cannot necessarily rationally explain, but leave just as much of a mark: an odd tone in an email, a comment on social media, being NFI (not f*ing invited) to a dinner, distance from your partner . . . Each of these is harder to directly link to a success or failure, yet bangs you up on the inside. Learning to roll with the punches, both tangible and intangible, prepares your body, mind, and life to achieve and preserve success.

The punches are the seeds to success; how you interact with them is the key to glory. Together—the punches and your attitude toward them—shape and create your victorious destiny. Roll with the punches, and you will crush it. Let yourself be bruised and abused, and you will lose.

The Retox cocktail for succeeding beyond your wildest dreams and Crushin' It helps you manage both the tangible and intangible punches, as well as your interaction with them. We start with the yoga, pushing and using the deepest layers and capabilities of your muscles and breath. We move on to nourishment, making sure you are not getting in your own way. And then with an easy mindset plan, we learn how to never get caught up in the punch, thus creating our own success from the inside out. This 360-degree approach to success reflects the multidimensional path that success itself rides upon, and can be applied to all stages of life, from parenthood to the boardroom.

YOGA

It's no secret that Retox and I.AM.YOU. yoga classes are hard—I have designed them specifically to be the hardest around. Do I get off on torturing you or am I a masochist? Neither. But I do love to make you feel the burn, which is the best training for rolling with the punches.

In the Retox plan for Crushin' It, I use the yoga poses and their sequencing as a physical manifestation of rolling with the punches. Basically, I provide the pain, so you can relish in all the gain. So, yeah, you may shake as I ask you to hold the poses or feel a little banged up the next day, but that's a good thing. It means you made it—you succeeded on the mat and can take on anything life throws you on your way to success.

Coincidentally, I have two clients with the same name, one a man, one a woman, both named Morgan. They did not know each other, but both were struggling with success. Morgan, the man, had gotten promoted to the highest level of his firm. Every deal he closed in the past

eighteen months was a huge success, and he and his fiancée were getting along better than ever. Yet he was panicked about it all unraveling; he feared losing his success and never being able to achieve the same level again. Morgan, the woman, was straight-up struggling. She was riddled with a series of bad bosses, all of whom created absurd bulwarks to her doing her job well or even just using her skill set to complete the tasks at hand. They were visibly blocking her success at the company every step of the way, leading her to believe that she would never win at anything in life and doubting everything about her capabilities. I gave both Morgans the same Retox yoga prescription. The man thought he was too inflexible and straight-up unable to do yoga. The woman thought she was not strong or in shape enough. I ignored them both and went to work.

During our yoga Retoxing, both Morgans sweat—a lot—and swore at me under their breath and via their fairly vicious glares, but I never let them give up. I threw them punch after punch, pose after pose, Chaturanga after Chaturanga. It was a No Pain, No Gain workshop, a lesson on not only yoga, but life. Both Morgans crushed the Retox yoga, and quickly realized that if they could do the yoga, day in and day out, they could take on and succeed at anything.

Retox yoga makes you strong in mind and body. It shows you that not only can you succeed, but you will. I throw you the yoga punches so that when you get out onto the stage of life, you are totally ready to rumble, and crush it just like you did on the mat not long before.

RETOX

DESK FIXES

VICTORY ARMS

Sit up tall. Reach your arms up alongside your ears and open them into a V. Now stay there, breathing, aiming for ten to twenty breaths. Repeat hourly.

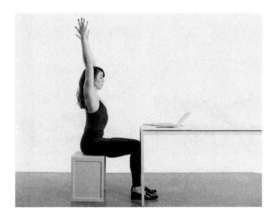

CHAIR

Stand up from your chair. Inhale fully and bend your knees. Bring your butt to hover over your chair. Stay here as long as possible. Maybe a moment, maybe for a whole call or email.

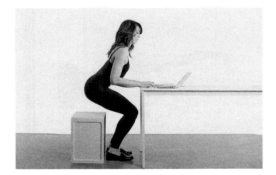

DESK PUSH-UP

Place your hands on the edge of your desk. Inhale, press into your hands and straighten your arms. Exhale, bend your elbows halfway, elbows straight back, like a mini push-up. Inhale, straighten your elbows. Repeat ten times.

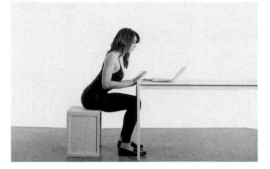

FLOATING SUCCESS

Come to the edge of your chair, and place your hands on the edge of the chair as well. Inhale, lengthen your spine. Exhale, press down on your hands and try to lift your butt off the chair and your feet off the floor, crossing your ankles if possible. Hover here for one to five breaths. Repeat one to five times.

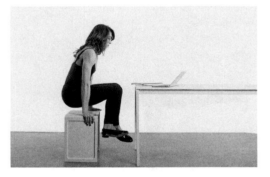

CRUSHIN' IT

QUICK FIXES

VICTORY VINYASA

Start in Plank pose, shoulders over wrists, legs straight, body parallel to the floor. Hold here for three breaths, or longer if you are up for it. On an exhale, bend your elbows straight back into Chaturanga. Hold here for three breaths. On an inhale, straighten your elbows and lift your left leg into Three-Legged Plank (page 224). Hold here one to three breaths. Exhale, bring your elbows straight back into a three-legged Chaturanga, keeping your right leg lifted. Hold here one to three breaths. On an inhale, come back to Plank pose.

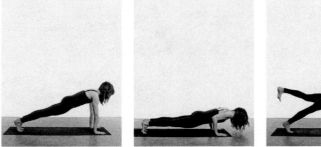 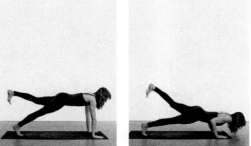

EXTENDED WARRIOR 3

Standing tall, inhale, lean forward, and take your right leg behind you, taking it parallel to the floor. Float your body parallel to the floor, balancing on the left leg. Place your fingertips on the floor or float your arms alongside your body or your ears. Balance here for five to ten breaths, then repeat on the other side.

TWISTED HALF MOON*

Start in Warrior 3, right leg in the air. Inhale, place your right hand to the floor. Exhale, lift your left arm up and twist. Take your gaze to the left thumb, keep your right foot flexed, and lengthen your torso. Hold five to ten breaths, then repeat on the other side.

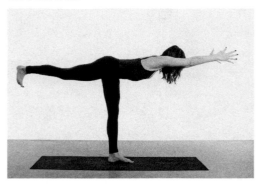 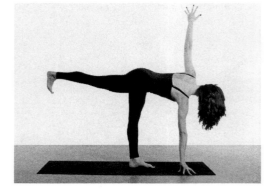

RETOX

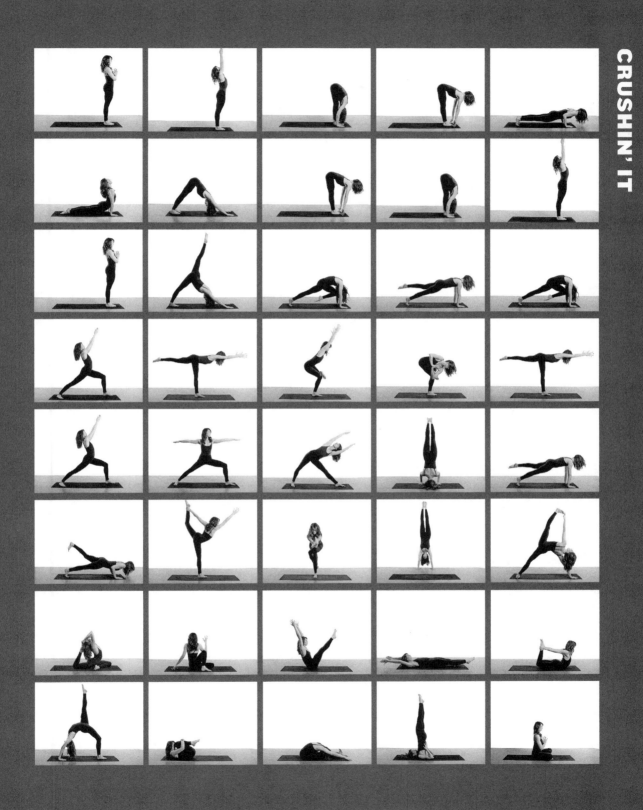

NOURISHMENT

There are already so many obstacles on the path to success that the last thing you need is to clutter it up even more, especially with something as delicious and essential as food. The key to Crushin' It in nourishment terms is taking out the foods that can obfuscate your victories and adding in the foods that can lock them in. But before we start salivating, let me give you three tips to eating your way to success.

3 RULES TO EAT YOUR WAY TO SUCCESS

1. **Eat Up.** Do not be afraid of food—it is a successful person's friend. Your brain and body need an inordinate amount of energy to function, so depriving them of it just so you feel or look thinner is not going to get you anywhere good for long. Eat, eat, eat throughout the day, choosing snacks and meals like the ones I suggest below, thus ensuring that you are never low on fuel and always ready to take on the next step.

2. **Break(the)Fast.** I can't lie, breakfast is far from my favorite meal of the day. I'd be infinitely happier with my croissant and almond milk cappuccino sometime around noon. But, like it or not, breakfast is the most important meal. Your body grows and repairs itself overnight as you sleep, requiring energy to do so. Breakfast, or the "break" in the fast that happened as you slept, is imperative to replenish the depleted energy from your body fixing itself up overnight. Think of it as a refueling of the tank before you take off (and maybe get punched) throughout the day. Without breakfast, it will be harder to accomplish everything you want and need to, let alone at the quality level you likely demand of yourself. Make sure you eat breakfast within three hours of getting up, even if you have to force a little something down. Your brain, body, and success will thank you.

3. **Share.** Eating and drinking with others is a must for crushin' it. Try to find a dining partner at least once a day, whether that means simply someone to walk with to pick up lunch, a proper dinner date, or a colleague to grab a drink with after work. Talking, sharing, and communicating as you feed yourself and indulge will help you internalize the day's activities, disseminate new information, and come up with new ideas and inspiration to guide you to success. If you eat and drink alone, you will be stuck alone in your mind, unable to really assess the surroundings or reaffirm your strengths. Find someone to talk it out with and your path to success will be that much clearer.

DETOX

Just like there are foods that can help aid your success, there are foods that can thwart it. Here is a list of foods to reduce or, ideally, eliminate entirely so that you can turn your mind and body into a clean, lean, Crushin'-It machine:

SODAS. They are just bad for you, especially the diet ones full of fake sweeteners that have been shown to cause cancer. Stick to water, or if you really have to have something with flavor, add cut up fruit, berries, or a small splash of juice to seltzer, make a homemade lemonade, or have some herbal iced tea without sugar.

FAST FOOD. Nothing will hold you back more than fast food. It is processed with low-quality ingredients and, quite frankly, should not even be considered real food. Feed yourself the real thing, fresh and easy, thus optimizing your fuel, function, and success.

FRIED FOOD. The fat in fried food bogs you down and is hard to digest. To stay nimble and on top of your game, swap fried foods for those baked or sautéed in olive oil.

CHOCOLATE. Yes, dark chocolate has antioxidants good for your brain and body functions, but most chocolate bars are laden with additives, sugars, and preservatives that will put you on another high and low roller coaster that you do not really need. Swap out your daily chocolate kick for a decaf cappuccino or piece of fruit.

SOY. Soy products bloat and have been shown to alter hormone levels. The last thing you need as you map out and own your success are your hormones going nuts on you. Scrap all soy products, from soy sauce to protein bars and beverages that use soy in them.

BEER. It can lead to a beer belly. Plain and simple. Pick another drink.

CIGARETTES. They are just gross and so 1960s. Not to mention, smoking these days is often seen as a blatant denial of (1) reality and (2) health. Avoid being seen smoking by colleagues and bosses by just not smoking at all.

CHICKEN. Do not get gobbled up in a chicken rut! So much of the chicken out there is nasty—injected full of antibiotics, hormones, and god knows what else to keep the profit margins and chicken breasts plump. Overdoing the chicken can mean that you are taking in all of these other substances that your body does not need, let alone know how to process. Swap it out for occasional high-quality chicken, or better yet salmon and tuna.

So now that you have some cardinal rules on the how, let's get down and dirty into the what. There are three genres of foods that will promote your success—those for the brain, those for vitality, and those for immunity. When you eat for these three, you create a bedrock for crushin' it.

RETOX

VITALITY FOODS

You can't get to the top if you don't have the energy to make the journey. Food is your body's fuel and you need all the right nutrients to keep you going strong.

BROCCOLI. Broccoli definitely needs a new PR agent. Aside from being full of vitamin A, calcium, folates for cell reproduction and repair, and phytonutrients that help prevent cancer, it is high in vitamin K, which is necessary for cognitive function. Sauté or steam a big batch every week, grab a container of it in the

321

cafeteria, and order it on your salad or as a side whenever and wherever you can.

BLUEBERRIES. A snack for success, blueberries have sugar coupled with a low glycemic index, making them perfect fuel for crushin' it. They are also high in antioxidants, which neutralize free radicals and protect the cells of the body from aging and disease. In addition, blueberries have been shown to improve memory and cognitive brain function. Snack on them throughout the day, grab a handful for breakfast, or blend them up into a grab-and-go smoothie.

TOMATOES. Tomatoes are rich in lycopene, an antioxidant shown to prevent cell damage. Eat them raw as a snack or in a salad, or for even more of a punch, cook down into a sauce or soup.

SAGE. This anti-inflammatory herb has been shown to improve both brain and body functions as well as improve the interconnectivity of different parts of the brain and body. Use it in your sautés or sprinkle it into soups or salads.

SPINACH. Popeye knew what he was doing. Spinach has been shown to slow the aging process, thwart mental decline, and prevent disease. It is high in iron, imperative for red blood cell production as well as your endurance and strength. Not to mention it is considered a functional food for its nutrients, antioxidants, and anticancer composition. Use it as a base in your salad, have it as a side with your main at dinner, or add a handful to your grab-and-go breakfast smoothie.

BRAIN FOODS

Your brain is the most critical instrument to your success. It demands twice as much en-

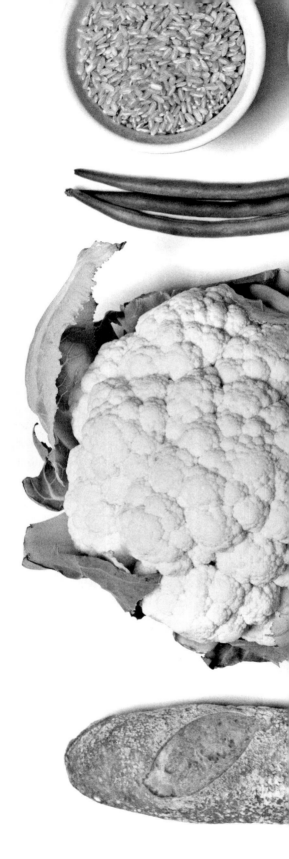

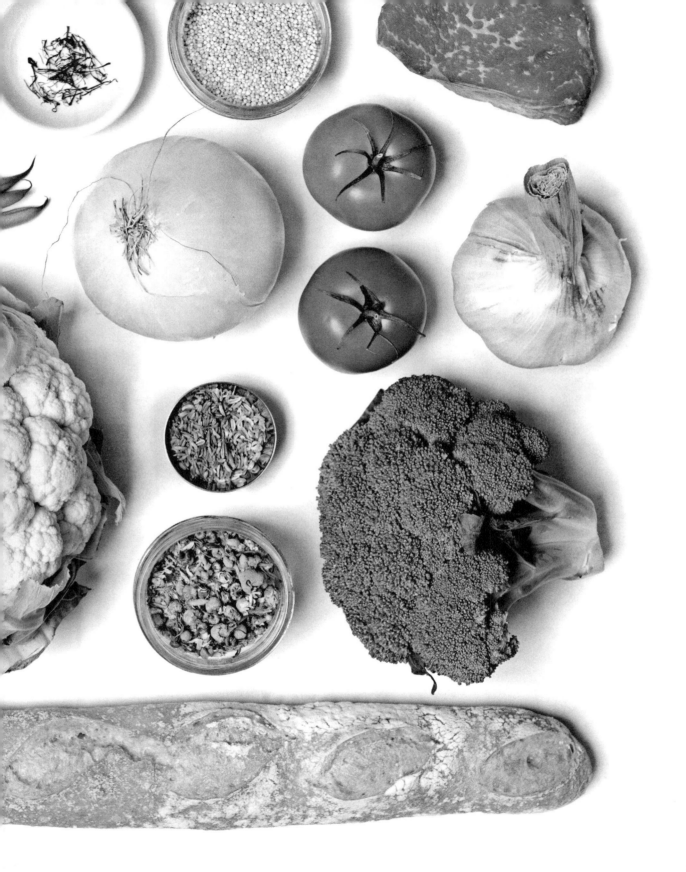

We all know that business dinners are inevitable, but what we tend to forget is that they are often the key to success. Sitting at a meal chatting with colleagues, bosses, clients, or fellow networkees can seem tedious, but it is precisely in this more relaxed, natural setting that we forge relationships, develop bonds, and embrace new concepts. If success is your goal, business dinners are your jive.

That said, you would not believe how many people—those already successful and those on the road to success—complain to me about business dinners. They whine about the drawn-out eating, the rich food, the unavoidable bread baskets and steaks, the endless wine, and they are always asking me for excuses to use to get out of them. Although I can commiserate, I have never been able to relate. Especially given that the whole thing is most often on someone else's dime!

I myself have sat through hundreds of business dinners, the bulk of which took place during my vegetarian years on Wall Street. Although I dreaded figuring out what and how I was going to eat at the sushi restaurant or steak house as the vegetarian female in the Boys Club, I knew that avoiding the dinners, professing self-imposed food dogma, or eating like a typical chick would get me nowhere. So I created a plan for eating at business dinners that has served me as a vegetarian on Wall Street and as a carnivore in wellness entrepreneurship, and has since helped dozens of others wine and dine themselves to the top, without gaining weight and feeling gross.

1. Water is your best friend. There will likely be drinks. That's fine. For better or worse, turning them down can often set you apart, and not in a good way. So drink with

ergy as any other organ in the body, using about 20 percent of your energy while only being about 2 percent of your body weight. It fuels itself with glucose and maintains itself with a combination of vitamins and minerals. You have to feed your brain if you want to be successful. There is no way around it.

FISH. The amino acids in fish create a feeding frenzy for your brain cells as they allow for the synthesis of neurons and neurotransmitters. Neurotransmitters are vital for keeping your brain sharp and on the ball. Of these, dopamine helps with immunity and the nervous system; serotonin guides moods, sleep, memory, and learning; acetylcholine helps with memory and recall; and norepinephrine keeps you alert and focused. Omega-3s and omega-6s are called essential fatty acids. DHA is the most abundant of these in the brain and is critical for cognitive and mental health. Eating fish and taking fish oil has been shown to prevent brain shrinkage and cognitive brain de-

324

your companions, but make sure you match each drink with water. For every alcoholic drink, be it a vodka tonic or a glass of wine, have one of water to match.

2. Keep it neat and clean. If you get to decide your drink, which I encourage, stick to the neat and clean bunch. Wine is your first choice, beer your second. If the dinner requires cocktails, go for vodka or gin with soda water or a whiskey neat or on the rocks. Once you decide on something, stick with it. Don't mix your drinks, as that is a recipe for disaster.

3. If you're out to eat, eat! Select real food options, not bird food, and then eat it. Pushing your food around in circles makes you seem indecisive. Making up excuses to not eat makes you seem fickle, untrustworthy, and boring. I am not saying to triple down on gravy and fried mozzarella sticks, but rather to pick a normal, full meal, one like your mom would have fed you when you were a kid, and just eat it. You can work it off tomorrow if you have to.

4. Eliminate the risks. Okay, so you may or may not want to be there, but you are, because you know it will help you crush it in the future. Now what do you order? Stick to items that are clear-cut and you know you should like. If you are at a sushi spot and know you do not like raw fish, pick from the black cod or teriyaki options. At the steak house, if you do not feel like red meat or do not eat it, go for the grilled fish. If you are a vegetarian at either, base your meal around the sides. Let others order first, if you can, so you can get an idea of the pace of the meal, and also don't stumble when it comes around to your turn. And really, even I, the number one salad lover in the world, am telling you this—do not just get a salad as a main for dinner. Get a proper, full meal, with a salad on the side or as a starter.

cline as we age. Try loading your diet with fatty fishes like salmon and tuna. On days you can't get it in your diet, pop a fish oil supplement.

EGGS. Eggs are a vital source of B12, a vitamin closely linked with the formation and function of the brain. Deficiency can result in impaired brain function, mental disorders, Alzheimer's, and dementia. Even slightly low levels can result in symptoms of poor memory and mental fatigue. Despite what anyone tells you, you cannot get B12 from vegetable sources. Eggs, followed by meat and fish, are your best bet. In addition, the yolk of the eggs has choline, a precursor for the neurotransmitter acetylcholine mentioned above. Eating eggs for breakfast or even during the day can help you improve your memory and sharpness on your path to success.

MEAT. Creatine provides energy to your cells for everyday activity, and especially fuels your brain for critical thought and endurance throughout the day. Although creatine is also found in fish, meat is the best source of it, with five grams in every 2.5 pounds of red meat, so it's sure to keep your brain going through all the punches. Slap a high-quality steak on the grill, go Mexican with beef tacos, Italian with beef sauce for a pasta, or all-American with a burger patty and side of veggies.

NUTS AND SEEDS. Not to turn you into a bird or anything, but feeding on nuts and seeds will help your brain health and function. The antioxidants and omega-3 fats protect against brain cell damage, and the protein gives you fuel to keep going. Walnuts are particularly known for improving mental ability and clearing thoughts, while flax, pumpkin, and sesame seeds add magnesium, zinc, and especially vitamin E to the equation. Keep some near you for snacks or toss them into your salads and breakfasts.

SUGAR AND CARBS. Glucose is chemically classified as a carbohydrate, but usually referred to as a sugar. Your brain will not—and cannot—function without glucose, which means that if you are on a sugar-free, carb-free diet, your brain is not functioning optimally. Try the fruits and veggies in the next section to feed, nourish, and protect your brain, and don't worry if you eat pasta, bread, and sugar. Your brain needs it, and thus so do you.

WATER. The brain weighs about three pounds and consists of roughly 75 percent water. To maintain healthy hydration levels, make sure you drink two liters of water a day, ideally flat and room temperature.

IMMUNITY FOODS

You can't crush it if you are sick all the time. Include an immunity-boosting food at least twice a day to keep yourself strong for battle. Try adding these foods to your diet regularly to boost your immune system and ensure that you are always ready to roll with the punches on the path to success:

GARLIC. Nature's best and original immunity booster. Slice it up and use it in a sauté, add a few cloves to your soup or sauces, and if you are really gangsta like my grandmother, straight-up munch on a clove every morning.

VITAMIN C. You know you and your immune system need it. Of course you can eat your orange, but kiwis, bell peppers (especially red), papaya, and broccoli all pack more immunity-boosting vitamin C in each bite.

HONEY. Honey has many antibacterial and anti-inflammatory properties. It has been used for thousands of years as an immunity booster and creator of strength and stamina. Add a dollop onto a piece of toast in the morning or have a teaspoon in your tea or as a snack.

SNACKS

Walnuts and almonds
Homemade trail mix: nuts, seeds, and
    dried raisins
Raw veggies: snap peas, carrots, bell
    peppers, cherry tomatoes
Blueberries
Dark chocolate
Half an avocado

326

RECIPES

Crushin' It Salad

3 cups baby spinach

1 red bell pepper, chopped

1 cup steamed broccoli florets

½ tomato, diced

1 (3-ounce) can all-white tuna packed in water

2 tablespoons pumpkin seeds

2 tablespoons walnuts

2 tablespoons extra virgin olive oil

1 tablespoon balsamic vinegar

Place all salad ingredients in a large bowl. Toss with olive oil and vinegar.

Success Smoothie

1 cup strawberries, sliced

1 cup blueberries

⅓ banana, sliced

1 teaspoon ground flaxseeds

1 handful spinach

1 teaspoon honey

Blend everything together and enjoy!

Salmon Crush Crunch

1 (6-ounce) salmon fillet

3 teaspoons olive oil, divided

2 cups baby spinach

1 cup diced broccoli

1 cup cooked quinoa or wild rice

1 teaspoon flaxseeds or sesame seeds (optional)

Rub salmon with 1 teaspoon of olive oil. Heat a skillet over medium heat. Add salmon and raise heat to high. Cook for 3 minutes, then turn and cook for another 4 or 5 minutes, until it is cooked through and flakes easily with a fork. Set aside. In the same pan, heat the remaining 2 teaspoons olive oil over medium heat. Add spinach and broccoli and cook until spinach is wilted and broccoli is tender. Add quinoa or rice and mix together. Sprinkle in flax or sesame seeds, if using. Add salmon to pan and flake it with a fork. Stir everything together and serve in a bowl or over a bed of lettuce.

Beef Sauce

1 tablespoon extra virgin olive oil

1 yellow onion, chopped

2 cloves garlic, minced

1 carrot, diced

½ pound organic ground beef

2 (28-ounce) cans crushed
   tomatoes

1 teaspoon oregano

Salt and pepper, to taste

Dash of red pepper flakes
   (optional)

1 (12-ounce) package pasta of
   your choice

Heat oil in a large skillet over medium heat. Add onion, garlic, and carrots and cook until carrots are soft. Add beef, breaking it up with the back of a wooden spoon, and cook until the meat is no longer pink. Add tomatoes, oregano, salt and pepper to taste, and red pepper flakes, if using. Cover and let simmer for 15 to 20 minutes. While the sauce cooks, bring a large pot of water to boil. Add pasta and cook according to package directions. When cooked, drain and add to pan with sauce. Stir together, serve, and enjoy!

MINDSET

Let's go back to the punches. Don't worry, I'm not going to beat you up . . . yet. I'll let the Tibetan yoga philosophers do it for now.

The fifth verse of the Yoga Sutra tells us that the mind works solely in ways where it is either afflicted or free of afflictions. The word for *afflicted* and *afflictions* in Sanskrit is *klesha*. It comes from the root *klish*, which means "a calamity, prickly, to disturb or bother, to obfuscate." Kleshas are mental obstacles, impediments to the path. They are the punches on your road to success.

Kleshas are categorized into six groups:

- Ignorance, a lack of knowledge and power to sustain understanding
- Ignorant liking, liking something for the wrong reasons
- Ignorant disliking, disliking something for the wrong reasons
- Lazy doubt, either being lazy or wavering on an action due to laziness
- Pride, conceit, and self-importance
- Wrong worldview, not understanding where things are coming from or how things really work.

Now take a moment and think about how many times you have blundered due to one of these kleshas. I, for one, can give you at least a dozen examples of each: thinking I was too good for something, dissing on someone without really knowing them, chasing something because I thought it would impress others, choosing not to make a move because I was too lazy to properly research it . . . These are all kleshas, punches that I encountered on my path to success.

The goal of crushin' it in the Retox mindset way is to learn to roll with the punches, slowly but surely moving past them, eradicating the kleshas and eliminating the obstacles, freeing yourself from them as you go. When you do, you will not only arrive at success, but you will own it for much longer than you thought possible. You will have thoroughly crushed it.

RETOX

This is a take on a Tibetan Buddhist practice called the Six Times Book. The original is a method for checking in on your mind six times a day, which, let's be honest, can be tough in a real-life setting. The Retox way, on the other hand, leverages the underlying technique but offers a realistic system to eradicate the six kleshas that may be hindering your success. In doing so, it creates a routine for you to roll through the punches and a framework for you to crush it.

Take out a calendar, planner, or your phone's calendar app. Write *ignorance* on today. Write *ignorant liking* for tomorrow. Write *ignorant disliking* on the day after that. On the next day, write *lazy doubt*. On the next, write *pride*, and finally, write *wrong worldview*. Repeat this order three more times for a total of twenty-four days.

Now, every day, one time a day, look at that calendar. If it says *ignorance*, write below it one way you failed or succumbed to ignorance. Below that, write what you would do better or change the next time. The next day, if it says *ignorant liking*, write one thing that drew you in ignorantly. Below that, write what you should have looked at or done differently. Repeat like this, klesha after klesha, day after day. Think of it as a symptom and an anecdote, or a punch and the relief.

If you forget a day, don't worry. Go back and do it when you remember. Try to complete a whole six-day cycle, and ideally all twenty-four you planned out, and you will almost miraculously see an easy, triumphant shift toward success.

Retox Soundtrack:
"I Won't Back Down" —TOM PETTY

Hitting the red carpet after bringing Retox and I.AM.YOU. to the Cannes Film Festival. France. >

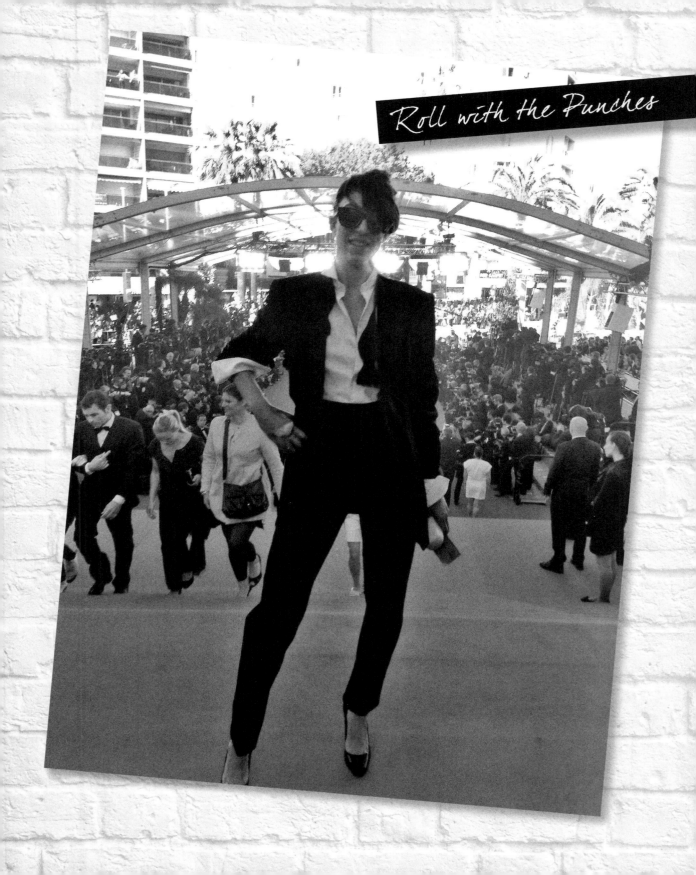

KIDS AT HEART

AN EXPLORATION IN FREEDOM AND FUN

Think less; live more

ON THE LIST AS LONG as Gisele's legs of why I could never be a supermodel, we must add my scars. You would not believe the number of scars I have. Left knee, four little circles from racing up an escalator. Left thumb, two-inch-long mark from trying to turn a chocolate bar into chocolate chips. Right knee, oval shape from falling while hurdling. Right shoulder, four marks from shoulder surgery caused by a high dive. Left calf, odd rectangle from getting whacked with a lacrosse stick. Right glute, four burn lines from going down a slide in a potato sack. Left eyelid, remnants of sixteen stitches to sew up a gash sustained on the basketball court. Right pinky, zigzag from falling out of a tree. The list goes on and on . . .

You would think after all those tangible reminders to be more careful, I would have been, but the kid in me never listened. Running around in the backyard, squealing with excitement for Santa, boiling over with enthusiasm for pizza night, playing baseball in the front yard with the neighbors until dusk, Rollerblading with a Popsicle . . . Sure, I got scarred up, but each scar served as a badge of honor, the gateway into a cool story or memorable experience. It was all *fun*! I was happy and free.

As I look at my scars now, I no longer feel invincible; instead, I worry about getting more. I'm just more careful. Maybe even a little scared. I have to wonder, what happened since my youth? When did we all become so serious? When did climbing a tree become dangerous, or camping out in a tepee become ridiculous? Why don't we find joy in these things anymore? Why can't we allow ourselves to roam without a plan? There was a thrill to everything during our youth, a pure exhilaration in living. Life was a series of adventures. For the most part, there was no obvious stress or reason to not be happy. Sure, there were rough times: fights with siblings, being made fun of, losing a game, getting scratched up on the playground. And some of us might have experienced real trauma: our parents divorcing, the death of a loved one, a serious childhood illness. Yet even in these circumstances, kids bounce back. They have an innate resilience that al-

334

RETOX

lows them to weather troubling times and pick themselves up and keep on going.

As kids, we may have been afraid of the dark or of the bogeyman, but we weren't afraid of life. We dared to go for it; we longed to see and try it all. Failure, sucking, injury, and stress were foreign terms, mere labels with unknown connotations, rarely ones perceived as risks. It is not that we did not care about falling, failing, or getting scared when we were young, we just did not let ourselves get preoccupied with these things and we never let them stop us. We cared instead about trying everything, being everything, going for it all. We were free.

Too often we look back on our time as kids and reminisce over our energy, freedom, desire, and sense of wonder. Yet the miracle of life is that our youth does not go away. It is merely hidden under layers of adult armor. This "go for it" persona, the one that smiles with awe and wonder, is the real you, the one naturally happy, energetic, and willing. If you cannot seem to find it, don't worry; I am going to Retox the kid out of you.

YOGA

I have been known to start many an I.AM.YOU. yoga class with cartwheels. Am I a gymnast? Far from it. But I do think that my serious, achievement-oriented I.AM.YOU.ers often need to remember to be kids.

On those days, I send everyone to the back of the studio and have them do a series of cartwheels to the front of the room. If I am really feeling frisky, I have them then cartwheel their way back to their mat.

You should see everyone's faces; maybe you are making one of them now. I know it seems embarrassing, but was it when you were ten? I think not. So what happened in those years? Why did something fun become something inappropriate and awkward? Why does the adult armor prohibit the youthful exuberance?

You can experience childhood's joy again. This is what Retox yoga is here to show you. With these poses and the longer sequence, I am going to help you manually take off your adult armor until you find the kid inside you, the one that looks forward to giggling and having fun, the way we were all born to do.

RETOX

DESK FIXES

BALANCING BACKBEND

Stand on your tiptoes. Lift your arms up. Inhale, grow taller. Exhale, try to find a slight backbend. Balance here for as many breaths as possible.

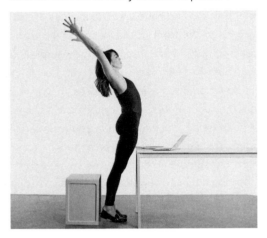

CHAIR DROPS

Come to the edge of your chair, and place your hands on the edge of the chair as well. Press down into your hands, straighten your elbows, and lift your butt up. Inhale here as you move your feet forward so your ankles are under your knees. Exhale, bend your elbows straight back, dropping your body lower than the chair. Inhale, straighten your elbows. Exhale, bend. Repeat three to ten times as it feels good.

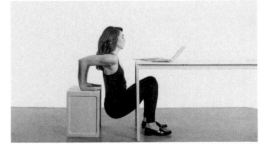

WIDE TWIST*

While sitting in your chair, spread your feet as wide as your desk will allow, toes pointing out. Place your left elbow on your left thigh. Inhale, lift your right arm up and look at your thumb. Exhale, press your elbow into your thigh to help you twist deeper. Hold five to ten breaths, then repeat on the other side.

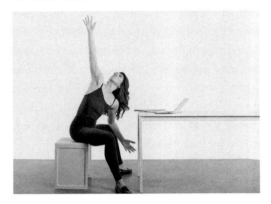

FLOATING CRADLE

While seated in a chair, cross your ankles. Place your hands on the armrests or on the seat by your hips. Inhale here. Exhale, press hands and feet down and lift your bottom up. Repeat one to five times.

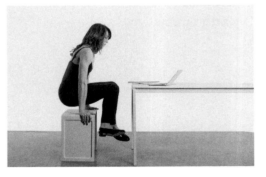

QUICK FIXES

CARTWHEEL

Do it just like when you were a kid. Place one leg forward, two hands down on the floor. Lift up. Flip over. Land. Repeat!

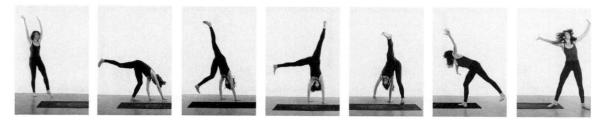

CROW

Start by squatting on the floor. Place your hands on the floor under your shoulders, fingers spread wide. Bring your knees as close to your armpits as possible. Inhale here, pressing your knees into the backs of the arms. Exhale, rock forward, and maybe lift your feet off the floor, balancing on your hands. Don't worry about falling unless you got a nose job this morning.

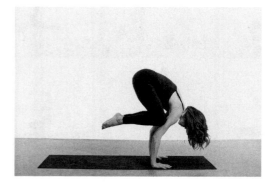

THREE-PRONGED SIDE PLANK

Start in Plank pose with your shoulders over your wrists, legs straight, and body parallel to the floor. Inhale, and move into Side Plank: Shift your weight onto your right hand and outer edge of your right foot, then lift your left arm straight up. Optionally, lift your left leg up as high as possible, grabbing the big toe with your left index and middle fingers. Hold five breaths, then repeat on the other side.

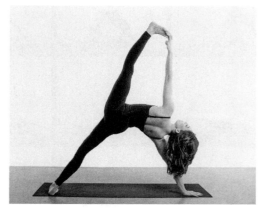

KIDS AT HEART

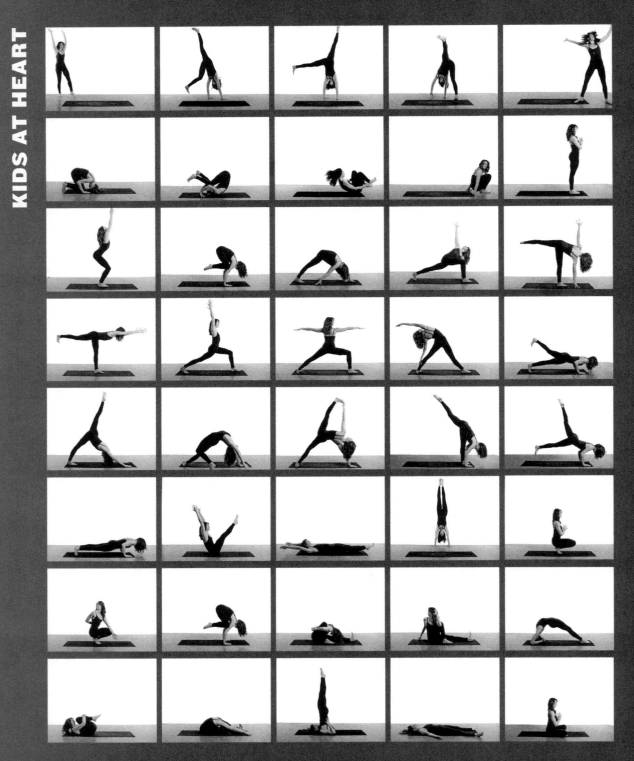

NOURISHMENT

I don't know about you, but when I was a kid, my sister and I would devour anything my mom put in front of us. A few bunches of green grapes, half a sheet of lasagna, a bucket of salad, and the best of all, tacos and quesadillas. On "Mexican night"—my favorite—my poor mom was chained to the stove, flipping tortillas on all four burners for an hour straight. Each time she came to the table with a round, we would scarf them all down and ask for more before she even got a chance to sit and join us.

Then one day right before high school, my friend Samantha told me I was going to get fat. Huh? I had just had a few bowls of minestrone soup, garlic bread, broccoli, and salad, and I felt happily and luckily full. Samantha explained to me that I was no longer a kid and could not get away with eating so many calories anymore. I did not understand. If I was hungry, and I felt good, what was the problem? Why would I have to eat less just because they took my braces off and shaped my unibrow?

I took the comment to my mom, who told me to ignore Samantha and have a cookie. Yet I have since realized that as we grow up, we generally do stop eating like kids and more like calorie-obsessed, health-obsessed robots. Over the years, we begin to approach eating like a science project, instead of blissful, succulent pleasure. We create endlessly long lists of no's—no gluten, no sugar, no carbs, no meat, no dairy, no dessert, no no no. And then we add a painful list of musts—supplements, portion control, cold expensive juices, and straight-up gross, unappetizing dishes. Why in the world do we do this to ourselves? Especially since, I am willing to bet, we were likely all healthier and happier as kids when we ate freely.

You cannot embody youth if you eat like a stodgy old adult. If you want to be free, happy, and feel like a kid, you need to freely eat like one. Here's how to eat your adult armor away and uncover your free-flowing happiness.

DETOX

1. **Don't Think About It.** Please, please stop turning every meal and snack into a scientific probe into the mysteries of wellness. Just notice what you are craving, then add some greens to it, whatever is accessible or you like, and sit down and eat. That's it. Overthinking eating takes all of the fun out of it, which takes me to my next point . . .

2. **Don't Indulge.** Seriously, do not "indulge." *Please*. Just enjoy it. *Indulge* is one of the most detrimental wellness words. Since when is a slice of pizza indulging? It is normal. Eat it. Stop thinking of good foods you have been eating your whole life as indulging. They are foods that you like. Shift the idiotic label and watch not only the guilt but the pounds disappear. (P.S.: You know processed junk food and fast food are still no-no's, right?)

RETOX

1. **Get Excited.** Create one meal a day at which you will have fun, and actually look

339

forward to it with excitement. Maybe that means dinner and drinks out at a new place, baking at home, or going for a walk with a friend to get a snack. But create space for fun while you eat. This is nourishment in and of itself.

2. **Eat the Faves.** We all have favorite foods, and I want you to eat them. Depriving yourself of what you love is akin to slapping on another layer of adult armor, for no reason. Eat what you like, but remember to have greens with every meal.

3. **Take It Back to Mom.** If you were lucky like I was, your mom made homecooked meals. I want you to reincorporate these into your life as an adult. Even if you did not eat like this growing up, try it now. Mom fed us to grow and to be healthy, happy, and strong, so there is no reason we should stop eating like that as adults! Have at least one meal a day resembling Mom's meal. A protein (fish, free-range chicken, or beef), two portions of cooked veggies, some rice or bread, and a side salad. After you eat all that, you can have dessert, too! In the Retox below, I offer you some straight-up original recipes, while others are my takes on my homey faves. And if you don't have time or don't want to cook, you can order these foods out at a restaurant or order in. So do not stress about not having Mom around to do the cooking!

SNACKS

Apple slices

Raisins

Unbuttered popcorn

Celery and carrots with dressing to dip

Retox Hot Chocolate: heated almond milk and 1 tablespoon good cocoa powder (you can add a bit of vanilla or cinnamon, if you'd like)

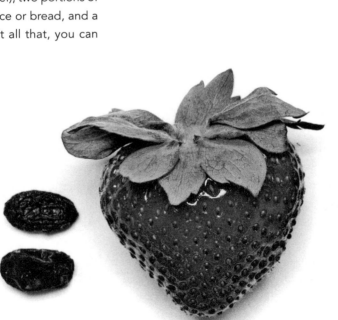

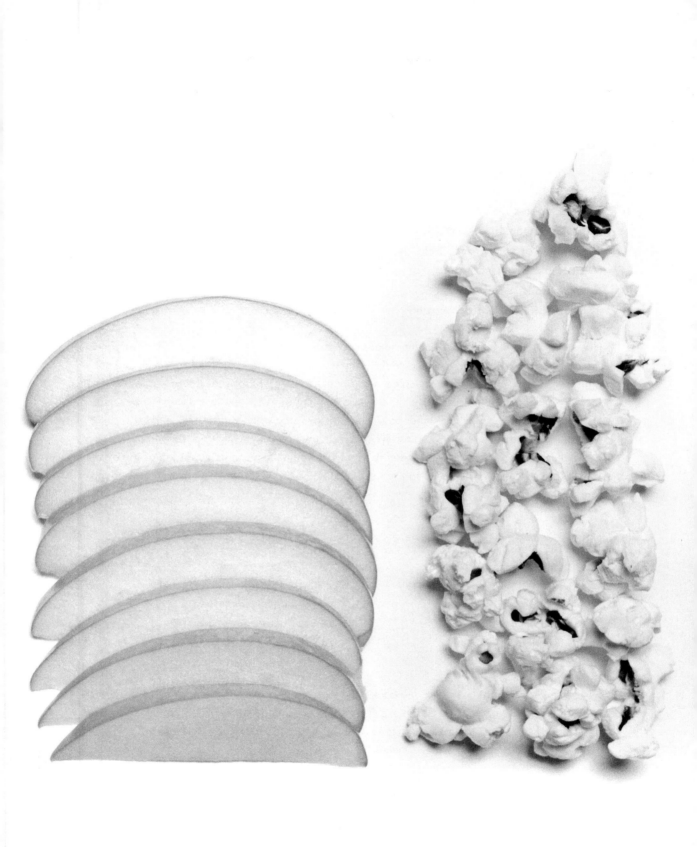

RECIPES

Taco Night Tacos

Tacos are great for you, easy, and fun.

1 teaspoon olive oil

1 white onion, diced and divided

½ pound organic ground beef

1 cup baby spinach

2 tomatoes, chopped

Handful fresh cilantro, chopped

1 jalapeño, diced (optional)

Salt, to taste

1 avocado

Juice of ½ lemon

8–12 corn tortillas

Heat oil in a large pan. Add half of the onions and cook until translucent. Add ground beef, breaking it up with a wooden spoon as it cooks. When beef is no longer pink, add spinach and cook until fully wilted. (You can cook the spinach and beef separately if don't want to have both in your tacos.) Place tomatoes, remaining half of the onions, cilantro, and jalapeño (if using) in a bowl. Add a dash of salt and mix well. In another bowl, mash the avocado with a pinch of salt and lemon juice.

When ready to eat, heat up the tortillas one at a time in a dry frying pan, or wrap in a damp paper towel and microwave for 30 seconds. Assemble your taco by spreading the avocado on the tortilla. Next place a line of meat and spinach in the center of a tortilla and top with tomato mixture. Roll and eat!

Harvest Stew

2 teaspoons extra virgin olive oil

1 onion, diced

1 zucchini, chopped

1 (28-ounce) can crushed
    tomatoes

Salt, to taste

1 (15-ounce) can corn

2 cups baby spinach

4 cups cooked quinoa or rice

Heat oil in a large pot. Add onion and cook until translucent. Add zucchini and stir. When the zucchini is soft, add tomatoes and a dash of salt. Stir, then cover and simmer for 15 minutes. Add corn and spinach and cover again, cooking for 5 minutes, until everything is heated through and spinach is completely wilted. Serve over quinoa or rice.

Retox Mac and Cheese

This recipe requires slightly more effort but is worth it!

- 1 tablespoon extra virgin olive oil
- 3 cloves garlic, minced
- 1 onion, diced
- 2 tomatoes, chopped
- 1 carrot, peeled and diced
- Salt, to taste
- ⅛ teaspoon red pepper flakes (optional)
- 1 (16-ounce) box of pasta of your choice (I prefer penne or rigatoni)
- 3 cups shredded Parmesan cheese, divided

Preheat oven to 350 degrees.

Heat oil in a large pan over medium heat. Add garlic and onion, cooking until onion is translucent and garlic turns golden. Add tomatoes, carrot, and two dashes of salt, as well as the red pepper flakes, if you like it *arrabbiata*, or a bit spicy. Stir, cover, and simmer for 15 minutes. While the sauce is cooking, bring a large pot of water to boil and cook pasta to al dente, about 10 minutes depending on your type of pasta. When pasta is cooked, drain and add to sauce pan, adding a handful of the cheese as you stir. (If pan is not big enough, then add the sauce to the original pasta pot instead.) Now take out a large casserole dish. Spread a layer of the pasta on the bottom of the dish. Add a layer of cheese. Add another layer of pasta topped by another layer of cheese, continuing like that until you get to the top of the dish. Finish by adding a top layer of cheese, especially in the corners. Place the dish in the oven until the cheese is melted and starting to bubble. Serve with a side salad and enjoy!

MINDSET

My dad taught me how to ski. It wasn't easy . . . for either of us. Poor guy—I literally ran him over the first time we went skiing. I was using the poles in a desire to go faster, yet I had no idea how to stop until he stopped me—with his body. We both plummeted into the soft snow, laughed, got back up, and headed immediately onto a real run. I had no idea what I was doing, but it did not matter. I believed I could, and I would. I was invincible. Plus, what was the worst that could happen?

Run after run, lift after lift, my dad taught me how to ski, encouraging me back up every time I fell, which, let me tell you, was often. A few days of Snickers bars on the lifts and a weird proud goggle tan later, I fell in love with the sport. It had an innate freedom to it, one in which falling was part of the beauty and fun. That was when I was ten. Fast forward to me at thirty-four, and suddenly I do not find those falls so fun anymore.

After fourteen years of not skiing at all—the same years I have been with my Colombian, warmth-adoring, winter-sport-avoiding husband—I headed out to the slopes to reclaim my powdery pre-Colombian love. Yet, as I looked down at the glistening slope ahead, I instantly noticed a drastic shift in attitude from my last time on skis: I was suddenly petrified of falling, and even more so of going fast, embracing the fall line, and hurting myself. After a solid fifteen minutes of staring at the fearless two- to six-year-old pip-squeaks no taller than my hips barreling down the mountain, I tentatively began my descent—jaw clenched, limbs rigid, body and mind tense on the inside and out. I focused on avoiding the fall line of the mountain, creeping horizontally back and forth, gripping my jaw, poles, and toes inside the boots. Deep down, I knew if I just let go and embraced the slope and the knowledge already inside me, I would be free to coast down, but the adult in me was filled with fear, all too cognizant of the potential risks and injuries. I analyzed every movement my body made, every bump in the terrain, every person passing me by. I was stuck in my head, thinking my way down the mountain, entirely obstructing my ability to actually glide down it. It was a miserable experience.

In the years I had gone without skiing, I had also grown up, bringing with me to the slopes all the baggage that comes with perceived maturity. I was suddenly a bogged-down, risk-adverse, bona fide adult. I had lost my childhood wonder, my ability to simply enjoy, my innate capability to go for it and have fun no matter what. I wanted to float freely, but I could not free myself enough to get there. I had forgotten about virya, and created an unsurmountable mountain in my mind.

Virya means "joyful effort" in Sanskrit. It is an enthusiasm for the world and everything that it offers—the good and the bad. Virya represents an unbridled desire to partake in life's activities, without judging or holding back. Living with virya is to rejoice in what is good, while simply observing and learning from what is bad. The ancient yoga philosophers believed that virya was necessary for a happy, successful, healthy existence. They saw it as the key to freedom. You have to engage with joyful effort or else the world will not happily engage you. They say that without virya, you will never be able to live out your intended path or discover your true nature.

Virya was so much easier when we were kids. If we were lucky, we did not know about bills or bosses, cancer or death. Our hearts had never been broken and we had yet to be fired. But now, as cognizant adults, virya often presents a challenge; our discerning, preoccupied, overanalytical brain gets in the way of the unadulterated joy we thrive upon. We must now peel away the adult armor and cultivate virya. We need to nourish the kid in us so we can be our true self.

RETOX

Being free and happy like a kid is simple if you let it be. Like with the nourishment and yoga elements, I do not want you to overthink this. Just make a note of these five things by your bed, on your desk, or in your phone and strive to do them, when you can, how you can, remembering to have fun with it. It is just life after all!

DARE TO SUCK

Go try something new and be willing to be bad, really bad at it. Maybe it is a dance class, maybe it is hot yoga, maybe it is cooking a meal. In merely trying you will be unearthing your inner kid.

LAUGH AT YOURSELF

When you suck, or even when you do not (lucky you), laugh at yourself! Stop taking ev-erything and everyone so seriously, and that also includes yourself! Have a chuckle. You will feel lighter afterward.

DO SOMETHING THAT EXCITES YOU

There is excitement everywhere if you let yourself in on it. Maybe it is going to shoot some hoops, trying a new bakery, experimenting with a new cocktail, cozying up with a movie. Do one thing that excites you every day, something you can look forward to and look back upon happily the next day.

MARVEL

Beauty is everywhere, you just have to see it. Make a point of noticing something small and wonderful daily. Perhaps it is the shape of the leaf or the sound of the people laughing next to you. Whatever, whenever—marvel in pure enjoyment and wonder daily. It will add years onto your life.

PERK IT UP

Life is not that bad, even when it is bad. Let yourself be perky, positive, optimistic, and excited. These emotions do not mean you are a slacker from Mars; they mean you are a happy kid at heart who is probably healthier and more successful than all the whiners and despondent adults out there. Let yourself be the happy version of you. What do you have to lose?

Retox Soundtrack:
"Fun Fun Fun" —THE BEACH BOYS

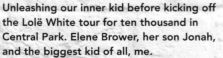

Think Less; Live More

Unleashing our inner kid before kicking off
the Lolë White tour for ten thousand in
Central Park. Elene Brower, her son Jonah,
and the biggest kid of all, me.

PURE ECSTASY

FINDING THE NATURAL HIGH

Deal in Truths, Not Twists

I LOVE ECSTASY. I HATE drugs. The ecstasy I am talking about is pure, ephemeral, effervescent; it is a tiny explosion of natural happiness and pleasure that feeds my energy, fuels my drive, stimulates the bounce in my step, and invigorates my inner and outer smiles. This is the ecstasy I have, and I want to give it to you.

The first time I encountered ecstasy I was bopping around my bedroom getting ready for my shift as a busser and waitress at the local café. In head-to-toe black, with leather bracelets and neon kicks, Oakenfold's techno tracks blaring from the stereo speakers, I barely heard my mom walk in my room. She turned off the music, dropped *Time* magazine on my desk, and asked if, like the girl on the cover, I was on ecstasy. *Thanks, Time*, I thought. No, I told my mom, I had never tried it. I was just naturally happy, loving, and excited. She looked at me, knew it was the truth, gave me a hug, and we all moved on.

That was in my early twenties and, let me tell you, a lot of life has happened since then. By *life*, I mean trials and tribulations, challenges and victories, fights and love. There have been epic battles and moments of sweet surrender, streaming tears and beaming optimism. In the past decade alone, I have suffered through every low emotion, yet have always managed to find the positive, even if just *a* positive, and grab ahold of it. This has allowed me to be happy, energetic, and hopeful throughout my life—the way we are all intended to be.

Yet life has a pesky way of getting in the way, making bona fide happiness challenging at times. Retox gives you direct access to the high; it offers a method to find and lock in the insanely good joyful madness that lies beneath all the rest of life's mumbo jumbo. Think of it as a prescribed dose of this pure ecstasy I thrive on, one you will get addicted to and should be proud of. Let me take you on my ride. Don't you want to be happy all the time, too?

YOGA

Yoga is so not about letting go or giving people hugs. It is about harnessing your inner powers, your innate energy, and your inherent nature, and using them to take you wherever you want to go. Yoga, real yoga, was designed to make you happy and successful all the time. And guess what? There are no heart doodles, *om shantis*, vision boards, or "Kumbayas" that will make this happen. There are just three things: the breath, the poses, and the dedication.

Before you do the Retox poses for pure ecstasy, let's revisit the breath. Take a moment and notice your breath, inhaling and exhaling through the nose, connecting the two so as to make one continuous stream. The breath is the most important ingredient in yoga. It is the secret sauce that ties it all together and makes it all work. Without the breath, the practice is nothing more than a series of random postures that—let's be quite frank—often look ridiculous. The breath is the link between the poses and the dedication, the connection between body and mind, you and your world. You have to breathe.

The second most important ingredient to yoga is the dedication. Doing it for you is not enough. Honestly, your butt looks fine. Close your eyes for a second and see the first person that comes to mind. Maybe it is someone who cannot seem to capture the high, someone unable to find happiness or is going through a rough patch. See them in front of you and decide to do your Retox yoga for them. Every time you feel the burn or your mind wanders, come back to that person and keep on going.

The third is the sequencing of poses. This is the trifecta combination that makes I.AM.YOU. yoga work. It is the recipe for pure ecstasy. So find your breath, pick a dedication, and let's get high.

RETOX

DESK FIXES

TIP-TOE MOUNTAIN
Stand up, if you can. (If not, do this sitting.) Come to your tiptoes. Lift your arms up. Open your palms wide. Hang out here as long as feels good.

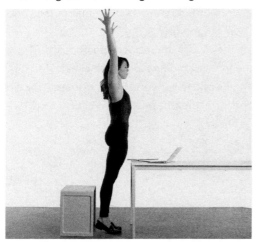

BACKBEND
Sit, inhale, grow tall in your chair, and place your hands on your chair, fingers down. Exhale, arch backward. Drop your head back. Hold five to ten breaths.

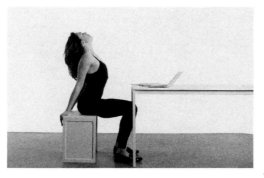

QUICK TWISTS*
Sit up tall. Inhale and extend your arms overhead. Exhale and bring your fingertips to the tops of your shoulders. Inhale and lengthen your spine. Exhale, start twisting left and right as fast as you can. Let your hair go wild in the wind. Do for ten to thirty seconds whenever you need a hit. Optional: Add the dynamic breath (khapalabhati) mentioned in the quick fixes.

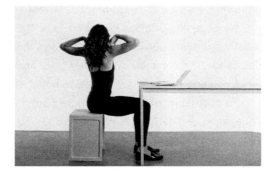

REVERSE BACKBEND TWIST*
Start sitting up tall. Inhale, lift your left arm up. Exhale, twist to your right and bring your right hand behind your butt. Inhale, grow long on your left side. Exhale, backbend and twist. Hold here five to ten breaths, then repeat on the other side.

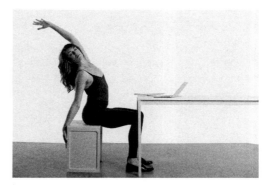

Bonus!
SMILE
C'mon, you know how to do this one.

QUICK FIXES

DYNAMIC BREATH*

Sit tall with your ankles crossed in front of you. Lift your arms up alongside your ears in a V. Close your eyes. Inhale to a comfortable level. Begin short, sharp breaths out of the nose, where the inhale is simply a reaction to the exhale, as the diaphragm pumps on the abdominal wall. It should feel somewhere between sneezing and blowing your nose. (If you are pregnant, skip khapalabhati.) Come to neutral and take three normal breaths. Repeat two more rounds.

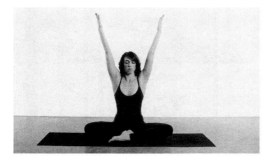

ROCK STAR

Start in Bent-Knee Down Dog Split (page 142), with you left leg in the air. Inhale here. Exhale, bend your left knee and open the pelvis. Inhale, drop the ball of the left foot on the floor behind you and lift the left arm up. Keep the right leg straight, left knee bent and weight on the ball of the left foot only. Drop your head back if it feels good and breathe here five breaths, then repeat on the other side.

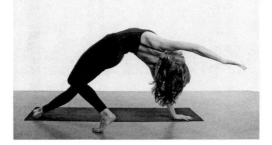

DANCER

Start standing. Inhale, bend your right knee, bringing the heel toward your butt. Exhale, grab the inner or outer ankle with your right hand, whatever feels best. Inhale, lift your left arm up. Exhale, pull the right leg up and reach forward with the left arm. Hold here five breaths, then repeat on the other side.

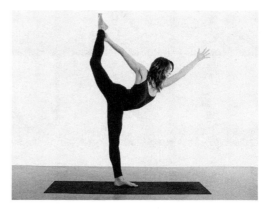

THREE-LEGGED WHEEL

Start with your back on the floor, feet to the floor, with your knees bent and hip distance apart. Place your hands by your ears. Inhale, lift everything up into Wheel pose. Exhale here. Inhale, lift your right leg straight up, pointing your toes. Hold here one to five breaths, then repeat on the other side. If this is too much for you, you can do this from Bridge pose, keeping your arms alongside your body and simply lifting your back and butt off the floor.

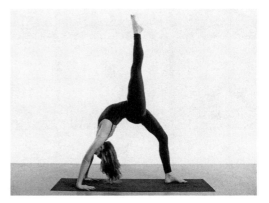

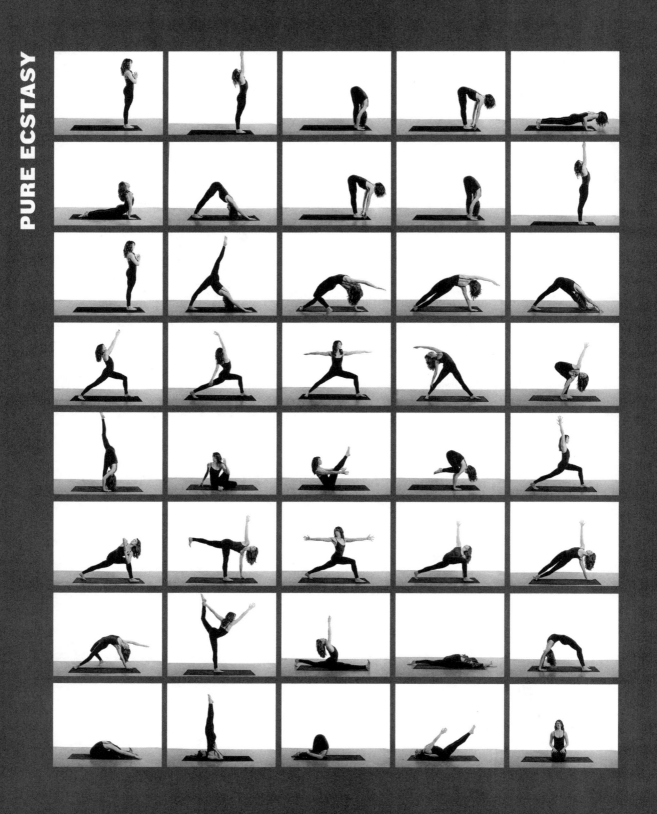

NOURISHMENT

Here's a crazy thought: Intellectualize food less; enjoy food more.

So simple, right? In the Retox pure ecstasy cocktail, it is not only possible, but the goal. We all want to be fit, and we know nourishment is a key ingredient. But wouldn't it be nice to just be able to *eat*, without turning every meal into a project? This is the crux of Retox.

Yes, eating well is essential, but if you honestly think that green juice is the key to making you ridiculously happy, you are seriously misguided. Food absolutely affects your mood, energy, routine, and outlook, as we have seen, but there is not one food, or food group, that can assuredly lock in the high you are longing for every time. If there were, every major corporation would have found a way to patent, package, and sell the bejesus out of it twenty times over.

There may not be a singular food, but there is one method to nourishing pure ecstasy. And like ecstasy itself, it is primal, basic, and straightforward. I am going to lay it out for you now.

You may notice that there is no Detox section here, nor are there specific food recommendations or recipes. That's because this chapter is all about not stressing over food. I want to bring back the enjoyment, the pleasure of eating. I want you to listen to your body and eat well so that you live well. Food is both fuel and fun for our body and our soul. Bon appétit!

RETOX

In numerology, six represents harmony, balance, healing, and protecting. I have thus outlined six nutrition guidelines for ecstatic happiness, which harmoniously link us back to where we started with the LSP.

ENJOY. Above all, allow yourself to enjoy food. Try to look forward to your meals, and thoroughly relish in not only what you are eating, but the experience of eating as well. Attempt to make it less of an angst-ridden experience, preoccupied with worry over what you are eating, and more of a cultural, nurturing occasion. In Italy and Spain, they regularly talk about food while they are eating food, reminiscing on the amazing pasta from the night before or planning the tapas that lay ahead. Food for the Mediterranean is not cause for guilt or stress; it is an instigator of delight. Which is part of the reason they are so healthy.

STOP FAKING. If you do not have a bona fide, clinically proven allergy, do not invent one. That is just silly. Sure, you can call your carb-free diet "gluten free," but why bother when gluten isn't a problem for you and carb free is not only nuts but a detriment to good health? Feed yourself what your body craves and what humans have been eating for thousands of years and just stop worrying about it.

SCRAP THE CRAP. Processed foods, fast foods, sodas, fake proteins, low fat snacks . . . cut them all out. Your body was not made to process them; it simply does not know how. They are laden with ingredients you probably do not even know how to pronounce, let alone explain, and provide little to none of the real nourishment you need.

DEFEAT THE ANTI-MEAT. Chowing down on low-quality, mass-produced meats or unsafely raised farmed fish is definitely not a

353

good idea. But neither is starving your body of essential proteins and vitamins that humans have survived on since the beginning of time. Eat meat, just choose it wisely. Instead of a roast beef sandwich at the deli, wait to enjoy a great steak; rather than tossing yet another chicken breast on a salad, decide to make a delicious one for dinner but with clean, antibiotic-free chicken; instead of picking up questionable tuna rolls at the supermarket, go out for sushi on a date night. I encourage you to strategically eat mainly beef and fish, always with enough veggie sides to turn the whole dish green.

WATER. You need it, more than you think. Water makes up 65 percent of your body content; without it, you cannot live. Drink normal, flat water, all day long, every day. Wet your insides with two to three liters a day and you will discover an instant high, one that will radiate through your eyes and skin and bring energy into every aspect of your life.

GREEN, GREEN, GREEN. Alas, green actually is critical to ecstatic health. The more green vegetables you eat, the better. Cooked or raw, snacks, sides or mains. Make sure two-thirds to three-quarters of your daily intake is green and you are good to go.

That's it. That is really all you have to do on the pure ecstasy trip. How can it get easier?

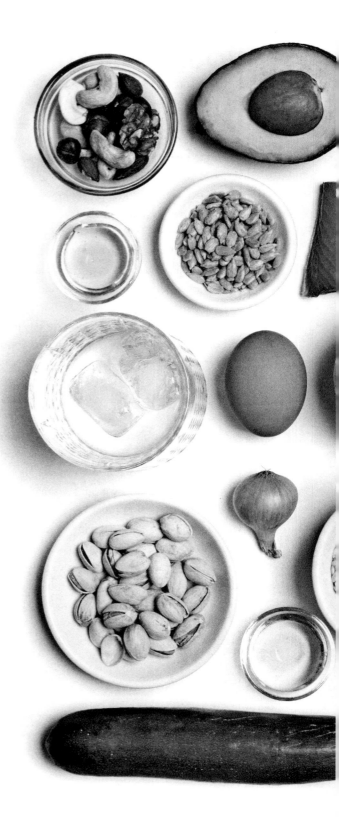

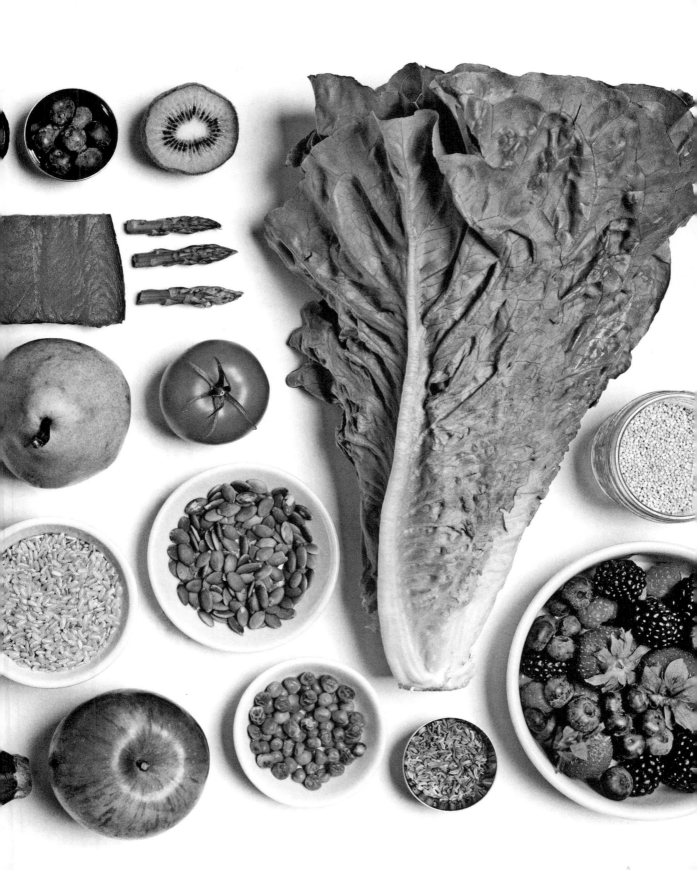

MINDSET

I am going to boil down the entire multibillion-dollar self-help, happiness-searching healing industry into one phrase:

Yogash chitta vritti nirodhah.
We become whole by stopping how the mind turns in the wrong way.

This is the second line of the first-ever book of yoga. Patanjali opens by saying he will now instruct us on how to become whole. He follows with this line—we become whole by stopping how the mind turns things in the wrong way—and goes on to say that if we do not stop the mind from turning in this way, we will become the twist, the anguish and misery, instead of the truth, the joy and elation that is your true nature and life itself.

You can get twisted up in the undercurrents of bitchiness, strife, and agony, or you can float on top of it into the ecstatic truth, not even knowing they are there. In the former, you sink and suffer; in the latter, you revel in your beauty, happiness, and success.

Too often Western yoga translates *yogash chitta vritti nirodhah* into "letting go and seeing what happens," or "stopping the chatter of the mind." But these translations remove the philosophy's power and almost force you to embrace an eternal path of mediocrity. That is not at all what the Tibetan philosophers intended.

You do not become happy or stay happy by letting go; your mind will chase you to whatever deserted tropical island to which you flee. You become happy, healthy, successful, and high on life by harnessing your mind, and teaching it to see the true nature of you and your world. The wisdom lies in understanding how your mind works. Every time you see something with your eye, your mind labels it in a complex femtosecond process of amalgamating past perceptions and experiences. In that minuscule amount of time between what your eyes see and what your mind labels, you create your reality.

The goal is to get into that tiny gap between seeing and perceiving, and ensure that you prevent your mind from twisting what you see in the wrong way, thus creating a perception you do not want to have. If you saturate your thoughts with positivity and happiness, you will create similar perceptions, and in doing so, you'll actually make yourself happy from the inside out.

Your eyes may see the world, but your mind perceives it. It is these perceptions that create your you, your world, your reality. It is up to you to decide how high on ecstasy you want to be. You are your own dealer. Should we pop a pill together?

RETOX

Every night before bed, or on your way home from work, I want you to take a moment to think about one thing that was good on that day. If you have three, even better, but one works. Even on the worst of days, I know there is always one, so find it. Maybe it is a text from friend you care for, a kiss from your partner, a great comment from your boss, the perfect blue sky, that deliciously foamy cappuccino, your smokin' I.AM.YOU. arms . . . Whatever it is, let it come to the forefront of your mind.

Inhale, think [your thought].
Exhale, say *Thank you.*

Thank you.

That's it. Say thank you for the good without focusing on the bad, and day by day, you will become the truth, not the twist. You will be your own dealer, pimp, and Retox ecstasy druggie combined. In doing so, you create the space for more good to come and lock yourself into a permanent pure ecstasy ride, happy, high, and free just like we all want to be.

Retox Soundtrack:
"Ask" —THE SMITHS

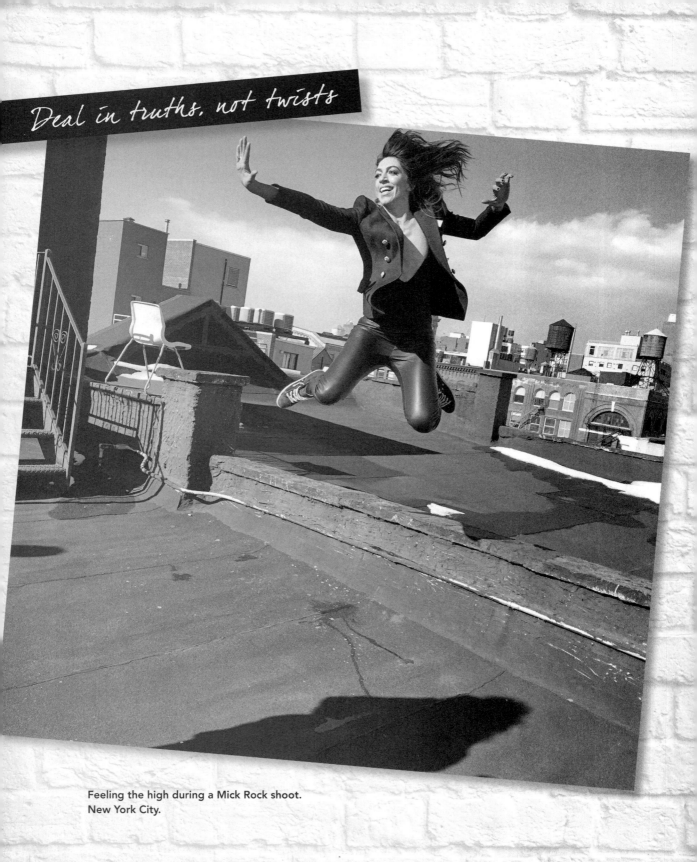

Deal in truths, not twists

Feeling the high during a Mick Rock shoot.
New York City.

GO LIVE IT

Live as if you were to die tomorrow.
Learn as if you were to live forever.

—GANDHI

EAT IT. DRINK IT. LOVE IT. LIVE IT.

Hopefully that is what Retoxing has inspired you to do. Yet I leave you and this book open-ended, without the need for a conclusion because life itself is a continuous cycle.

Learning is a process; living is an experience. It is not how much you have learned throughout the course of Retox, but rather how much you have lived.

Remember that today is happening to convert itself into the past. Tomorrow will happen so you can live in the present. Yesterday happened so you can do it all even better.

You can and will be everyone and everything you have ever dreamed of, every single moment of every day. You will be at the top of your game; maybe you already are.

Everything you need you have inside you already, and now you have the Retox tools to keep pointing you in the right direction. Just make your passion you, and you will become your best you.

If you take your dream and add some hustle, you will achieve success—whatever *success* means to you. Simply be adaptable, live it all to the max, and do not be afraid to dive in and get dirty. When you feel like you are drifting away from where you want to be, how you want to feel, and who you are, just revert to the basics:

Did I Retox today?

We are all one, but only you can change you. Sweat, rock out, and feed yourself what you need to become all of you.

That's Retox. That's you. That's I.AM.YOU.

And if you ever forget it, just take a moment and, like I am doing right now, say:

Thank you, Life.

xx

Lauren

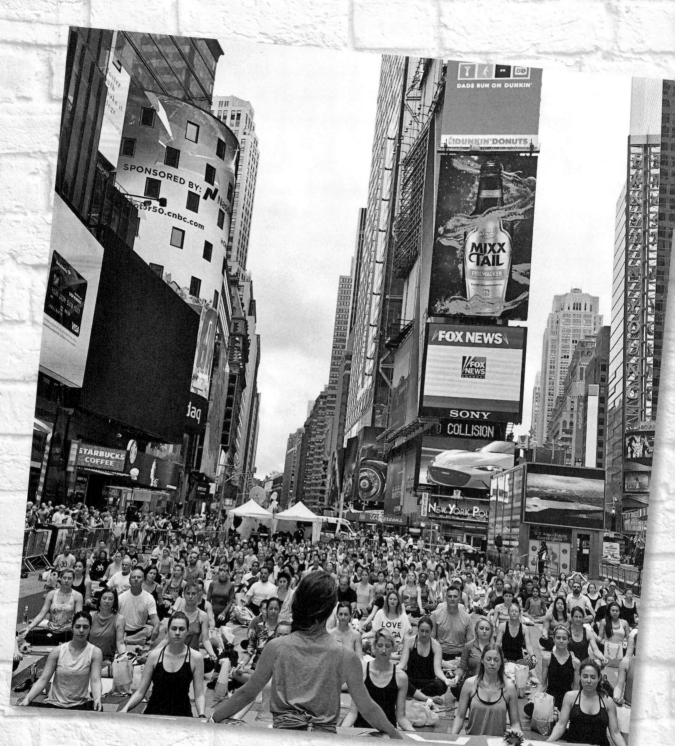

If you can make it there, you can make it anywhere. It's up to you. I.AM.YOU. Times Square takeover for two thousand with Athleta. New York City.

ACKNOWLEDGMENTS

A TOAST:

To my friends, colleagues, advisors, editors, students, teachers, and family—your inspiration has guided me through the RETOX and the I.AM.YOU. journey.

To my mother, for giving up her dream career so I could achieve mine one day in the future. From cheering me on every rebound, race, and recital to showing me what a good cappuccino really tastes like, you are the most elegant, erudite person I know. Thank you for teaching me to be smart, to listen to my body, and to be patient.

To my father, for giving us everything, literally, and never holding back. I would not be here without your generosity, patience, and sacrifices. Let alone my passion for reading, writing, and running.

To my sister, for being a fearless pistolette of a warrior. For teaching me that being me may not always be the coolest, but is always cool.

To Mick Rock, the definition of a true rock star and guru. Your professionalism and talent are beyond words. Thank you for believing. You captured the real me.

To my literary agent, Linda Lowenthal, for always having my back, ready for battle, and believing the world needs to Retox. To my editor, Denise Silvestro, for putting up with my vision and desire for perfection. To Walter Zamora, for getting me and I.AM.YOU. before I even did, from the logo to the infamous "one quick shot" while I was still at Morgan Stanley that now graces the cover of this book. See, you do like yoga and wellness. ☺ To Brittany Wright, for your uncharted, incomparable talent and creativity. To Joshua Rosenthal and the Institute for Integrated Nutrition, for providing the well-rounded education I needed to fulfill my dreams and complete I.AM.YOU.

Most of all, to you I.AM.YOU.ers across the globe and the growing New York City team for embodying the brand and straight-up love for life. You are my daily inspiration, my teachers, my motivation to get up every day. Thank you for being YOU and wanting to RETOX I.AM.YOU. style, no matter where, no matter when. You are the reason I.AM.YOU. is what it is. Thank you!!!

And above all, to my husband, aka I.AM.YOU.'s ResidentMixologist and my number one penguin, without whom this journey would have never started. From your beats to your wisdom, you have created a garden for me and my dreams to blossom. Thank you for believing in me and I.AM. YOU., for being my sounding board in every sense, and for inspiring me to be a better person every day. You are my best friend, partner in crime and life.

And now, we have a drink.

Cheers, Salud, and Salute!

INDEX

Page numbers in **bold** indicate figures; those in *italics* indicate photos.

INDEX

369

INDEX

370

INDEX